The Young Deaf
or Hard of Hearing Child

The Young Deaf or Hard of Hearing Child

A Family-Centered Approach to Early Education

Edited by

Barbara Bodner-Johnson, Ph.D.

and

Marilyn Sass-Lehrer, Ph.D.

Gallaudet University, Washington, D.C.

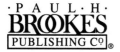

·P A U L·H·
BROOKES
PUBLISHING C⁰ ®

Baltimore • London • Sydney

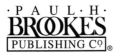

Paul H. Brookes Publishing Co.
Post Office Box 10624
Baltimore, Maryland 21285-0624

www.brookespublishing.com

Typeset by International Graphics Services, Newtown, Pennsylvania.
Manufactured in the United States of America by
Victor Graphics, Baltimore, Maryland.

Most of the stories in this book refer to real-life experiences. In these cases, the individuals' names and other identifying features have been changed to protect individuals' identities. Stories involving actual names and details are used by permission.

The photographs on the front cover and throughout this book were taken by Dr. Barbara Bodner-Johnson.

The list appearing on pages 87–89 is from FAMILIES, PROFESSIONALS, AND EXCEPTIONALITY: COLLABORATING FOR EMPOWERMENT 4/E by Turnbull/ Turnbull, © 2001. Adapted by permission of Pearson Education, Inc., Upper Saddle River, NJ.

The lists appearing on pages 192–193, 195, 197, and 198 are from Mertens, D.M., *Research Methods in Education and Psychology: Integrating Diversity with Quantitative and Qualitative Approaches*, pp. 231, 233, 234, copyright © 1998 by Sage Publications, Inc. Reprinted by Permission of Sage Publications, Inc.

Library of Congress Cataloging-in-Publication Data

The young deaf or hard of hearing child : a family-centered approach
to early education / edited by Barbara Bodner-Johnson, Marilyn Sass-Lehrer.
    p.   cm.
Includes bibliographical references and index.
ISBN 1-55766-579-6
    1. Deaf children—Services for.   2. Parents of deaf children—Services for.
3. Deaf children—Education (Early childhood).   4. Hearing impaired
children—Education (Early childhood).   5. Early childhood education—
Parent participation.   6. Deaf children—Means of communication.
7. Deaf children—Family relationships.   8. Communication in the family.
I. Bodner-Johnson, Barbara.   II. Sass-Lehrer, Marilyn, 1948–

HV2391 .Y68 2003
371.91/2 21   2003052482

British Library Cataloguing in Publication data are available from the British
Library.

*To our families whose love and
support helped us find our place in the world*

Contents

Section One: The Family

Section Two: Program Foundations

Section Five: Research Models

About the Editors

Barbara Bodner-Johnson, Ph.D., Professor, Department of Education, Gallaudet University, 800 Florida Avenue, N.E., Washington, D.C. 20002

Dr. Bodner-Johnson holds degrees from the University of Iowa and Creighton University; she earned her doctoral degree in education at Syracuse University.

She has directed research projects focusing on families who are hearing who have deaf or hard of hearing children and is the author and co-author of chapters and articles on family learning environments, family dinnertime conversation, family life experiences of deaf college students, parents as adult learners, and best practices in family-centered early intervention programming.

Dr. Bodner-Johnson's current focus in the Department of Education at Gallaudet University is on preparing teachers to work with young deaf children and their families. She taught preschool at the Iowa School for the Deaf, middle school at the Ohio School for the Deaf, and secondary-level students at Oak Lodge School in London, England. She directed and taught in a parent–infant program for deaf children and their families in Syracuse, New York, and held a faculty position at Syracuse University.

Marilyn Sass-Lehrer, Ph.D., Professor, Department of Education, Gallaudet University, 800 Florida Avenue, N.E., Washington, D.C. 20002

Dr. Sass-Lehrer received her master's degree in deaf education from New York University and her doctoral degree from the University of Maryland in early childhood education and curriculum and instruction. Dr. Sass-Lehrer is the coordinator of the family-centered early education teacher education specialization in the Department of Education at Gallaudet University, focusing on the preparation of graduate students to work with families with deaf and hard of hearing children from birth through 5 years of age. In 1990, she received the Outstanding Graduate Faculty Member Award from Gallaudet University. Dr. Sass-Lehrer has worked with deaf and hard of hearing children and their families in public schools as well as special schools for deaf children in New York, Maryland, and Mississippi.

Her research and writing address teacher competencies and guidelines for best practice, diversity, family–school partnerships, early intervention, and family support and involvement. Dr. Sass-Lehrer is a co-author of *Parents and Their Deaf Children: The Early Years* (Gallaudet Press, 2003) and has authored chapters and articles focusing on deaf and hard of hearing children and their families. She is actively involved in professional organizations that advocate for programs and services for deaf and hard of hearing children and their families.

Contributors

Beth Sonnenstrahl Benedict, Ph.D.
Educational and Family
  Involvement Consultant
Germantown, Maryland 20874

Laura A. Blackburn, Ph.D.
Postdoctoral Research Fellow
Cognitive Science Program
University of Arizona
Tucson, Arizona 85724

Carol Jackson Croyle, M.S.
Educator
Gallaudet University
800 Florida Avenue, N.E.
Washington, D.C. 20002

Brandt Culpepper, Ph.D.
Associate Professor
Department of Communication
  Sciences and Disorders
Towson University
8000 York Road
Towson, Maryland 21252

Linda Delk, Ph.D.
Program Evaluation Coordinator
Laurent Clerc National Deaf
  Education Center
Gallaudet University
800 Florida Avenue, N.E.
Washington, D.C. 20002

Carol J. Erting, Ph.D.
Professor
Department of Education
Gallaudet University
800 Florida Avenue, N.E.
Washington, D.C. 20002

Janice C. Gatty, Ed.D.
Lecturer
Smith College
Morgan Hall
Northampton, Massachusetts
  01063
Director
Harriette Smith Short Center for
  Parents and Young Children
The Clarke School for the Deaf
Round Hill Road
Northampton, Massachusetts
  01060

Jan Christian Hafer, Ed.D.
Associate Professor
Department of Education
Gallaudet University
800 Florida Avenue, N.E.
Washington, D.C. 20002

Julie K. Jones, Ph.D.
Project Director
Academy of Educational
  Development
1825 Connecticut Avenue, N.W.
Washington, D.C. 20009

Thomas W. Jones, Ph.D.
Professor
Department of Education
Gallaudet University
800 Florida Avenue, N.E.
Washington, D.C. 20002

**Kathryn P. Meadow-Orlans,
Ph.D.**
Professor Emerita
Gallaudet University
800 Florida Avenue, N.E.
Washington, D.C. 20002

Donna M. Mertens, Ph.D.
Professor
Department of Education
   Foundation/Research
Gallaudet University
800 Florida Avenue, N.E.
Washington, D.C. 20002

Barbara Raimondo, J.D.
Consultant
American Society for Deaf
   Children, Conference of
   Educational Administrators of
   Schools and Programs for the
   Deaf
Gallaudet University
800 Florida Avenue, N.E.
Washington, D.C. 20002

Nancy Rushmer, M.A.
Language Consultant/Family
   Program Coordinator
Deaf-Hard of Hearing Services
Columbia Regional Program
531 S.E. 14th Avenue
Portland, Oregon 97214

Patricia E. Spencer, Ph.D.
Professor
Social Work Department
Gallaudet University
800 Florida Avenue, N.E.
Washington, D.C. 20002

Arlene Stredler-Brown, M.A.
Director, Early Education
   Programs
Colorado School for the Deaf and
   the Blind
Department of Speech, Language,
   Hearing Sciences
University of Colorado
Campus Box 409
Boulder, Colorado 80309

Lisa Weidekamp, M.S.W.
Research Associate
Council on Social Work Education
1725 Duke Street
Suite 500
Alexandria, Virginia 22314

Foreword

The beginning of the 21st century is an exciting time for educators and other professionals working with families of children who are deaf or hard of hearing. For the first time in the history of deaf education, we, as professionals, have the opportunity to begin intervention in the first few months after birth for the majority of the population of children with congenital hearing loss. In order to provide the highest quality of service, it is critically important that professionals gain skills in providing a family-centered approach to the education of children who are deaf or hard of hearing.

The Young Deaf or Hard of Hearing Child: A Family-Centered Approach to Early Education provides valuable information about how to design, implement, and evaluate a family-centered approach to the education of children who are deaf or hard of hearing, beginning in the infant period and continuing through the early education of the child and the development of literacy. Woven throughout the book are the voices of families reminding the reader about the importance of listening to these voices in the development and implementation of educational services.

The beginning chapters identify characteristics that are similar and unique in the parent–child interactions of hearing children of hearing parents, deaf children of deaf parents, and deaf/hard of hearing children of hearing parents. Accommodations that can be made in the home during everyday interactions between parents/caregivers and their children illustrate the importance of expertise about the impact of deafness and hearing loss on communication access. It is critically important that at the very beginning of the journey families make from identification of deafness and hearing loss to successful development of language, literacy, communication, and social-emotional development, expert knowledge is available to them for support then and throughout their child's educational experience.

The development of equal partnerships between parents and professionals now begins shortly after birth and depends upon a high level of respect and value for the unique and important role that parents play in the development of their deaf or hard of hearing children's communication, language, and literacy. Families acquire these skills through knowledge about how their communication may need to be adapted and modified in order to allow the child full access to the information in the world in which they are enveloped.

This book illustrates a variety of family supports, including the role of other parents and families as well as members of the Deaf/deaf and hard-of-hearing communities, and knowledge about family rights, legislation, and policies. Readers will gain information about how families can actively participate in developmental assessment/evaluation of their children's progress through interviews, questionnaires, and videotapes. The role of Deaf/deaf individuals providing shared reading experiences to families with very young children and how that may enhance the children's road to literacy are exciting models to consider for implementation.

The Young Deaf or Hard of Hearing Child deals with important and timely issues regarding considerations about inclusion, the services that are designed and implemented for children with multiple disabilities, and the role of technology with its remarkable advances. Early intervention program and system models are described as well as a model for the evaluation of the effectiveness of the program. The book explores issues related to mode of communication, the interaction between language and literacy, and the role of the teacher as an ethnographer.

Our teaching or intervention techniques are assisted by developments in technology and insights from parents, the Deaf community, individuals who consider themselves hard of hearing, individuals who are deaf and hard of hearing, those who use American Sign Language, those who use conventional amplification and cochlear implants, those who are predominantly speakers of Spoken English, and those who use a manually coded or sign-supported communication system. We are also informed by successful inclusion and center-based programs, insightful evaluation through ethnographic models and team approaches, and the need to collaborate with health systems and the medical home. I read this book from cover to cover with almost no interruption. It is a valuable resource for beginning professionals and for experienced professionals. I have no doubt that families will also gain valuable information from this book. It is a treasure chest of knowledge from a host of families, teachers, and researchers to help guide us all as we discover better ways to work with families and together educate the next generation of children with congenital deafness and hearing loss. It is our job to support them in their journey to find the way to fulfill their family and children's dreams and overcome the challenges in life that they will encounter.

Christine Yoshinaga-Itano, Ph.D.
Professor, Department of Speech, Language & Hearing Sciences
University of Colorado, Boulder

Acknowledgments

We are honored to thank many people who helped us with *The Young Deaf or Hard of Hearing Child*, and we are grateful for this opportunity. First, we want to acknowledge the "voices" of family members (especially parents and their children), practitioners, and deaf adults, who helped to enrich the concepts we have tried to communicate in this book. We are most grateful to the many contributors who accepted our invitation to prepare state-of-the-art reviews of their areas of expertise, to develop practical strategies for application, and to propose future directions for the field. Numerous discussions with the authors over the years and our conversations regarding the conceptualization of their chapters have been challenging, lively, and always so satisfying. Funds from the Department of Education at Gallaudet University were instrumental in helping us gather these expert contributors together early on in developing the scope of the book and in shaping the content of the chapters. We are grateful also to our colleagues in the department and our families and friends for understanding our need to be focused on this work. We want to thank Gail Solit and the Clerc Center at Gallaudet for allowing us to spend time there taking the photographs for the book. We acknowledge the highly capable and thorough assistance and support of Heather Shrestha and Mackenzie Cross, our editors at Paul H. Brookes Publishing Co. Their ability to enhance the clarity of meaning and expression of ideas and to work for consistency within and across chapters has contributed significantly to the overall quality of the work.

Introduction

Parents who discover that their infant or toddler has a hearing loss are confronted with a range of possible interventions and advice on how best to raise a deaf or hard of hearing child. Professionals, parents, and adults who are deaf or hard of hearing advise parents to pursue different approaches. Their advice may take into consideration the individual characteristics of the child and family; but it is often more strongly influenced by their understandings and perspectives of what it means to be *deaf*.

For new parents who have no experience with people who are deaf or hard of hearing, their children's hearing loss is often viewed as devastating, shattering their dreams and expectations for their children's future. Adults who are deaf or hard of hearing often are puzzled by this reaction. For them, hearing loss may create some difficulties from time to time but mostly it is experienced as a difference that presents unique experiences and opportunities, not a disability.

Paul Ogden, the author of *The Silent Garden* (1996), wrote, "Deafness is not about hearing but about communication." To those who can hear, deafness is understood as a "lack" of hearing; for those who cannot hear, deafness has little to do with how much or how little one hears and has everything to do with how easy it is to communicate. *The Young Deaf or Hard of Hearing Child: A Family-Centered Approach to Early Education* is about early communication, language, literacy, and the academic and social opportunities for people with hearing loss. This book is not about how much or how little damage there is to the hearing mechanism or about what needs to be done to restore or rehabilitate hearing. In this book, we try to provide a perspective that is not found in many other works; that is, we present our content based on the premise that hearing loss is a communication and socio-linguistic experience that begins with the family. We invited the contributors to work on this book not only because of their shared perspective but also because of their range of knowledge and diverse experience with families and children. The wisdom of this selection of authors is in the difference in perspectives the authors bring based on their work with deaf and hearing families, their experience in clinical and school settings, and their expertise in promoting communication via visual and auditory/oral approaches.

Rationale for Family-Centered Focus

Early education programs for children who are deaf or hard of hearing develop needed services for children from the foundational assumption that the development of the young child can only be fully understood within a family context and that, in turn, the family interacts within a larger social system. This contextual framework—beginning with the family system and extending outward to include the immediate environments with which the child interacts—sets the stage for implementing programs and practices that establish the well-being of the individual family as a priority goal, which is integral to planning for the child. A family-centered approach is sensitive to family complexity, responds to family priorities, and supports caregiving behavior that promotes the learning and development of the child (Shonkoff & Meisels, 2000). For deaf or hard of hearing children with hearing parents, it is likely that full access to the language being used in the family is not available. Early language acquisition and communication development, therefore, as well as the development of child–family relationships are primary early intervention focus areas for these families. The deaf or hard of hearing child's ability to communicate with his or her parents or caregivers and siblings is key to developing intimate and enjoyable family relationships that benefit everyone. Furthermore, family engagement patterns support the child's ongoing social development. For example, how deaf children make and keep friends and how they develop their identities are directly influenced by the relationships experienced within their families as well as by the quality of the communication within their families.

Family-centered early education programs emphasize the families' roles as collaborators and decision makers with early education professionals and promote the self-efficacy of families, their individual strengths and resources, and the strengths and resources of their various communities. Collaborative, family-centered early education supports family–professional partnerships that strengthen families' abilities to nurture and enhance their children's learning, development, and well-being. Furthermore, services developed for each family derive from an interdisciplinary, team-based approach in which audiologists, social workers, medical practitioners, speech-language pathologists, and deaf consultants, for example, coordinate with early education specialists and families to develop individualized programs unique for each family.

Strengths and Challenges of Early Education

The promise of universal newborn hearing screening and early intervention has raised expectations for children who are deaf or hard of hearing.

Prior to the mid-1990s, young children entering the educational system were, more than likely, already exhibiting delays in one or more areas of development. With early identification, competent professionals, and comprehensive family-centered early education, it is now realistic to expect that many children with hearing loss will experience few delays by the time they reach school age.

A hearing loss creates a difference in the way in which individuals communicate and acquire information, but hearing loss is not disabling provided there is full access to communication. The widespread use of American Sign Language (ASL) and the recognition of Deaf communities reflect a sociological, cultural, and linguistic view of deafness that is in sharp contrast to a disability perspective. In addition, a wellness model of deafness has gained popularity, underscoring the recognition that individuals who are deaf or hard of hearing are competent, productive, and successful and lead fulfilling lives (National Association of the Deaf, 2000).

This book emphasizes a family-centered approach that recognizes that children's developmental opportunities lie within the context of their families and the children's early environment. Early education professionals develop relationships with families and strive to promote each family's strengths, natural caregiving roles, and competence. Family involvement is a primary goal of family-centered early education. Families with children who are deaf or hard of hearing need professionals, parents of other deaf or hard of hearing children, and adults who are deaf or hard of hearing to help them understand their children's unique abilities and needs. At the same time, families need to develop skills to communicate with their deaf or hard of hearing children, not only to promote the acquisition of language but also to ensure a sense of belonging and a place in the family.

The importance of early communication for children with hearing loss and the essential role of their parents was recognized as early as the mid-17th century when parents were urged to fingerspell to their infants (Dalgarno, 1680, cited in Moores, 2001). The first early intervention program in the United States (a "family" school established by Bartlett in New York City in 1852) incorporated many of the characteristics that are considered "innovative" today (Moores, 2001). Early intervention programs for children with disabilities did not attract public attention or resources until the mid-1960s with the establishment of Head Start and the Handicapped Children's Early Education Act (PL 90-538; Bailey & Wolery, 1992). In 1968 the Bureau of Education for the Handicapped of the U.S. Department of Education established the Handicapped Children's Early Education Program to develop and evaluate models for serving young children with disabilities and their families (Bowe, 2000).

Recognition of the successes of these early programs and the importance of family involvement and the home environment (Bronfenbrenner, 1975) led to the expansion of early intervention programs in the 1970s. A decade later, the Education of the Handicapped Act Amendments of 1986 (PL 99-457), in effect, assured services for preschool children with disabilities and established the framework for early intervention services.

The field of early childhood special education emerged from the contrasting perspectives of early childhood education and special education (Bruder, 1997). Early childhood education is rooted in a developmental and constructivist view of learning that emphasizes a child-centered approach in which adults are responsive to child-initiated interactions and interests (Bredekamp & Copple, 1997). Special education tends toward a functional/behavioral perspective that emphasizes more direct instruction and the acquisition of functional skills that are carefully designed by adults. These paradigms for learning (developmental and behavioral) and their respective practices (responsive, child-directed; directive, teacher-centered) represent the continuum of teaching and learning contexts evident in early education programs (Bailey, 1997). Early education for children who are deaf or hard of hearing and their families continues to seek its place amid these two disciplines (Sass-Lehrer, 1998; Sass-Lehrer & Bodner-Johnson, 2003).

Characteristics that make each child and family unique are significant for program planning. Children with hearing loss are very heterogeneous, differing from each other not only in how they use sight and sound to acquire language and communicate (i.e., visual abilities and extent of hearing loss vary widely), but also in rates of development and special learning characteristics and aptitudes. No two children share the same developmental profile, and many children with hearing loss have needs that may require a more functional or directive approach. Family situations also shape the nature of services provided. For example, family differences in hearing status (whether parents themselves are deaf or hard of hearing), home language, cultural perspectives, and economic situation will influence parents' expectations for their child and the services they choose (Meadow-Orlans, Mertens, & Sass-Lehrer, 2003; Meadow-Orlans & Sass-Lehrer, 1995). Collaboration with professionals from different disciplinary perspectives and areas of expertise are more likely to result in services that are appropriate and tailored to achieve the best outcomes for each child.

The opportunities and services available for young children with hearing loss and their families have never been greater. Not only has the widespread implementation of newborn hearing screening provided the opportunity for an early start for early intervention for the majority of infants born with a hearing loss and their families, but also, technological advances provide options for improved access to sound. At the same time, challenges exist that may deter these opportunities for some children and families. For example, almost one half of all infants referred for further testing from newborn hearing screening do not receive hearing evaluations and follow-up services (*Sound Ideas Newsletter*, 2003). Of those children and families who enter the early intervention system, a majority receive services from professionals who do not have preparation in education of the deaf (Stredler-Brown & Arehart, 2000). In fact, families report that many medical and health care professionals have little understanding of the cultural experiences, language, and successes of Deaf adults. And yet, strong recommendations from these professionals often lead parents to choose surgical interventions and communication approaches that may do little to advance their child's opportunities or help their child to achieve his or her potential.

How Unique and Useful Is this Book?

Each chapter in *The Young Deaf or Hard of Hearing Child* reflects a family-centered philosophy and is considered a resource for communication across the different disciplines that contribute to family-centered services. Designed as a core text for anyone interested in young children who are deaf and hard of hearing, this book seeks to address the needs of a wide array of audiences, including pre-service professionals and faculty and practitioners associated with teacher preparation programs, program development, and evaluation efforts. Those individuals who provide direct services to young children who are deaf and hard of hearing and their families and those involved in carrying out research programs and policy development would also benefit greatly from this book. Families may also find selected chapters of this book informative.

The Young Deaf or Hard of Hearing Child provides a comprehensive and developmental understanding of the early educational experience for young children who are deaf and hard of hearing and their families. Families' experiences and communication are central themes that appear throughout the book. We advocate for comprehensible and clear communication among family members and their young deaf or hard of hearing children. We argue that the communication methodology selected is less important than full and accessible communication and that the options selected for communication and hearing technologies are as important as the process by which these decisions are made. This book purports that families who are well informed of the range of options available and appropriate for their children and receive quality support provided by professionals, other parents, deaf or hard of hearing adults, and their own families and communities are more likely to be strong families, well-informed, and competent advocates for their children.

Structure and Organization of the Book

The book is divided into five sections. The first section, "The Family," focuses on the deaf or hard of hearing child in the family. These chapters discuss deaf children's family experiences growing up with hearing parents and siblings, how the changing world and different cultures have influenced needed support services for parents, and strategies for family involvement and advocacy from a legislative and policy perspective.

The second section, "Program Foundations," provides a comprehensive discussion of programs and systems that serve deaf and hard of hearing children and their families—beginning with early identification through universal newborn hearing screening—and describes the array of family-centered early intervention assessment and curricular models available. This section concludes with a chapter on program evaluation using an inclusive evaluation model.

In the next section, "Challenges in Early Education," three particular challenges for family-centered early intervention are explored: programs for hard of hearing infants and young children, inclusive programming, and educational programs that serve young deaf children with multiple disabilities.

The fourth section of the book, "Language and Communication," explores the areas of language and communication from both a theoretical and an applications perspective. The chapters here include information on the foundational concepts for language and literacy development and for parent–child interaction. These chapters also examine the implications for intervention and development when a child is born deaf and needs a visually accessible communicative and linguistic environment to develop to his or her full potential.

All of the chapters in Sections One through Four in *The Young Deaf or Hard of Hearing Child* review or highlight the available research for their particular content. The fifth section of the book, "Research Models," offers descriptions from a more detailed perspective of three research models that explore important aspects of family-centered early education. Each of these research designs is based on the value that families are an important source of information and that unobtrusive research methodologies can effectively gather that information. The first chapter describes a participant–observation model that examines the lived experience of a bilingual, bicultural family (deaf and hearing). The second chapter describes a survey, interview, and focus group approach to understanding families' early experiences with their deaf and hard of hearing children. The final chapter in this section describes an ethnographic, longitudinal, and collaborative approach to the study of language, literacy, and cultural development of young deaf and hard of hearing children.

Each chapter in Sections One through Four begins with a vignette or quote that poignantly introduces the particular focus of the chapter. The theoretical foundations and research findings related to the chapter content are reviewed early and then applications of the knowledge base and recommendations within the context of future perspectives are presented. At the end of each chapter, a parent or practitioner presents an essay or reflection piece prepared as a response or reaction to the content of the chapter. These essays highlight the writers' own unique perspectives and experiences and are considered an important vehicle for including diversity of thought and viewpoint throughout the book.

Notes:

1. Throughout this book, "deaf" with a small "d" is used to refer to an audiological status, whereas "Deaf" with a capital "D" is used in reference to the linguistic minority that makes up the Deaf community, shares Deaf culture, and is composed of individuals who identify themselves as Deaf people (Marschark & Spencer, 2003).

2. American Sign Language (ASL) is a complete signed language with distinct grammatical rules, word order, and idioms. It is the primary language of many Deaf people in the United States of America. Signed English systems are manually coded systems that use signs from ASL and invented signs for spoken English words, prefixes, and endings (e.g., –ing, –ed). Signed English systems are not languages but are used to support spoken English. Examples of Signed English systems are Seeing Essential English (SEE I), Signing Exact English (SEE II), and Signed English. Cued Speech is a visual, gestural supplement to speech reading; it is a communication tool using eight hand shapes positioned close to the mouth, chin, neck, and side of the head.

REFERENCES

Bailey, D. (1997). Evaluating the effectiveness of curriculum alternatives for infants and preschoolers at high risk. In M.J. Guralnick (Ed.), *The effectiveness of early intervention* (pp. 227–247). Baltimore: Paul H. Brookes Publishing Co.

Bailey, D., & Wolery, M. (1992). *Teaching infants and preschoolers with disabilities.* New York: Merrill/Macmillan.

Bowe, F. (2000). *Birth to five: Early childhood special education* (2nd ed.). Albany, New York: Delmar Publishers.

Bredekamp, S., & Copple, C. (Eds.). (1997). *Developmentally appropriate practice in early childhood programs* (Rev. ed.). Washington, DC: National Association for the Education of Young Children.

Bronfenbrenner, U. (1975). Is early intervention effective? In B. Friedlander, G. Sterritt, & G. Kirk (Eds.), *Exceptional infant: Assessment and intervention* (Vol. 3, pp. 449–475): New York: Brunner/Mazel.

Bruder, M.B. (1997). The effectiveness of specific educational/developmental curricula for children with established disabilities. In M.J. Guralnick (Ed.), *The effectiveness of early intervention* (pp. 523–548). Baltimore: Paul H. Brookes Publishing Co.

Education of the Handicapped Act Amendments of 1986, PL 99-457, 20 U.S.C. §§ 1400 *et seq.*

Handicapped Children's Early Education Act of 1968, PL 90-538, 20 U.S.C. §§ 621 *et seq.*

Marschark, M., & Spencer, P. (Eds.). (2003). *Deaf studies, language, and education.* New York: Oxford University Press.

Meadow-Orlans, K., Mertens, D., & Sass-Lehrer, M. (2003). *Parents and their deaf children: The Early Years.* Washington, DC: Gallaudet University Press.

Meadow-Orlans, K., & Sass-Lehrer, M. (1995). Support services for families with children who are deaf: Challenges for professionals. *Topics in Early Childhood Special Education, 15*(3), 314–334.

Moores, D.F. (2001). *Educating the deaf: Psychology, principles, and practices* (5th ed.). Boston: Houghton Mifflin.

National Association of the Deaf (2000). *NAD Position on Cochlear Implants.* Silver Spring, MD: Author.

Ogden, P. (1996). *The silent garden* (2nd ed.). Washington, DC: Gallaudet University Press.

Sass-Lehrer, M. (1998). Current perspectives as guidelines for best practices. In A. Weisel (Ed.), *Insights into deaf education: Current theory and practice* (pp. 210–219). Tel Aviv: Tel Aviv University, Academic Press, School of Education.

Sass-Lehrer, M., & Bodner-Johnson, B. (2003). Early intervention: Current approaches to family-centered programming. In M. Marschark & P. Spencer (Eds.), *Deaf studies, language and education* (pp. 65–81). New York: Oxford University Press.

Shonkoff, J.P., & Meisels, S.J. (2000). Preface. In J.P. Shonkoff & S.J. Meisels (Eds.), *Handbook of early childhood intervention* (pp. xvii–xviii). New York: Cambridge University Press.

Sound Ideas Newsletter. (2003, February). *5*(1). Available from http://www.infanthearing.org/newsletter.

Stredler-Brown, A., & Arehart, K.H. (2000). Universal newborn hearing screening: Impact on intervention services [Monograph]. In C. Yoshinaga-Itano & A. Sedey (Eds.), Language, speech, and social-emotional development of children who are deaf or hard of hearing: The early years. *The Volta Review, 100*(5), 85–117.

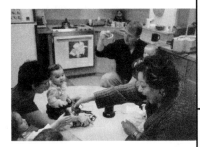

The Family

CHAPTER ONE

The Deaf Child
in the Family

BARBARA BODNER-JOHNSON

t is graduation day at Gallaudet University, and families gather across
campus preparing for their sons' and daughters' big day. Walking
behind one family—in this case the parents and brothers and sisters are
hearing—I notice the ease of the communication; everyone was signing
with great enthusiasm, reflecting the importance of the day. As this scene
unfolded before me, I wondered how this family was able to communicate
so well. What story could their son, who was deaf, tell me?

Early childhood education is based on a number of underlying assumptions and beliefs; significant among these is the belief that the development of young children can only be fully appreciated and understood within a broad ecological context, beginning with a core understanding of the family as a dynamic system (Shonkoff & Meisels, 2000). This contextual framework sets the stage for early intervention programs to establish family-centered philosophies and to develop practices that focus on the well-being of the family as well as that of the child.

The very word *family* has significant meaning for most people. Families generally provide a foundation for everything we are or do. Families are the source of our greatest anticipated love and understanding. We believe that if we can fit into our families, we can fit into our friendships, the community, and the world.

Many of us, for example, can recall family experiences when the adults gathered—friends of our parents, aunts and uncles—and reminiscences were told and retold. As infants and toddlers, we were included in this family interaction—sitting on an adult's lap and eventually drifting off to sleep in the midst of the stories and the company.

As children, we sat quietly, maybe out of sight, hoping we could stay up and listen to the stories and feel the excitement in the conversation. As adolescents and young adults, our parents wanted us there among them so we could learn about our family's life and our heritage and so that we would be able to tell our children these same stories. Elizabeth Stone (1988) described the role family stories have for shaping us, fashioning our identities, and helping us become part of our families. For most children, access to this kind of family event is inclusive and welcomed. But for many deaf children who do not have full access to the language being used among their hearing family members, the joy of being part of these intimate family interactions and the substance of those conversations are likely not fully available.

Sometimes with my family, they'd sit around and talk about things that happened when we were young, late into the night. And I'm interested in that kind of information, but I can't be involved in the conversation.

— *Adam*

My brother (hearing and 4 years younger) would go and listen to the conversation . . . at the same age, I didn't get involved . . . as adolescents, I would leave and my brother would stay. And my parents understood when I left. They felt like, "Sorry, we can't interpret all the time." But . . . they gave me the responsibility to watch the kids.

— *David*

Given that we understand the importance of the family context and child–family relationships for the developing child, this example of inaccessible family interaction can raise concerns for professionals working with young children who are deaf because it may point to a lifetime of such events.

This chapter presents the everyday family life experiences of five deaf college students (Adam, David, Cynthia, Marie, Noel) who grew up in hearing families and largely in hearing communities. The information on which the chapter is based was obtained in interviews with these students.[1] The purpose of the interviews was to learn how young adults who are deaf think about their lives growing up in hearing families and their beliefs about their place in their families. The chapter identifies the major topics, issues, and concerns that emerged from the interviews and describes the family experiences that "tell the story" behind these topics and concerns.

For professionals who work with families with young deaf children and for the families themselves, an important outcome of this effort is an increased awareness of what specific family events and family life experiences mean for these deaf individuals and what implications they might have for young children who are deaf with hearing families. The perspectives of these young adults can provide insight into the deaf child's attitudes, beliefs, and behaviors regarding his or her family and "transactions with his or her ecology" (Calderon & Greenberg, 2000, p. 171). Their perspectives also direct attention to parental strengths and challenges, family relationships, and how families and caregivers adapt their behaviors in unexpected ways when they discover that their child is deaf or hard of hearing. There is the assumption that the students' perspectives are meaningful, knowable, and able to be made explicit. Their lived experiences and critical observations make them an important resource for information and for lessons to be learned about life for deaf children in a hearing family environment.

The quotations in this chapter are excerpts taken from the interview transcripts. Stories emerge from the "hands and voices" of the five students that are poignant and clear; these are the primary contributions to the chapter and to the field of early education for deaf children and their families. For example, the following excerpt is from a discussion Cynthia and others are having about how their parents were involved in

---

[1]It was a privilege to hear the stories and be a part of the interviews with these five university students. Of course, as their stories about growing up in hearing families unfolded, there was a realization of how "in the midst" (Clandinin & Connelly, 2000, p. 187) of the family experience they all still were and how their perspectives would continue to change as they constructed new meaning out of each experience.

their schooling. In her description of leaving home to attend a residential school, Cynthia depicts a caring mother and worried daughter experiencing new feelings:

If you go to a public school, then you see your parents every day since you go back and forth from home to school. But at a school for the deaf, you stay for the week and see your parents only on the weekends. The first time I was taken to the school for the deaf, about 1 hour from my home, I wasn't used to being sent to school for a whole week. I was so young, and I cried because I was going to the deaf school. My mother would call the school and ask how I was doing. I wasn't used to not seeing her for a whole week. It's funny, it is such a different feeling being at home and being in the dorms at school. You realize that mom is not there . . . mother was not watching over me everyday like before.

— Cynthia

This is a good example of the quality of the communication the students provided in the interviews, from which the themes or recurring content patterns (Patton, 1990; Spradley, 1979) described in this chapter were derived. Three major themes emerged from the content of the interviews; a discussion of each theme forms the basis for the organization of the chapter:

- Theme 1: Family conversation provides access to family life.
- Theme 2: Deaf children face choosing a deaf identity.
- Theme 3: Deaf children want their parents to know what it means to be deaf.

The recommendations at the end of each discussion are meant to provide early childhood professionals and parents with a conceptual framework from which to develop more specific programs and activities in order to meet the needs of individual families with deaf children. They are intended to assist all parents and families who want to enhance the visual aspects of their communication and who are interested in Deaf culture and in developing relationships within the Deaf community. Although it is assumed that the deaf child and family members acquire American Sign Language (ASL), the recommendations do not preclude stressing the importance of oral/auditory skill development and the acquisition of English.

After exploring these themes and recommendations, the last part of the chapter focuses on possible applications or "lessons to be learned" from the interviews for early intervention practice and for families with young children who are deaf and hard of hearing. This chapter is intended to offer context for the family focus that is woven throughout this book.

THEORETICAL CONTEXT AND CONCEPTUAL FRAMEWORK

An understanding of what a family is and how families work is imperative for professionals who work with children and their families. For early intervention specialists who serve young children who are deaf and hard of hearing and their families, this knowledge can transform their thinking about such related concepts as family development, stress, and adaptability.

This chapter was developed with the perspective that family and individual behavior should be understood within an ecological and family social system theoretical framework. First, the ecological perspective, after Bronfenbrenner (1979), locates individual behavior in its social context; the child develops within the family and the broader contexts of his or her community and school environments. Both child and context shape and accommodate one another as they interact, and the process of accommodation is greatly influenced by the larger settings in which it is embedded. To understand an individual child, parent, or family, you have to understand their worlds. The ecological perspective rests on the idea that development relies on the child's capacity to understand and shape the world he or she experiences; the ability of children to communicate effectively with those in their environment is a critical influence on that capacity.

The family system perspective has come to be accepted widely by social scientists because it offers insight into family interaction patterns and how each family is unique. Systems thinking is grounded in the notion that what defines a system are the relationships among its parts and not the individual parts themselves. A Calder mobile, with each part in a critical place and in perfect balance with the whole work, comes to mind.

Family systems theory views the family as a social unit that, in order to survive and thrive, constantly accommodates to developments within individual family members and their relationships to one another and to external influences (Walker & Crocker, 1988). The application of the systems metaphor for the family directs our attention to the interaction within families and to that which contributes to the uniqueness of each family. From this perspective, it becomes clear that the interrelationships among family members, more so than the individual family members, are central to understanding the complexity and diversity found in each family. At the same time, family systems are characterized by their wholeness; that is, the individuals in a family together form a unitary whole that functions structurally to support a shared life that meets the needs of each family member.

Knowing that a child who is deaf lives in a family with hearing parents and brothers and sisters, for example, tells us very little specifically about day-to-day life inside that family or what to predict regarding the child's development and learning. To understand that life and how it works for the deaf child, we must come to understand the individual child and the individual family. What are the various subsystems (e.g., parents, brothers and sisters, father and son)? How do they interact with one another? What are the relationships that occur among them?

The students interviewed knew well the significance for them of family interaction and discuss at some length wanting access to their family conversations when they were growing up. They clearly convey the belief that their ability to communicate with the members of their family and have in-depth discussions with them, as well as quick exchanges of conversation in the car or while watching television, was key to developing intimate relationships with their parents and brothers and sisters.

Family systems theory, like the ecological perspective, is a resource or tool for early intervention professionals. It encourages professionals to look beyond the individual mother or father sitting across from them at the kitchen table to explain behavior within the family. It encourages professionals to consider the multiple influences on a child's and family's life and how they interact with personal characteristics, such as values and coping styles, as well as characteristics of the family, such as their culture and resources, in order to understand the families with whom they work.

FAMILY CONVERSATION PROVIDES ACCESS TO FAMILY LIFE

For me it was not specific times, it was all day. All the time that I was with my family it would happen. Anytime there was communication, whether it was at dinner or if we were in the living room, or watching TV, or going out shopping, I would always be left out. It was an everyday thing for me. It was frustrating.

— Marie

Access to the conversation that occurs naturally throughout a family's day at home around the television, at mealtimes, or in the car means access to family life. Regardless of the communication mode chosen by their hearing parents, the deaf students interviewed indicated that they were not able to participate fully in the language used in their homes, and like many deaf children, felt left out of family life (Foster, 1998). For Marie, being "left out" was not episodic or limited to one situation; it was pervasive and left her feeling like an outsider in her family. Without a shared language, conversation or reciprocal dialogue among family members is a challenging, often frustrating task.

My family is hearing, and most do not sign. Those who know the most are my mother and sister. I was left out . . . if my sister was with her friends, they would talk and I would ask what they were saying. With deaf people, I'm not just sitting there. But with a hearing family, it's easy to get bored. They might have to write out what is being said, like at church. My mother would write out what is being said, or sometimes she would interpret. . . . But, really you are just left out. I'd tell my mother that I wanted to go out with my deaf friends so that I'd have something, anything, to do. The captions on television were sporadic. I'd have to ask what was being said and get an explanation. Or, I'd ask questions. I could only really talk to my mother and my sister. That was it.

— *Cynthia*

Having Voice and Access "In the Moment"

Communicating in a shared language with our parents and siblings is the primary means by which we become a part of our families and have our "voice" included in family decisions and events. By sharing our ideas, we become part of each other's thoughts and feelings and share who we are—building relationships that daily contribute to lifelong family ties. In all families, communication is key to developing alignments or close relationships among family members (Tannen, 2001), and communication influences overall family functioning, such as how a family manages conflict and plans tasks needing to be done together (Weiss & Jacobs, 1988). As family members discuss the news of the day, plan for an outing, or take care of household tasks such as paying bills, the deaf child experiences great difficulty contributing to and sharing in the information and feelings being conveyed. Interacting with family members is also an opportunity for young deaf children to take in and synthesize new information and to struggle with new concepts and perceptions.

The differential family communication interaction that hearing and deaf children experience is evident during the early childhood years and continues throughout childhood (Schlesinger & Meadow, 1972). David tells of his experience as a 10-year-old at home with his parents and brother:

They signed if talking to me, but not if they were talking to each other—even if I was sitting in the room. I would ask, "What did you say?" They would give me a condensed version of the discussion. They would tell me, for example, "We were talking about financial matters," which meant they didn't want me to know. Or they would say, "We're paying bills." And wouldn't tell me any of the details. Or they'd say, "We're talking about your brother" or "We're talking about school." But they wouldn't tell me exactly what they were talking about. I didn't realize that was wrong . . . until I went to college.

— David

For Noel and Marie, being "the last person to find out anything" and "never the one who is doing the talking" meant their participation was limited and could not be simultaneous with other family members or "in the moment" with the conversation. It meant it was difficult to have their ideas fit into the flow of ideas; in fact, it meant their ideas probably did not get into the conversation and, therefore, what was happening in their family did not reflect their input.

I was always the last person to find out anything . . . Everyone would be laughing and I would be the last person to laugh. I felt left out.

— Marie

Sometimes it's frustrating because you always have to ask what they are talking about. You are never the one who is doing the talking. You are just trying to get someone to fill you in. Therefore, you are never involved in the conversation, you're just always trying to find out what is being said, and you are too busy doing that.

— Noel

Family Mealtime

Sitting down together as a family for meals occurs less frequently in today's overscheduled households than in previous generations. Still, when it does happen, the family mealtime remains a golden opportunity for sharing ideas, for socialization, and for family members to keep current with each other's lives. For young children, family mealtime is an opportunity to learn about family rituals, the rules of sharing, and to practice basic communication skills such as turn taking and initiating conversation topics. These lessons are lost to young deaf children unless parents and other family members make a special effort to set the stage so that they can happen.

For the students interviewed, mealtime with their families was singled out as a particularly challenging experience. This family event emerged again and again as the arena of exclusion that gave focus to their feelings of failure and disconnect from their family. The mealtime scene repeatedly reaffirmed their inability to communicate with members of their family and their inability to feel fully included in their family's life. The following excerpts describe these frustrations and what the students did to make the best of the situation.

In my family, the four of us always ate dinner in the family room. Sometimes they would have conversations and if I couldn't follow—I was an oral child—I would just ignore them and go back to my plate of food. Sometimes my mother would catch me up. I know that I did feel left out of course, but it was always a fact of life that I am this way and that's the way it would be for me for the rest of my life. I just had to make the best of it. I can't sit and complain about it all of the time.

— Adam

My dad made it a rule that all four of us had to have meals together, and I always had a problem with that because at mealtime I felt left out. My mom and dad and brother would always talk without signing. I often had to ask them to repeat what they were talking about. Sometimes they were talking about something that they didn't want me to know about, and then they would tell me they were talking about "nothing." I got upset. It happened at almost every meal, really. It got to the point where I got so sick of it, I would finish my meal quickly and leave the table as soon as possible. My mother complained about me not staying at the dinner table or wanting to spend time with the family.

— David

At dinner, I wanted to be the first to finish because I could then watch the talking. I felt that communication was important in my family and that I shouldn't just ignore them. I should make some effort to communicate with them.

— Noel

There is no sense in any of these conversations that parents assumed a "gatekeeper" role for their child. That is, neither parent monitored the conversation in order to guide their deaf child's active participation; the students assumed the responsibility of trying to gain access.

Holiday Family Gatherings

Holiday visits to relatives' homes and family reunions, like family mealtimes, can also challenge a deaf child's access to family life. The inability to participate in meaningful conversation can be amplified by the presence of greater numbers of people with whom the child does not share a language. These rituals of family life, a rich source of enjoyment and learning about our family's heritage and how we fit in, may not be the most exciting experience for any child or teenager, hearing or deaf, but for very different reasons young deaf people may choose to excuse themselves from the holiday dinner table. Wendy Lichtman, a hearing mother of a deaf teenager, tells the story of how her daughter volunteered to exclude herself from the company of 19 people at Thanksgiving dinner when room was tight at the table:

I know it's not only deaf teenagers who might prefer to skip a large holiday meal—hearing teens, too, can feel disconnected from their families, and, at a table without peers, get bored or annoyed. But for deaf teens, 90% of whom have hearing parents, there's usually something else going on as well: There's a good chance that before they've had the opportunity to make the natural adolescent choice of bowing out of the conversation, they've already been shut out of it. There's a good chance that a deaf kid who says no thanks to sitting at the family table isn't rejecting the scene so much as feeling rejected herself. (Lichtman, 1998, p. 16)

The following excerpts from the students' conversations about large family gatherings reflect similar strong emotions:

At Christmas and Thanksgiving, when there would be 10 people sitting at the table, I could not keep up. There were so many conversations happening at once that it got to the point where I would just eat and leave. My parents and all my family members would ask me what was wrong and I'd tell them, "I just have no one to talk to," and so they would excuse me from the table. It's not their fault. I asked them to please be more sensitive to my needs. They'd want to talk to me but once conversation started up again, they forgot. And I got tired of always reminding them, so I just gave up. I remember last Christmas I went home [from school], and we went to my aunt's house for dinner. I left the table early and went down in the basement to watch uncaptioned television. It was more acceptable to watch TV without captions than to deal with my family with no captions. Other times, I would go read a book. It was an escape. Now when I go home and visit my family, at the dinner table I try to have one-on-one conversations with people. I don't get involved with the general table talk.

— Adam

I hated going to my grandmother's or my aunt's house. My own family thought it was rude that I didn't want to go. I didn't want to because I couldn't enjoy myself. I didn't feel part of the family. I just sat there. Everybody was talking. I didn't know what was going on. I hated being there . . . I didn't really know what the problem was, until I got older, and then I realized it was communication. I thought it was me—my problem. I thought I just wanted to get attention . . . when I look back now I know why.

— *Marie*

Basically, I was left out of family gatherings most of the time. When the conversation was about me, then everybody was involved, but . . . if I wasn't the topic, then I was left out. It was unintentional. Sometimes my grandmother or aunt would ask me a question. They had all learned to sign a little for me when I was a baby, and today, they try to remember what they've learned. Now when I go to a family gathering, I may leave the room or watch television because it's too difficult to follow the conversation.

— *David*

Seeking a Solution for Family Access

Oftentimes, as deaf children get older, they begin to seek solutions to the communication barriers they experience in their families. For example, as David and Adam got older and went off to college, their lack of access to family conversation when they came home to visit was no longer an acceptable situation. They tried to resolve it and find a way for their families to accommodate their communication needs. David pleaded with his parents, asking them to join in the solution to his problem of being left out of family conversations and not knowing what was going on around him.

Watching television and making comments, my parents and brother never signed. That bothered me a lot; I used to get angry. When I started college, and I came home, I told them how I felt very much ignored, they were making me feel left out, and we had a big fight about it. They were telling me they didn't understand that I had felt like this. I told them, "All I want is that you sign in front of me. If I'm reading a book and you're talking, sign so that if I happen to put the book down I know what you're talking about, and I don't have to ask. My mother took it very hard. She said, "I won't sign if I don't want to." She had a hard time dealing with this. She was very upset because she thought it was her fault. She was the one who raised me. She thought she was doing the right thing and I was saying, no, I didn't like what she did. My dad and brother agreed to sign. So now when I go home, my family tries to sign . . . it's not that they always do it, but I see them trying. We really had a hard time trying to resolve this problem; it took 3 or 4 years of our lives.

— *David*

Adam tells a story about how his father came to understand at last his son's communication frustrations:

In my house, signing was uncomfortable when I first started coming home from college. My parents would ask me what I was talking about with my deaf friends. I remember one incident clearly. My father had a Deaf roommate in college, if you can imagine that. How ironic. My father was surprised to know that I knew this Deaf man, so he invited his old college roommate over, together with his wife. We were sitting drinking coffee . . . my father and his girlfriend and the two guests. My father would speak, and his old college roommate didn't understand, and I interpreted between the conversations. And then the Deaf man would ask me a question and, without even thinking, I would respond in sign without my voice because I was talking to a Deaf person. I didn't think about my father at all. My father would say, "What did you say?" And, I'd have to interpret what my conversation had been with this Deaf couple. Then the Deaf couple left and my father said, "I finally understand what you felt like growing up." I can't believe you put up with that experience your whole life, always having to ask, "What did you say? What did you say?" My father finally understood. He finally saw what I was trying to get through to him, that I was not understanding the conversation.

— Adam

David and Adam also discuss their need to explain to their parents how they felt—wanting their parents to understand without blaming them, wanting to be part of their families. They talk about how they approached their parents and their parents' reactions:

David: *My parents never said, "Oh I understand how you feel." My parents said, "Well, I understand how you feel and that's life. And, if I were in your shoes, I would be frustrated, but we'll try to do our best. Okay?" And I couldn't argue with that. I got to the point where I got them to think about how I was feeling, the frustrations and the anger, that I wanted to know what was going on in the family.*

Adam: *For my father it took time to try and explain how I felt and my father would say, "Well, I can't change anything." And I was telling him, "I don't want you to change anything that happened, I just want to tell you how I felt so you know. I don't want to hide anything from you. I just want you to hear me out. Let me tell you about it. And if you want to know what my experience is like, ask me. If you want to know anything about me, let me tell you."*

David: *Right. I just felt that they should know this is how I felt and this is how it was for me. I'm not blaming anyone; I just wish it hadn't happened this way.*

Although they recognize their families' efforts to sign and to include them in regular family mealtime as well as holiday dinner conversations—even with aunts and grandparents—these students indicate a deep dissatisfaction with the access to communication they have had over the years with their families. It is as though their level of involvement in family dinnertime conversation is a metaphor for their level of participation in family life.

These challenges associated with communication have been observed and reported in the literature (Bodner-Johnson, 1991; Foster, 1998; Lichtman, 1998). In her research, Foster noted how special family events most associated with family camaraderie—when the whole family gets together—are frequently the most difficult in the lives of deaf people. Some of their worst memories were of conversations around the dinner table. In my own analysis of family dinnertime, I found how specific patterns of parental conversation elicited different results in interaction with their 10-year-old children. Family conversation around the dinner table was most inclusive of the deaf child when parents paid attention and took interest and extra time to "listen" to their child's communication efforts. When parents responded to their child's initiation of a conversation topic by asking leading questions and incorporating wait time in order to keep the conversation going, their deaf child contributed more to the conversation. Also, both open-ended questions (what? how? why?) and two-choice (yes/no) questions were effective in eliciting and sustaining contributions from deaf children.

The students in these interviews said they wanted a chance to be involved "in the moment" and to share their ideas. Getting condensed versions of family discussions was not acceptable. And as they said, they wanted to be the ones doing the talking and not always last to find out anything. They wanted their parents to know their dissatisfaction and so they told them. For example, as beginning college students returning home at break, Adam and David, in different ways and for different reasons, were compelled to confront their parents and siblings with their feelings about missed communication. They don't blame anyone but admit that they wish it had been different for them growing up.

Recommendations for Using Family Conversation to Provide Access to Family Life

If the whole family participates in communicating with the young deaf child, Schlesinger and Meadow (1972) observed, the child will feel like an accepted member of the family. Early childhood educators are in a good position to discuss, model, and practice visual communication strategies with family members; they have established a relationship with the family and can observe and build on already existing strengths in their communication practices. Discussions can occur informally as professionals and parents focus on communication and plan together the activities and goals they want to pursue.

For example, professionals can suggest several strategies that family members might use to provide their young deaf children access to the family conversation. The following are various strategies.

Adopt a Visual Way of Thinking About Communication   Whenever the deaf child is present, and even when he or she is not, family members can practice using visual communication strategies in order to build a foundation of family sensitivity to all aspects of visual communication. Effective visual communication strategies include gently waving a hand within the child's line of vision or his or her peripheral vision, using tactile techniques such as tapping on the child's shoulder, and being responsive to the child's focus of attention (see Chapter 11; Mohay, 2000). Although these strategies are designed for parents and young deaf children, they can be readily modified to family communication for children of all ages who rely on vision.

Take Advantage of Family Mealtime   Family members have each other's attention at the dinner table; if they know that active participation is expected, children are at the ready for communication. Family members should wait for or get the deaf child's visual attention by seeking eye contact or by lightly tapping his or her shoulder or the table. When the child is engaged and then looks away, family members should "hold" or pause the conversation for the few seconds needed to regain the child's attention and to resume the conversation. Using these and other strategies that work for the family, the deaf child will likely grow up knowing his or her attention is expected and that inattention will not be tolerated because important information will be missed. Also, family members can make it a practice to invite Deaf friends to join the family at meals from time to time: These could include the child's playmates as well as adults in the parents' support group. Monitoring the child's visual attention and participation can be the responsibility of everyone present at the dinner table.

Facilitate Access to Large Extended Family Gatherings   Holidays, family reunions, and weddings, for example, can be particularly challenging communication environments for deaf children. Extended family members and friends spend much less time around the deaf child than parents and siblings do and so get little opportunity to learn about and practice visual communication strategies. Parents should find a way to discuss the deaf child's reliance on visual communication with people beyond the immediate family who occasionally spend time with the family, and they should always model effective visual communication practice. For large family gatherings, parents and caregivers should make it a practice to prepare the child for the particular event. For instance, parents and caregivers can show pictures of what the child might expect, including the people he or she will likely see there, or they can give the child a role when company comes over—even a 3-year-old can pass around a plate of cookies—so that he or she can participate in family rituals. So the child learns from an early age that family gatherings can be fun, parents and caregivers can invite a friend or two to join the family event. If possible, the seating of those at the table—from the child in a high chair to the teenager wanting to "split"—should be arranged so that the deaf child is near more fluent signers. Also, in these family gathering situations, family members can share being available to interpret for a time.

CHOOSING A DEAF IDENTITY

Deaf people experience the world and structure their lives in fundamentally different ways than hearing people. "A shared life experience structured around vision creates community among deaf people" (Erting, 1994, p. 5). Like many children who are deaf, the students interviewed identified themselves as Deaf (Becker, 1980). Choosing Deafness, the process of developing individual Deaf identity, emerged as a major theme in the conversations of these five young adults. Being deaf played a significant role in the lives they constructed for themselves with their hearing families and hearing peers and in how they structured their lives toward the Deaf community and Deaf culture. They preferred to be somewhere where they could be Deaf, be the way they are. Their experiences as children, their friendships as adolescents, and their lives today reflect the meaning they made of the fact that they are deaf.

"That's When I Realized What I Was Missing"

The memories the students shared were vivid; they revealed how they came to choose Deaf culture and align with the Deaf community and how the day-to-day realities of being deaf affected their identity development. The conversations about their identity seemed to be triggered by and parallel to their conversations about realizing how much of the communication and information they were missing with their families and how much family life was being lost to them. The students indicated they had no idea of the enormity of the loss and the stories they tell seem to reflect some regret. Whether that realization was a gradual process or a "eureka" moment, they speak of it as though it was an integral part of the process of constructing their identity.

I was with my girlfriend who could hear, and she heard everything my parents were talking about. My girlfriend was interpreting what my family was saying, and she told me what was going on, and my parents were upset about that. Wow! That's when I realized what I was missing, that I was being left out of all of the things they were talking about.

— David

I always thought I fit with hearing people because my family was hearing, but at school the more I was with Deaf people the more I realized that I belonged with them. It was difficult because at the same time I wanted to be part of my family. But I had to separate them. I don't think they understand our culture. I don't socialize with hearing people now. I can communicate with them just fine, but I feel more comfortable with Deaf people and I identify with them. You can try to go back and forth and be in both worlds or you can separate them. This worried my mom because she always believed that we should make a bridge between worlds—and I still believe that, but it's not an easy thing to do.

— Noel

Once I got into college and started to sign, I realized Deaf people can have real discussions and debates and understand what everybody else is saying. I never knew that could be. I didn't know that's what it was really like. And I became rebellious at my parents. I became angry.

— Adam

Living in the Deaf and Hearing Worlds: Separate or Back and Forth?

Individuals who are deaf often describe their lives as moving between the hearing world and the deaf world. The students describe their experiences of trying to live in both the hearing and deaf worlds. Some recall how it was a process that started early in their lives as they met Deaf individuals, and they discuss how that process continues to develop. They recognize and talk about how their use of sign language and certain behaviors, such as stomping their feet, set them apart from hearing people, even from their families.

In the following conversation between Noel and Marie, the issue of dual affiliation with the Deaf and Hearing worlds comes up. Dealing with this issue was challenging for them and seems to have been part of constructing a Deaf identity for Noel and Marie.

When I was little, deaf or hearing didn't matter. I liked my deaf friends at school; they signed with me. When I went home, I had hearing friends and I talked with them without any signs. I didn't know that there was Deaf culture or a Deaf world until high school when I had a deaf teacher. I became immersed in the Deaf world. I fell in love with the Deaf world. But I did not reject hearing people.

— Noel

When I first came to Gallaudet University and met all these Deaf people, I was really overwhelmed but it was a relief. It took me a long time but I realized that I fit in with the Deaf community. I identify with the Deaf. A long time ago, I wanted to be like hearing people. Not any more. I experienced both worlds. . . . When I go home, I bring my Deaf friends with me and some Deaf culture too. Like in the Deaf community, we can't hear so we eat loudly and it bothers my parents but I say, "Well, we're deaf; we can't hear it." They feel like I don't have any manners but it's not that. It's just that here, nobody can hear you so you don't have to worry about that. Or I'll walk loudly, stomp my feet. My mom gets mad at me but I don't mean to be rude. Sometimes I'll pound on the table and my mom will say, "What's that? Why don't you call my name?" And I say, "Oops, sorry!"

— Marie

Rejecting or Just Moving On?

The students' discussions about the dual influences in their lives—their hearing families and their Deaf peer group—and how, after experiencing both, they feel they belong to the Deaf community, can be understood within the context of their fulfilling the key developmental task of adolescence—the search for a separate definition of self, or an identity (Erikson, 1968).

In the following excerpts, the students discuss leaving their families to be on their own at the university. David describes his feelings of rejection toward his family. Although Adam discusses the separation he felt from his hearing family when he was in high school and now in college, only David uses language of rejection; he believes he had to reject his family in order to be a healthy person. Adam finds he must try to understand his parents' motivations and decisions in providing him with only an oral education experience growing up. After he entered college, he tried to come to grips with his feelings of lost opportunity as he came to meet and identify with Deaf people.

When I started college I didn't want to have anything to do with my family. I totally rejected them. I didn't want to talk to them; I didn't want to write to them. My parents had a hard time with that. It was awful. I rejected my family because I had this anger about being left out of many different things. After a few years I found the need to reconcile with my family just so I could feel better.

— David

In terms of rejecting my family, I don't think so. No, I moved on. I kept in touch with them. I wrote to my mother every week for 5 years. I just did what I needed to do for myself, for my own personal growth and to start my life here in Washington.

— Adam

I think in order for me to be healthy, I had to reject them. I think it was part of the growth process.

— David

When I came home from college at Christmas time, and I was signing and very involved with Deaf people, I remember thinking, "Wow, I have to go back to this. I was very angry at my parents. I wondered why they had never given me the Deaf experience growing up—to give me that opportunity, that chance. I used to ask my mom, "Why didn't you send me to deaf school? Why didn't you teach me sign language? Why didn't you ever think of what I needed? Why, why, why?" My parents were so overwhelmed they started to wonder if they raised me wrong. We had fights all the time. My father and I fought about the Deaf issue. For example, my father would complain about my friends coming over and he'd always ask, "Are they deaf or hearing?" I would say, "Why do you want to know?" And he'd say, "Because I want to know if I'll be able to communicate with them or not." I told him it didn't matter; if they were hearing, it would be all right and if they were deaf, it would be all right. My mother was very understanding, she learned sign language and I knew she would fit into the Deaf world. Then I thought, "Why should I be mad at my parents. I was happy growing up. I'm fine." Life is pretty much okay now. My life and family are here—in the Deaf community. But I feel connected to my family.

— Adam

I love my family but I'm here [at school]. I don't get too involved with them in their lives because they don't understand me. Sometimes I wonder if my staying so far from my parents is because I'm Deaf. When I go home I lose my Deaf identity, and I don't want to do that. I prefer to be somewhere where I can be Deaf, be the way I am. And if I go closer to my family, and if I do things in the Deaf way, or want to talk about being Deaf, my parents don't want to hear it. And I think that applies to a lot of other Deaf people.

— David

Identity is described by Grotevant (1992) as a framework or cognitive structure out of which individuals interact in the world. This identity structure is continually updated as the individual encounters new experiences and information. Eventually, this framework provides a sense of coherence and continuity in the perception of the self—it permits a deep sense of unity to develop (Erikson, 1968).

The students identified themselves as Deaf—as Deaf individuals whose shared language, American Sign Language, and similar life experience create community, the Deaf community (Erting, 1994; Padden & Humphries, 1988). The students, like most deaf people, each met Deaf people and encountered Deaf culture outside of their hearing families at different times in their lives; these experiences over the years eventually resulted in the students adopting the conventions of the culture and choosing to be Deaf. They described how they came to identify with Deaf people: They fell in love with the Deaf world, they no longer wanted to be like hearing people, they found their identity with Deaf people. Their opportunities to meet Deaf people—especially Deaf role models, but peers too—increased when they came to Gallaudet University. Gallaudet University is a liberal arts university for deaf and hard of hearing undergraduates; it also has many faculty and staff who are deaf. The sociolinguistic environment at Gallaudet is characterized by the predominant Deaf culture and the use of American Sign Language as well as spoken English. This experience seems to have "clinched" the Deaf identity structure for these students. Nevertheless, they recognize the need, and the desire, to live in both Hearing and Deaf worlds.

Although, as many deaf people do, the students feel they have experienced a tremendous loss of certain aspects of family life growing up due to "not hearing," they talk about their love for their families. In fact, generally they seem determined to remain a part of their hearing families and to work to make that happen. Perhaps their discussions about their struggle to live as members of their hearing families and to live as Deaf people really represent a struggle to integrate two competing and conflicting identities—one formed out of the need for community with others who share fundamentally similar experiences and a language, and the other a result of the power and influence of the parent–child bond (Erting, 1994).

Recommendations for Supporting the Development of Identity

Identity, similar to other constructs of development, is thought to occur through the course of typical maturational processes within appropriate, supportive social contexts (Erickson, 1968); family relationships, as social context, are key to this development for the individual (Markstrom-Adams, 1992). Markstrom-Adams reported that certain family system characteristics, such as connectedness and permeability, provide the bases for identity formation as opposed to either too little or too much cohesion and affection. Individual family relationships characterized by separateness give the child permission to develop his or her own point of view; and a family context characterized by connectedness among family members provides the child a secure base from which to explore the world outside the family.

For deaf children with hearing parents, the task of identity formation is more complex than it is for their hearing peers. From early on, deaf children who rely primarily on information presented visually, consistently confront issues of language difference as well as behavioral distinctions within the two communities in their environments—their hearing families and the Deaf community. A challenging communication experience between the deaf child and his or her family members due to the language difference can be a distancing factor that affects the nature of the relationships that the deaf child develops within the family, and, therefore, can impact the child's development of identity.

Professionals and parents of young deaf children should be aware of how each of the child's environments (i.e., family, school, and community) might work together to support the child's identity formation and facilitate this complex and often conflicting developmental process.

Do Not Underestimate Parental Influence   Parents may underestimate the impact their beliefs and behaviors have on their deaf child. If deaf children go to residential schools during the week, and are home only on weekends, or if deaf children prefer deaf friends to hearing children as playmates and later develop relationships with their deaf teachers and others within the Deaf community, parents should not think their influence in the parental role is somehow diminished. In fact, family support for the child and a sense of stability within the family are foundational to their child's exploring outside the family and developing their own identity.

Develop a Bicultural or Multicultural Family Identity   Hearing parents early on in their child's life can adapt their family culture(s) to align with Deaf culture. Most families, however, are not prepared to make this change alone; with the assistance and resources of the early childhood specialist, this process of transforming the family cultural identity to include a Deaf culture dimension becomes partly a process of education and also one of developmental change. To facilitate this process, early childhood education programs should encourage hearing parents of young deaf children to meet Deaf adults and Deaf adolescents, to learn ASL, and to introduce their deaf children to adult role models who are deaf; in this way both parents and children learn about Deaf culture and the Deaf community together. Parents can then model the ability to navigate more than one culture and, thus, perhaps find a way to "bridge the two worlds." Hearing families can be encouraged to incorporate into their communication some of the visual/tactile communication strategies common to Deaf culture, such as waving, tapping on the table, or even stomping their feet; once included into the family's way of communicating, extended family members and friends will recognize them as valid attention-related strategies rather than strange behaviors that should be avoided.

DEAF CHILDREN WANT THEIR PARENTS TO KNOW WHAT IT MEANS TO BE DEAF

My parents don't know who I am. If they knew who I was they would know that I'm a very open person, that I'm a very fun person to be around . . . I think if I had the communication with my family, they would know who I am. Once that communication was there, if they could communicate with me like I am today, I think everything would have been fine.

— David

Each of us has a great desire to be known, of having the experience of being totally understood as an individual by those we love and to whom we are closest. Establishing a close emotional relationship or attachment with another human being, usually our mothers, is the primary social task during the first 12–18 months of life (Ainsworth, 1973). The quality of that relationship depends on the infant's experience in interacting with his or her mother or primary caregiver. The mother's ability to be sensitive to her infant's signals and to respond appropriately is significant for the development of attachment. In order to ensure healthy attachment relationships, mothers with deaf infants and toddlers have to recognize how their young child understands the world, and they must embrace how their child is different regarding his or her visual communication needs. Throughout this discussion, the students linked being known by their parents to their parents' understanding of Deafness and to their parents' ability to communicate with them.

Through communication with others we come to create relationships and come to know one another (Tannen, 2001). Deafness gives many individuals outsider status in their families by not having a communication system that enables relationships to develop fully. Outcomes of the lack of fully developed relationships within families are that parents and brothers and sisters do not get to know who deaf individuals are, what their ideas are, or what kind of people they are. Their life experiences are different because they are deaf, and they believe that the people who should be closest to them in their lives do not know what those experiences are or what they mean to them.

"What I'm Like with My Deaf Friends"

The following excerpt of a conversation with Adam and David develops the third theme. Here they compare and contrast what they are like with their deaf friends with what they are like with their hearing families. They reveal their belief that it is because their friends are deaf that a reciprocal relationship develops and so does the foundation for being known.

Adam: *I would like my parents to know what I'm like with my Deaf friends. My mother said one time that she wanted to follow me around with her own interpreter who could tell her everything I was signing. She didn't want me to use my voice. She wanted to see me with my Deaf friends to see what I was like.*

David: *I completely close up when I'm at home. Here, I am comfortable about being myself and being open and emotional. But at home I'm very closed. I'm more open with my wife's family because they understand me; they're Deaf. And that's tough on my mother. My mother doesn't want to lose me to my wife's family because they're a Deaf family.*

Adam: *I had some Deaf friends over at my house and my father was standing in the kitchen, looking into the living room, and he saw me having such a good time with my friends. He didn't understand what was going on, but he knew I was happy. And he made a comment about it. He said, "I notice you look happier with your friends. You're very involved; you're very lively." And I had to tell him, "Yes, that's who I am. That's what I'm like." I want my parents to understand what I'm talking about, what the conversation is about. I want them to know, not just watch what's going on, but to know what's going on. Having a conversation with Deaf people is just so much different; we talk about everything in the world, and I would like for my father to know that.*

"You Have to Be Deaf to Understand"

A deaf person who aligns with the deaf community experiences a way of life with particular customs and values different than those in the hearing majority (Parasnis, 1998). These deaf students believe the differences to be at the core of who they are, and they believe that the differences impact the degree to which their parents, who are hearing, can come to know what it means to be deaf.

I think of the phrase, "You have to be deaf to understand." That applies to my parents. They love me. They accept me, but they don't understand what I go through. The everyday things that I experience. My mom thinks she does, but from my perspective she really doesn't.

— Noel

In an early interview with David, he talked about his parents' understanding what it was like to be deaf. In part of that conversation, given below, he links the level of his parents' knowledge about deafness, their ability to communicate with Deaf people, and their views regarding American Sign Language with their ability to understand him as a Deaf person. The use of ASL is considered one of the significant characteristics that defines and unifies members of the Deaf community (Higgins & Nash, 1987); for David, if his parents deny that ASL is a language, then they are denying the legitimacy of the Deaf community.

To this day I don't think they [my parents] understand what it is like to be deaf. For example, when I try to talk to them about American Sign Language as a language, they deny that it is. They still don't accept that ASL is a language. They say it is a short-cut form; it is a quicker way to communicate. I try to tell them that that's not true. My parents have tried to interact with other Deaf people, but it's difficult because of their sign language skills. It's difficult for them to try and convey their views. They made the effort much more when I was a young child. But they don't truly understand the way Deaf people are and Deaf culture. My mother will listen and say she understands, but I don't think she really does. And that's the problem, they're not trying to work with me and understand who I am. They know I'm deaf, but they're not willing to see my perspective. They say I'm just not different from anyone else. I happen to be deaf. And that's a good opinion, but they have to understand that I am Deaf and that I am different.

— David

David thinks his parents see him as no different than anyone else—that he just happens to be deaf. That perspective, he believes, ironically sets up a barrier that prevents his parents from knowing him. They are, in effect, denying that he is Deaf. David feels this denies the very essence of who he is. For David, this may reflect the ultimate example of how his parents do not know him.

What stands out in these conversations is that, for deaf children of hearing parents, the reason for that lack of knowing is not attributed to an adolescent separation from family, or a generation gap, or a geographic separation—rather, it is attributed to a lack of shared communication from an early age that has persisted through adulthood. These students have high expectations for the kind of communication and intimacy in their families that comes with understanding Deafness and with knowing what they are like as Deaf people; these expectations have not been met. Perhaps, as the students said, it is not possible for a hearing person, even their most loved ones and those closest to them bound by family ties, to cross that boundary and to understand Deafness. This cannot happen because how Deaf people see the world and their everyday life experiences are unknowable by anyone who hears and is not governed by vision (Erting, 1994).

Recommendations for Parents Getting to Know Their Deaf Children

In the book, *We Want to Be Known* (Hubbard, Barbieri, & Power, 1998), teacher researchers write about their efforts to understand girls—who they are, their culture—and how they came to change their perspectives and teaching practices as well as the classroom learning environment as they watched and listened to girls in specific ways. Professionals can encourage parents with deaf children early on to make similar efforts to understand their children by watching and listening carefully. Such efforts may include the following.

Using Parents as Family Observer-Researchers   When Adam's mother said she wanted to follow him around for a day, she was talking about being able to observe her son just as he is so she could learn what he was like. This is a very good idea. Parents can be encouraged to take on the role of observer-researcher. This means that they need to step back and objectively look at and reflect on a particular situation—a piece of their child's family life. What they learn can be used to help them broaden or change their understanding of their children as individuals. For example, when their child is playing with a friend who is deaf, parents can observe how their child uses language to communicate, how he or she relies on the visual and tactile elements of communication, how the children use auditory input in the interaction, and what kind of social interaction skills their child uses. Early intervention specialists can suggest this kind of activity when appropriate for a particular family. The professional can be especially helpful in guiding a family discussion about what the parents observed, by asking leading questions about any changes in perspective that occurred, and by asking whether the family might make any specific changes in behavior due to insights that were gained by the parents. An important outcome for the family is that they develop objective and evaluative ways of thinking—and find their own starting point for understanding—within a parent–professional supportive relationship.

Sustaining an Active Parent–Professional Relationship Over the Child's School Years   David said that his parents made the effort to learn and use sign language when he was a young child. It is doubtful that parents give up learning how to communicate with their child when he or she enters school. However, at this time their involvement in their child's educational program and their relationship with his or her teachers change dramatically. Parents of school-age deaf children most often are on their own if they want to find ways to improve their communication skills (Calderon & Greenberg, 2000). The early education literature has made parallel but related observations regarding how parents continue to be faced with making significant decisions for their deaf child as the early intervention phase ends but with increasingly less information and support from professionals in school-based services (Calderon & Greenberg, 2000). Given the schools' decreased efforts on behalf of families, it is challenging for parents seeking ways to sustain an active level of family support throughout the child's schooling years because institutional resources are not available. Just as parents are encouraged to be assertive and persistent in advocating for services for their deaf child and their family (Calderon & Greenberg, 2000), they need to be similarly encouraged to be active in advocating for continued support and informational services during their child's school years. Parents should be offered opportunities to learn about advocacy during their years in the early intervention program and during transitioning times over the child's school years. Identifying ways to work together with schools and maintaining a teacher–parent partnership model are important functions of the parent-as-advocate role.

Recognizing that a Family with a Deaf Child is a Deaf Family   Parents can come to know their deaf children better, that is, to come closer to understanding what it means to be deaf and to experience life as a deaf person, when they come to know themselves as parents of a deaf child and their family as a family with a deaf child. In the late 1980s, Luterman (1987) observed that hearing families who have a deaf child are deaf families. A deaf child in a hearing family influences family dynamics, how a family lives its life, how family members spend their time, and often where the family lives. Professionals working with families can incorporate practices that encourage opportunities for reflection and understanding regarding how their deaf child, because he or she is deaf, contributes to family life. Parents can be offered opportunities for direct interaction with other families (with both hearing and deaf parents) who have deaf children. Also, by developing relationships with deaf parents, other deaf adults who are important in their child's life—such as his or her teachers—and hearing parents of older deaf children, parents gain first hand knowledge of how families with deaf children work and what it means to be a parent of a deaf child.

RECOMMENDATIONS FOR PRACTICE

What is it we might learn from these students' experiences? More specifically, what did the students tell us that they wanted us to learn? They recognized that prior experience and knowledge about deafness are factors influencing how parents live with their deaf child. They told us that they wanted to get closer to the people they loved. They told us that they wished their families could have joined with them and other Deaf people and shared in their Deaf cultural, perhaps bicultural, identity development. As David said,

I would have liked them to take a class in Deaf culture when I was a baby . . . they knew how to sign, but only between myself and them. That's important . . . But also they should have knowledge of Deaf culture. You have to know about it to be a member of our community. . . . If my parents had known and understood these things when I was a young child . . . then maybe I could have been more involved with my family.

— David

The students provide examples of what the author has suggested (2001) as the process parents experience as they "become parents of a Deaf child." When parents become aware of and critically reflect on what being deaf means to their child, to themselves as parents, and to their family, and their perspectives and behavior regarding deafness change, parents will have experienced a transformative learning process that allows them to become parents of a Deaf child. Adam's father, for example, seems to have gained a new awareness when he found himself in a social situation with Adam and a deaf couple and he could not understand the communication. He came to realize what Adam's communication experiences had been like growing up in their family. But we never know if Adam's father takes action and joins his sons' Deaf culture. David told us that he thinks it was very difficult for his mother to be a mother of a deaf child. His words are moving:

I get the feeling that my mother was disappointed that I was deaf. It bothered my mother. I think because she worked so hard and tried so hard to be a good mother. It was like a criticism of her. And because I was sent to the residential school, my mother wasn't there to take care of me. She wasn't able to see that I was doing okay, and she wasn't able to do her job as a mother. To this day, from time to time, it still bothers her. It reflects on her being a mother.

— *David*

In a course I teach, "Families with Deaf Children," one of the assignments requires the students to meet with a family in order to get a first hand glimpse into that family's life with their deaf child. After her meetings, one student observed: "Hearing parents of deaf children have responsibilities they never even knew existed for parents." From the parents' perspective, knowing this could be overwhelming; for the young deaf child, living in a family that has integrated these responsibilities into their life could make all the difference in their life; and for the early childhood professional, this knowledge is foundational to their work with families with deaf children.

SUMMARY

We assume in our discussions about families and the relationships between parents and children generally, that young children will have access to the family life experiences that occur in their individual families, that they will share a language and, thus, that participation in family communication will be accessible. It is also assumed that children will construct their lives and their self-identities jointly with their families and within the cultural/social context of their families and the communities in which they grow up. But the distinctive lives of Deaf children with hearing families sometimes offer a contrast to these assumptions. When they do not have access to their families' language, there is a disconnect, a setting apart from family (Padden & Humphries, 1988). The life experiences of these five students as "outsiders" (Becker, 1980; Higgins, 1980), included an inability to share ideas, feelings that their families cannot know them, and the development of identity aligned with those outside the family. They allow us to witness how crucial access to family communication is at every stage of development. Communication has a unitary function in the family system.

The stories of lived experiences the students selected to share reflect their interpretations of family life events that occurred; these involved primarily the interactions and relationships they had with their parents and siblings. The themes that emerged capture and label the foundational concepts of these interpreted stories about deaf children growing up in hearing families. Their stories are poignant. As the students talked about their family experiences, they said they felt cherished by their families. They wished things had been different and point to some specific ways their lives might have been better. They said they didn't get the chance in their families to fully experience being the person they are, a Deaf person. They wonder why not. They didn't get a chance to practice and develop their Deafness—who they are—right from the start as infants and toddlers. Their words and stories indicate how they coped; they do not blame their families—indeed, they credit their parents' care and love in raising them. Their voices have much to teach us about the needs of young deaf children growing up in hearing families and communities.

FUTURE PERSPECTIVES

A number of developments have contributed to changes in how the field of early childhood education for deaf children conceptualizes and offers services to deaf children and their families. Family-centered programs based on empowering parents through strength-based strategies and parent–professional partnerships have replaced most child-centered, teacher-as-expert models of early intervention. Information emerging from data based studies of hearing mother–deaf child interaction, language acquisition, and family–professional relationships is changing specific practices in the day-to-day work of early childhood specialists.

Universal newborn hearing screening and diagnosis of hearing loss made within the first few weeks of life make earlier access to information and support possible for families with deaf and hard of hearing children and, when considering optimal learning periods for language acquisition, result in significant advantages for the child. Earlier diagnosis also raises new questions for early intervention specialists used to meeting hearing parents who discovered that their child is deaf after months and sometimes years of thinking he or she was hearing. What are the implications for program development and for working with hearing parents and families—understanding their needs—when, right from the start, they have a deaf child in the family?

One area of knowledge that lags far behind in the field's research efforts is the study of families with deaf children. The first sentence in this chapter refers to the centrality of understanding the family as a dynamic system and context for understanding the development of young children. Although early childhood education for deaf children and their families has included concepts of family systems with speculations about the impact of the deaf child on the hearing family, the field has not yet generated a comprehensive study of the family life experience of those families. Knowledge about family structure, family relationships, family functions, the family life cycle, and related concepts in families with deaf children would provide the conceptual framework professionals need to understand the complexity of family interaction and the day-to-day issues faced by the parents and family members they meet.

Implications for the family life of deaf children are often drawn from studies of important components of family life. Information derived, for example, from studies of stress in families with deaf children (Greenberg, 1983; Meadow-Orlans, 1994), studies of attachment or the quality of the early mother–child relationship (Greenberg & Marvin, 1979; Lederberg & Mobley, 1990), studies of mother–child interaction (see Chapter 11), studies of bilingual families (Blackburn, 2000), and those that focus on social support (Meadow-Orlans & Steinberg, 1993) and family–school relationships (Mertens, Sass-Lehrer, & Scott-Olson, 2000) has provided a significant knowledge base. Also, studies that give voice to children and adults who are deaf to tell their own stories about their life worlds and experiences growing up have made important contributions (Sheridan, 2001; Steinberg, 2000). All of these have advanced the implementation of more appropriate early intervention strategies that meet the unique needs of individual families.

A major challenge to the research community is to devise procedures that enable the study of families with deaf children that is comprehensive and recognizes the great heterogeneity in families. Accomplishing that and then linking the major findings to the practical needs of professionals who work with families, parents, and others would enhance the likelihood that deaf children would be able to sit with their families, late into the night, and be involved in the conversation, reminiscing about things that happened when they were young.

REFERENCES

Ainsworth, M.D. (1973). The development of infant-mother attachment. In B.M. Caldwell & H.N. Ricciuti (Eds.), *Review of child development research* (Vol. 31, pp. 1–95). Chicago: University of Chicago Press.

Becker, G. (1980). *Growing old in silence.* Berkeley: University of California Press.

Blackburn, L. (2000). The development of sociolinguistic meanings: The worldview of a deaf child within his home environment. In M. Metzger (Ed.), *Bilingualism and identity in deaf communities* (pp. 219–254). Washington, DC: Gallaudet University Press.

Bodner-Johnson, B. (1991). Family conversation style: Its effect on the deaf child's participation. *Exceptional Children, 57,* 502–509.

Bodner-Johnson, B. (2001). Parents as adult learners in family-centered early education. *American Annals of the Deaf, 146*, 263–269.

Bronfenbrenner, U. (1979). *The ecology of human development.* Cambridge, MA: Harvard University Press.

Calderon, R., & Greenberg, M. (2000). Challenges to parents and professionals in promoting socioemotional development in deaf children. In P. Spencer, C. Erting, & M. Marschark (Eds.), *The deaf child in the family and at school: Essays in honor of Kathryn P. Meadow-Orlans* (pp. 167–185). Mahwah, NJ: Lawrence Erlbaum Associates.

Clandinin, D., & Connelly, F. (2000). *Narrative inquiry: Experience and story in qualitative research.* San Francisco: Jossey-Bass.

Erikson, E. (1968). *Identity: Youth and crisis.* New York: W.W. Norton.

Erting, C. (1994). *Deafness, communication, social identity: Ethnography in a preschool for deaf children.* Burtonsville, MD: Linstok Press.

Foster, S. (1998). Communication experiences of deaf people: An ethnographic account. In I. Parasnis (Ed.), *Cultural and language diversity and the deaf experience* (pp. 117–135). New York: Cambridge University Press.

Greenberg, M. (1983). Family stress and child competence: The effects of early intervention for families with deaf infants. *American Annals of the Deaf, 128*, 407–417.

Greenberg, M., & Marvin, R. (1979). Attachment patterns in profoundly deaf preschool children. *Merrill-Palmer Quarterly, 25*, 265–279.

Grotevant, H. (1992). Assigned and chosen identity components: A process perspective on their integration. In G. Adams, T. Gullotta, & R. Montemayor (Eds.), *Adolescent identity formation* (pp. 73–90). Thousand Oaks, CA: Sage Publications.

Higgins, P. (1980). *Outsiders in a hearing world.* Thousand Oaks, CA: Sage Publications.

Higgins, P., & Nash, J. (1987). *Understanding deafness socially.* Springfield, IL: Charles C Thomas.

Hubbard, R., Barbieri, M., & Power, B. (Eds.). (1998). *"We want to be known."* York, ME: Stenhouse Publishers.

Lederberg, A., & Mobley, C. (1990). The effect of hearing impairment on the quality of attachment and mother-toddler interaction. *Child Development, 61*, 1596–1604.

Lichtman, W. (1998, November 22). A place at the table. *The Washington Post Magazine,* pp. 15–27.

Luterman, D. (1987). *Deafness in the family.* Boston: Little, Brown.

Markstrom-Adams, C. (1992). A consideration of intervening factors in adolescent identity formation. In G. Adams, T. Gullotta, & R. Montemayor (Eds.), *Adolescent identity formation* (pp. 173–192). Thousand Oaks, CA: Sage Publications.

Meadow-Orlans, K. (1994). Stress, support, and deafness: Perceptions of infants' mothers and fathers. *Journal of Early Intervention, 18*, 91–102.

Meadow-Orlans, K., & Steinberg, A. (1993). Effects of infant hearing loss and maternal support on mother-infant interactions at 18 months. *Journal of Applied Developmental Psychology, 14*, 407–426.

Mertens, D., Sass-Lehrer, M., & Scott-Olson, K. (2000). Sensitivity in the family–professional relationship: Parental experiences in families with young deaf and hard of hearing children. In P. Spencer, C. Erting, & M. Marschark (Eds.), *The deaf child in the family and at school: Essays in honor of Kathryn P. Meadow-Orlans* (pp. 133–150). Mahwah, NJ: Lawrence Erlbaum Associates.

Mohay, H. (2000). Language in sight: Mothers' strategies for making language visually accessible to deaf children. In P. Spencer, C. Erting, & M. Marschark (Eds.), *The deaf child in the family and at school: Essays in honor of Kathryn P. Meadow-Orlans* (pp. 151–166). Mahwah, NJ: Lawrence Erlbaum Associates.

Padden, C., & Humphries, T. (1988). *Deaf in America: Voices from a culture.* Cambridge, MA: Harvard University Press.

Parasnis, I. (1998). On interpreting the deaf experience within the context of culture and language diversity. In I. Parasnis (Ed.), *Cultural and language diversity and the deaf experience* (pp. 3–19). New York: Cambridge University Press.

Patton, M. (1990). *Qualitative evaluation and research methods* (2nd ed.). Thousand Oaks, CA: Sage Publications.

Schlesinger, H., & Meadow, K. (1972). *Sound and sign: Childhood deafness and mental health.* Berkeley: University of California Press.

Sheridan, M. (2001). *Inner lives of deaf children.* Washington, DC: Gallaudet University Press.

Shonkoff, J., & Meisels, S. (Eds.). (2000). *Handbook of early childhood intervention* (2nd ed.). New York: Cambridge University Press.

Spradley, J. (1979). *The ethnographic interview.* New York: Holt, Rinehart and Winston.

Steinberg, A. (2000). Autobiographical narrative on growing up deaf. In P. Spencer, C. Erting, & M. Marschark (Eds.), *The deaf child in the family and at school: Essays in honor of Kathryn P. Meadow-Orlans* (pp. 93–108). Mahwah, NJ: Lawrence Erlbaum Associates.

Stone, E. (1988). *Blacksheep and kissing cousins: How our family stories shape us.* New York: Times Books.

Tannen, D. (2001). *I only say this because I love you.* Boston: Houghton Mifflin.

Walker, D., & Crocker, R. (1988). Measuring family systems outcomes. In H. Weiss & F. Jacobs (Eds.), *Evaluating family programs* (pp. 153–176). New York: Aldine de Gruyter.

Weiss, H., & Jacobs, F. (Eds.). (1988). *Evaluating family programs.* New York: Aldine de Gruyter.

A Mother's Reflection

Rosaline Crawford

Every child and every family is unique and has its challenges. Children who are deaf or hard of hearing and their hearing families have special challenges. The stories told in this chapter reflect the experiences of young adults who grew up in hearing families and have identified themselves as Deaf. All young adults who are deaf or hard of hearing do not share that identity, but many of them share similar experiences. The details of those experiences illustrate the isolation that can exist for any child who is deaf or hard of hearing growing up in a hearing family. The recommendations in this chapter can help strengthen the family and foster inclusion by improving access to communication within the family and by extending the family in new directions.

I confess that I approached this chapter with some trepidation. I was afraid that I would see my family reflected in less-than-happy stories about growing up in a hearing family told by young adults who are deaf. At the same time, I told myself that times had changed, and the experience of my hearing family with a child who is deaf would be different. It is, and it isn't.

When my daughter was an infant we learned that she had a "significant" hearing loss. I cried because I feared that I would not be able to communicate with her. I believed then, as I do now, that communication is an integral part of the parent–child relationship. We did not and could not know how much she could hear, even with the hearing aids we bought for her. We were unwilling to invest her precious early years for language acquisition on the auditory/oral method alone. We wanted to provide her with access to language and a means to communicate that we knew had at least some guarantee of success. We began to learn sign language and practiced what we learned when we talked to her. Unlike many other families, we had access to good resources. We enrolled in several early intervention programs (state, county, and then local) to ensure that our daughter would have better sign language role models than we could provide ourselves.

I recall, vividly, a time when she was a toddler and a group of parents were discussing some new research findings about language and the brain. That research suggested that stimulating residual hearing might reduce the brain's ability to allocate its resources to acquire visual sign language. One of the mothers in that group had outfitted her child with hearing aids, had enrolled her child in speech and auditory therapy, was learning and using sign language, and had placed her child in a sign language based educational program. Like me, she was doing her best to provide her child with every possible opportunity to access two languages, spoken English and sign language. She was outraged that someone would now suggest that what she was doing was not the best thing for her child. In response, she stated emphatically that, when her child is 16, she does not want him to be mad at her because she cannot communicate with him. She wants him to be mad at her for not giving him the car keys. That mother has since become an interpreter.

I, on the other hand, have not become an interpreter. At best, I am "conversant" in sign language. Learning another language as an adult has not been easy or quick. It took several years of almost daily exposure to and use of sign language for me to feel comfortable having a conversation with another adult who signs well. It was impossible to have a conversation with another adult who was also learning sign language—my husband. This is a hard truth. When our daughter was 4 years old, we each felt comfortable enough communicating in sign language with her, and we were able to expose our newborn hearing son to both spoken English and sign language. Still, the conversations we had between us were in spoken English, sometimes sprinkled with the signs we knew.

On this home front, my daughter had more to contend with than just parents who could not communicate with each other in sign language. When she was 7 years old, her father died after fighting an extended battle with cancer. It was important to him that she knew what was happening. Using the sign language he knew, he talked to her about his illness, his surgeries and treatments, and his love for her. Because of his absence, she misses out on ambient adult family conversation. Also, she has a lifelong challenge of missing him.

My now 12-year-old daughter switches between the sign language she uses fluidly at school and the sign language that I and her 8-year-old brother are capable of at home. The differences between us can still be felt almost daily. For example, her hearing brother goes to a neighborhood school and has friends whose families live nearby and visit our home frequently. My daughter's friends and their families are widely scattered, and we visit with them less frequently. Unlike her brother and me, my daughter does not have passing casual conversations with the neighbors, postman, librarian, or store clerks because they do not sign.

I cannot change the world. For my daughter, I wish I could. Instead, my focus has been centered on our immediate family, trying to build strong ties here at home and giving my children room to grow. Part of my job as a hearing parent of a child who is deaf is to explore and develop my own and my family's identity, and ensure that my children have the opportunity to explore their own.

Some people say that my daughter is lucky. In addition to her mother and brother who can sign, her grandmother, aunts, uncles, and cousins can sign a little. They live in another state and hired a sign language tutor for weekly family group lessons. We include my daughter in our annual family gatherings to the best of our abilities, as good as they are and as insufficient as they may be. Our extended family also includes two families with parents who are deaf and children who are deaf and hearing. We help each other with child care occasionally, and we get together just to visit and for birthdays and other special occasions. We have gone camping together, vacationed for several years at the beach together, and recently all went to Disney World together.

There is no doubt that my daughter has a Deaf identity. She prefers to be with people, peers and adults, who are deaf and/or can sign fluently. This is understandable and natural. She is involved in after-school sports activities and a monthly book club. She invites friends to visit and stay overnight because it extends the time for interaction and is generally more convenient.

Perhaps it is because of my less-than-fluent sign language skills that the communication between my daughter and me is less than what I would like it to be. Perhaps it is because I am not Deaf and cannot fully understand and appreciate her life experiences. Perhaps it is because my daughter has been practicing to be a teenager for years. Not only am I not Deaf and do not sign as well she can—I am her mother. She has never been very responsive to my attempts to initiate conversations with her, but I will never stop trying. The moments of her impromptu information sharing with me are treasured. I, too, do not want my daughter to be mad at me because I cannot communicate with her. I want her to be mad at me for not giving her the car keys.

Postscript: I shared this commentary with my daughter. I wanted to share my thoughts with her, and I wanted her permission to share them with others. She scoffed at the notion that she has been practicing to be a teenager for years. Then she demanded the car keys.

CHAPTER TWO

Support for Parents

Promoting Visual Attention and Literacy in a Changing World

KATHRYN P. MEADOW-ORLANS

I t was very helpful to have the early intervention person who could come and help educate us about deaf children. [She could tell us] What does that mean? Why is she having trouble here? What's the prognosis for this? What should we be doing? . . . We were totally [ignorant]. We had no idea. So that was really good, having somebody. She kind of held our hand through all the early trauma of it. (Interview conducted for Gallaudet National Parent Project, Meadow-Orlans, Mertens, & Sass-Lehrer, 2003)

Support for families of children who are deaf or hard of hearing has been a cornerstone of early intervention for many years. It is widely accepted that professionals can provide appropriate services and support to parents as they adjust to the identification of hearing loss in an infant or young child, plan for the present and the future, or deal with financial and child care pressures (Meadow-Orlans & Sass-Lehrer, 1995). However, as population characteristics have changed and new social patterns create different pressures for families, the nature of needed support services has shifted. This chapter describes the changing world of families, especially related to parent or caregiver involvement in children's education and acquisition of literacy. This discussion is followed by suggestions for promoting visual attention and book sharing at home.

SPECIAL COMMUNICATION NEEDS

Communication is the foundation of literacy. It is the key to expressing and understanding feelings about oneself and others; through communication children learn the rules of social behavior needed to operate effectively at home and at school. Literacy is typically acquired during early childhood, and the importance of children's early years is recognized by folklore and common sense as well as by practitioners and researchers.

Those concerned with the early years of children who are deaf or hard of hearing pose a recurring question: What effect does restricted auditory ability have on the children, their hearing parents, other family members, their schools, and their communities? In the most general sense, limited hearing requires a child to rely on vision to perceive and interact with the world. Thus, children who are profoundly deaf must learn to communicate using visual attention, and those who are hard of hearing must learn to augment their residual auditory skills.

If hearing parents are to influence their child's literacy, they will probably try to become fluent in Signed English, American Sign Language, or Cued Speech (Meadow-Orlans et al., 2003). Parents need also to understand and incorporate the broader habit of using vision rather than sound for comprehending the world. They must grasp the processes and the demands of managing their child's divided attention: A child who does not hear must gaze first at the object and then at the speaker in order to understand the subject of a discussion about an object. Parents must learn to wait until their child is attending to them before presenting a visual message and then allow time for the child to gaze at a conversational object before returning his or her gaze to the parent's face and hands. It is difficult for hearing parents to replace the lifelong habit of simultaneously discussing an object while maintaining eye contact with a communicative partner. Even the habit of talking while performing a task with one's hands is difficult to break. Along with an individual family's unique needs, these special communication needs for parents or caregivers and their deaf or hard of hearing children must be considered within the broader context of the social patterns and pressures that influence all parents in the 21st century.

THE CHANGING WORLD FOR PARENTS AND CHILDREN

Changes in the United States since the 1980s, such as more mothers working outside of the home and more single-parent families, have placed increasing demands on the time parents have available to spend with their children. Time management is a central issue for all families, but it becomes even more difficult for families of children who are deaf or hard of hearing. It takes time for parents and siblings to learn sign language, to go with a child to extra medical checkups and to audiological tests and hearing aid checks, and to communicate appropriately to a child who must divide his or her visual attention between person and object.

Working Mothers

Among the general population in the United States, family life has changed dramatically in a relatively short time. For example, 12% of mothers with preschool-age children were working in 1950, compared with 47% in 1980 and 67% in 1997 (Hofferth, 1999). It is difficult to obtain comparable family-based data for children who are deaf. One of the few available sources, the Gallaudet National Parent Project (NPP), included a survey of American parents of 6- and 7-year-old children with a hearing loss. Those data showed that 60% of hearing mothers of those children were working outside the home, compared with 67% of all American mothers of preschoolers (Meadow-Orlans et al., 2003).

As more and more families rely on two incomes, economic pressures for mothers to work outside the home increase. Those who opt to stay at home may feel community disapproval similar to that directed toward working mothers in the 1950s. These pressures and ambiguities are compounded for working mothers of children with special needs. A hearing mother of two young children who are deaf expressed the resulting ambivalence poignantly:

Financially, we're really struggling . . . I don't know if I should sacrifice the signing . . . [and] being able to communicate, and go back to [work] . . . I really feel that communication's important. If I go back to work they're going to miss out on the communication. But if I don't . . . we're getting the bare necessities and sometimes not them. Then I can honestly admit that there's

*a strain on the marriage. Because he's like working constantly, and I'm
feeling guilty . . . I'm caught in a situation where I feel guilty that I'm not
working and helping him out to support us, yet I'll feel guilty if I go back
to work because [the children] will be lacking [communication]. (Meadow-
Orlans, 1995, p. 355)*

A sociologist found that working mothers in the general population
experience a great deal of stress (Hochschild, 1989). They work a full
day before going home to work a second shift performing household tasks:

> For women as well as men, work in the marketplace is less often a
> simple economic fact than a complex cultural value. If in the early
> part of the century it was considered unfortunate that a woman had
> to work, it is now thought surprising when she doesn't. (Hochschild,
> 1997, p. 198)

The conflicts for working mothers with deaf and hard of hearing
children are multiplied, and family and community pressures are esca-
lated, because these mothers, in addition to attending to everyday stres-
sors, need to attend to a child with special needs. Like the mother quoted
previously, families of deaf children often have additional demands, such
as learning sign language, arranging for special accommodations in school,
or advocating for their child's inclusion.

Presser, a sociologist, has identified an additional emerging trend
that affects many working mothers and is likely to influence more families
in the future. She reported that "Americans are moving toward a 24-
hour, 7-day-a-week economy. Two fifths of all employed Americans
worked mostly during the evenings or nights, on rotating shifts, or on
weekends" (1999, p. 1778). Parents often work two jobs or work different
shifts so that one is available to care for children while the other is on
the job, with new strains placed on marital and family relationships.
Among couples with children, divorce is three to six times more likely
if one spouse is employed nights, the other days (Presser, 1999). Despite
these increasing pressures, a mother averaged 5.8 hours per day with
her children, which is slightly more than the average mother spent with
her children in 1965. This was managed by "stealing" time from other
activities such as recreation, housekeeping chores, and sleep (Milkie,
Bianchi, Mattingly, & Robinson, 2002).

Single-Parent Families

There have been a few attempts to investigate what relationship, if any,
there is between caring for a child who is deaf and marital discord and

divorce, and results are inconclusive. Some families are drawn closer together as they cope with special needs; others are driven apart by the additional strain (Koester & Meadow-Orlans, 1990). The NPP survey found that slightly more than two thirds of children surveyed lived in a "traditional" family with two biological parents, and 32% lived with one parent only or with step, adoptive, or foster parents (Meadow-Orlans et al., 2003). *USA Today* (1999) reported that 42% of U.S. children without hearing problems lived with one parent only or with step, adoptive, or foster parents. Although these percentages appear to be favorable for deaf and hard of hearing children, it is important to remember that these percentages reflect only a moment in time and do not reflect the parental separations, divorce, and death that occur as children age.

Data from studies on children in one-parent families show that, on average, these children tend to have fewer economic advantages compared with their peers living with two parents, because a one-parent family tends to have less disposable income. Single parents may experience more stress and therefore be unable to provide optimal attention to family matters. Children living with single parents may exhibit more academic, health, and behavioral problems; complete fewer years of education; and typically enter lower-income occupations (Hernandez, 1993). However, it is important to remember that many single parents cope successfully with increased stress and demands and that many of their children perform extremely well.

Of 22 three-year-old children with hearing loss enrolled in an early intervention program in Seattle and participating in a research project, five (23%) lived in homes in which the father was absent. Language and academic-related test scores of children in those homes were significantly lower than the scores of children in homes in which fathers were present. However, of equal importance is the finding that maternal involvement and social-emotional adjustment were no different in the two groups of mothers (Calderon & Low, 1998). Many single mothers enlist friends or relatives to serve as male role models for their children.

The Changing Role of Fathers

Another cultural trend observed in American families is what one author has called "the modernization of fatherhood" (LaRossa, 1997). He believes that the revolution in fathers' family roles began around 1930, with growing expectations that fathers would participate in child care. Young fathers increasingly place priority on their families. A 2002 survey found that 70% of men in their twenties and thirties were willing to give up some of their pay in exchange for more time with their families (Grimsley, 2000).

Nevertheless, there is a good deal of documentation that fathers are less involved than mothers with their children who are deaf, and fathers tend to have more difficulty and (perhaps) less motivation to learn sign language than do mothers (Gregory, 1995; Meadow-Orlans, 1990). The NPP survey found that 75% of mothers and 61% of fathers reported using signs or cues. Parents were asked to rate their signing or cuing skills as "excellent," "good," "fair," or "poor." Sixty-four percent of mothers versus 37% of fathers rated their skills as either "excellent" or "good" (Meadow-Orlans et al., 2003). This means that intervention specialists must pay special attention to the needs and the schedules of the fathers of families participating in their programs (Vadasy, Fewell, Greenberg, Dermond, & Meyer, 1986).

Diversity and Deafness

The increasing diversity of the American population as a whole is a social demographic trend with special importance for those concerned with the welfare of deaf children and their families. These families, like all others, come from many different cultural, linguistic, socioeconomic, and educational backgrounds. Too often people assume that deaf children and their families represent a homogeneous group; this is far from the truth. Although it is convenient to refer to "deaf" children, more than half of those receiving services are hard of hearing. The NPP survey also found that 30% of all children were identified as having a disabling condition (other than deafness), 7% were said to have a behavior problem, and 9% were said to have an attention deficit. These subgroups of children have special needs that require extra time from their parents.

Parents of children who are deaf are also heterogeneous. Prominent differences among these families are their racial and ethnic backgrounds. An analysis of racial and ethnic backgrounds of deaf and hard of hearing children reported to Gallaudet's Annual Survey found a decrease in those categorized as "white, non-Hispanic" from 71% in 1977 to 58% in 1997. In the same 20-year period, children from Hispanic backgrounds increased from 9% to 18%, and those from Asian/Pacific Islander families increased from 1% to 4%. Proportions from African American and American Indian families remained stable at 17% and 1%, respectively (Holden-Pitt & Diaz, 1998).

Other differences among these families may include language, socioeconomic status, and education. Parents whose native language is not English often find it more difficult to support English literacy skills in their children. Parents who are struggling financially may have less time and energy to devote to book sharing and other literacy-promoting activities. Families with limited education whose own backgrounds do not include a "culture of literacy" may be less able (though no less motivated) to read with their children. Children from these homes will need additional support from skilled and sensitive intervention specialists.

Because families with children who are deaf or hard of hearing are heterogeneous, educators must focus on serving the needs of these families across a broad spectrum of race, ethnicity, socioeconomic status, and education, and should recognize the increasing presence of these children and parents in intervention programs.

PROVIDING SUPPORT FOR FAMILIES

Parental time constraints are important because they may bear directly on the parent or caregiver's ability to be involved in educational activities with their children. One study of deaf children, conducted 9–53 months after their completion of an early intervention (birth to three) program, found that mothers' early involvement was closely related both to their own communication skills and to their child's early reading skills (Calderon, 2000). Support professionals struggle with assisting families in which parents' time limitations often interfere with their ability to fully attend to the special needs of their children. On the one hand, it is the defined role of the professional to support families in performing the tasks that promote the child's development. On the other hand, many professional intervention expectations can escalate the guilt that some parents feel. Professionals constantly need to be aware of parents' competing obligations, acknowledge the demands on the parents' time, and perhaps work with parents to prioritize the tasks related to their child with a hearing loss. Could a sibling, babysitter, grandparent, or aunt read with the child on a regular basis? Could time management strategies be incorporated into parent meetings? In today's family-centered programs, professionals and parents often collaborate to develop strategies that build on families' strengths, resources, and preferences, thus enabling greater parental involvement and more frequent learning opportunities for children.

Dealing with Guilt

American parents, especially mothers, have habitually received guilt-inducing advice from a variety of well-meaning professionals. In the 1990s, there were arguments about what makes a "good" mother:

> Americans are divided on whether mothers should stay home with their children, and on whether a "good" parent would spank a child.

We even disagree about what age a "good" mother should be. Most of us agree it's bad to be a mother too young, but at what age does a new mother become too old? Does allowing a baby to sleep in your bed build a more secure child or an overly dependent one? Is it bad to breast-feed a toddler—or to give a newborn a bottle? . . . [A]dvertisers make mothers feel bad if they don't buy the right baby products, while advice givers say a sure sign of a "bad" mother is a woman who buys her child too much. (Ladd-Taylor & Umansky, 1998, pp. 2–3)

Parents whose child is born with a disability sometimes feel they are to blame in some way (Harvey, 1989). Some cultures and religions see disability as a punishment from God for past sins of a parent (Steinberg, Davila, Collazo, Loew, & Fischgrund, 1997). Guilt can be induced by conflicting advice about appropriate communication modes or about choosing hearing aids and cochlear implants (Harvey, 2001; Schwartz, 1996). A plethora of choices and guilt about proceeding in the "right" direction can induce a sense of powerlessness in parents of deaf and hard of hearing children. Schlesinger suggested that these conditions might produce "families where mothers are temporarily or permanently unable to use effective communication strategies with their children . . . [and] the children in turn develop passive stances toward learning" (1992, p. 39). Professionals certainly do not want to add to whatever burdens of guilt or blame parents may already be carrying. Most are sensitive to the dangers of parental guilt and powerlessness, but the line between motivation and action, paralysis and inaction, is fine. When in doubt, professionals should remember to ask parents, "What can I do to help you?" (Meadow-Orlans et al., 2003).

Maintaining Professional Flexibility

Flexibility may be the most important characteristic for success in working with families and young children, but it is a difficult one to acquire. Professionals may need to be flexible to accommodate working parents' schedules. Conferences by telephone or e-mail—arranged for early morning, evening, or weekends, before or after working hours, or offering alternative dates—may encourage more parental participation. Meetings held in the community or in families' homes might save parents driving time. Meetings held over dinner can also save time. Some schools establish voice-mail systems that enable educators to record messages with news and assignments. Time management discussions in parent groups can be helpful, and provision of opportunities for child care sharing and carpooling or ride sharing may be practical aids for parents. Many support professionals use modern technology, such as e-mail, web sites, or CD-ROMs. Videotaped sign language and speech lessons or hearing aid demonstrations enable parents to proceed at their own pace and in accordance with their own schedules. Sometimes a "low-tech" strategy, just listening to parents with a sympathetic ear or recognizing families' time constraints, can be comforting and enable a stressed parent to manage the next day's schedule.

VISUAL ATTENTION, SYMBOLIC PLAY, AND LITERACY

Much research has been devoted to deaf children's difficulties in developing literacy (Musselman, 2000). "Since the very beginning of formal approaches to deaf education, the development of literacy has been a priority issue" (Power & Leigh, 2000, p. 3). Reading skills are related to visual attention skills, the development of symbolic play, and prereading activities, each of which is examined in the following sections.

Visual Attention: Entry to the Literate World

The importance of visual attention cannot be overstated in relation to the development of children with a hearing loss. These children quickly learn how closing their eyes can control unwanted information. Since 1990 there has been a good deal of research investigating the intuitive techniques used by deaf mothers for socializing their deaf infants in the appropriate and efficient use of visual attention (Swisher, 1993, 2000). These techniques include increased use of touch, signing on the child's body, exaggerated facial expressions to draw the child's attention to the face, signing in the child's line of vision or in the peripheral field of vision, kinetic and tactile contact, and increased use of positive facial expression. Many deaf parents use fingerspelling very early with their children (Erting, Thumann-Prezioso, & Benedict, 2000). These techniques serve to support the development of visual attention skills. Analysis of data from the Gallaudet Infancy Project videotapes found that 18-month-old deaf infants and their deaf mothers engaged in significantly longer periods of joint attention than either deaf infants with hearing mothers or hearing infants with deaf mothers (Meadow-Orlans & Spencer, 1996).

In England, Wood, Wood, Griffiths, and Howarth (1986) were among the first to emphasize the problem created by deaf children's need to divide their attention between the acts and the objects of communication. This means that communication proceeds more slowly than when a child can attend visually to an object while he or she listens to an observation about it. Wood and his colleagues believe that mastering these techniques of visual attention create the basis for all future learning, including reading and writing. Many studies have demonstrated the higher reading achievements of deaf children with deaf parents, compared with those with hearing parents (Marschark, 1993; Meadow, 1980). These findings may be explained by the fact that deaf mothers "are more sensitive to the ebb and flow of their young child's attention and, hence, are more contingent upon her actions" (Wood et al., 1986, p. 173). Thus, future achievement may rest not only on sign communication skill, but also on attentional empathy.

Book Sharing: Early Window to Literacy

Research with hearing children shows that those with early and extensive exposure to print have a head start on learning to read (Paul, 2003). One study has shown that the value of naming activities decreases in relation to the achievement of literacy at later developmental stages (Wells, 1985). This study found that the preschool activity most closely associated with reading comprehension at age 7 was "listening to stories." The author of this study proposed that early reading is more likely to result from being given opportunities to become aware of the symbolic properties of written language than from simple vocabulary building. Likewise, early book sharing with deaf and hard of hearing children can facilitate the ability to engage in prolonged periods of joint attention, give them exposure to print, and provide a head start on literacy, especially if combined with storytelling.

One deaf child with deaf parents demonstrated joint attention skills very effectively on videotape when she was 18 months old. She had learned to start at the front of a book and work toward the back and to turn one page at a time and absorb the new information on each page. She had learned to divide her attention between the information on the page and the information supplied by her mother. As an active participant in the interaction around the picture book, she recognized that the objects pictured in the book had names, the names had signs, and that there is meaning to be found in the pages of a book and enjoyment in the learning process. When these skills are broken down into their small components, the achievements of this child, guided by her mother, were very impressive. A mother of a child who is hard of hearing described reading to her 3-year-old:

One thing we always noticed [before her hearing loss was identified] was how much she would watch our mouths . . . and when we would read a story to her it was like she would turn around and read my lips . . . I just thought she was interested in watching me while I was reading the story. But I think she was . . . compensating very well. . . . She was our first child, and I spent loads of time with her. . . . We read to her and sang to her, and I think she just compensated really well as I heard deaf and hard of hearing children can. (Interview conducted for Gallaudet National Parent Project, Meadow-Orlans et al., 2003)

Children enjoy having the same story read to them again and again (Schleper, n.d.). Adults usually find this repetition boring, but children get pleasure in the repetition of familiar narratives. Stories heard over and over become children's own. Pretending to read books is one way that children explore literacy (Elster, 1994). Two 5-year-old hearing children gave these explanations of how they learned to read by frequent exposure to the same stories (Sulzby, 1985, p. 459):

> First Child: Well, my sister and my mom read me Sherman and Herman lots of times, and then I started knowing it 'cause she reads a good line lots of times. And The [Very] Hungry Caterpillar, she read it lots of times, too.
> Second Child: When my mother reads me stories, I learn how to read. I can even remember one of the books. I have one of the books at home I know how to read, and I can read it. I can read most of the pages without even having the book with me.

As children gain familiarity with the words, situations, and meanings of stories, the prelearning that leads to literacy takes place.

SUGGESTIONS FOR PROFESSIONALS: SUPPORTING VISUAL ATTENTION AND BOOK SHARING

Parents whose time is limited will still recognize the need for structured time with their children in order to promote visual attention and preliteracy skills. Setting aside a specific time of day (e.g., after breakfast, before bed, Sunday mornings) can lead a child to expect and enjoy a quiet time together with a parent. Concrete suggestions and demonstrations can empower parents with specific techniques and strategies to use with their deaf or hard of hearing children. Several options are available, two of which are described here.

Mohay's Demonstration Strategies

Based on her observations of deaf mothers' interactions with their young deaf children, Heather Mohay in Australia has developed a program to demonstrate strategies to facilitate visual attention for hearing mothers of deaf infants (Mohay, 2000). She trains teams of deaf mothers to go into homes of hearing parents. Here are some of the strategies for gaining and directing attention and making language salient that are demonstrated for hearing parents:

> Breaking the child's line of gaze and gaining attention using movements of the hands and body . . . Using touch to gain the child's attention . . . Using pointing to direct attention while still permitting

language input . . . Reducing the frequency of communication so that it is recognized as worthy of attention . . . Using short utterances . . . Positioning self and objects in the child's visual field . . . Moving hands or face, or both, into the child's visual field. (pp. 155–157)

Shared Book Reading Project

Gallaudet's Laurent Clerc National Deaf Education Center has a Shared Book Reading Project, initiated by David Schleper, Jane Fernandes, and Doreen Higa (Schleper, 1998a, 1998b). Helpful tips for parents are included in the program. Although the tips are aimed at parents who use sign language, they can be adapted by parents who are sign beginners, or by those whose children are exposed to "speech only":

1. Choose books both you and your child like.

2. Make sure your child can see your face, your signs, and the print at the same time.

3. Don't be limited by the words. Expand on the book's ideas.

4. Talk about the story with your child as you read. Ask your child questions. Connect ideas in the story with your experiences. Have your child predict what will happen next.

5. Be dramatic. Play with the signs and exaggerate your facial expressions to show different characters.

6. Vary where you make the signs. Sometimes sign on the page; sometimes sign on your child; sometimes sign in the usual place.

7. If you don't know some signs, don't panic. Use gestures, point to pictures, and act out that part of the story. Later you can ask your child's teacher for the sign.

8. Keep attention by tapping lightly on your child's shoulder, or giving your child a gentle nudge.

9. Let your child guide you through the story. For very young children, this may mean letting the child turn the pages as you briefly describe the pictures. When your child is older, you can actually read the story.

10. Act out the story after you have read it.

11. Read the story over and over if your child asks. This is an important part of language development.

12. Have fun! Make your time together a positive experience.

Expanding the Family Circle

In order to give all children a head start on achievement, those outside the immediate family can be involved as well. Connecting with extended family and the community is important in this era when parents are often overwhelmed with work and other responsibilities. Older siblings, grandparents, aunts, uncles, cousins, friends, and neighbors or babysitters can be encouraged to read to a young deaf or hard of hearing child, and this can multiply the child's exposure to early literacy activities. Having outside support also can help to deal with family time constraints.

There are numerous additional community avenues that can be explored. For example, local public libraries might sponsor signed storytelling hours. High school or college students enrolled in sign language classes might volunteer (or be assigned) to sign storybooks for children on a regular basis. Public notices calling for Deaf adult volunteers to read to children who are deaf might be an option. These activities require a great deal of organization, but there are many community volunteers, especially in senior citizen and church groups, who could be excited about participating in such projects.

CONCLUSION AND FUTURE PERSPECTIVES

Young children with a hearing loss need increased time, attention, language, and communication from their parents or caregivers early in their lives if they are to develop the communicative and preliteracy skills that lead to adequate reading achievement and positive social-emotional development. However, their parents, like all American parents, are caught in a time-bind, with fewer resources at their disposal for meeting their children's needs.

Professionals in the field of early childhood education for children who are deaf or hard of hearing have taken some positive steps toward meeting the needs of families. Those who collaborate with parents in family-centered programs find that parents expend enormous amounts of time and energy advocating on behalf of their children. Many programs to help parents and young children improve communication skills and promote literacy are in place throughout the country.

A broad perspective may be needed to make further progress toward family involvement in early literacy development. One parent group crafted a Parents' Bill of Rights, with impressively broad objectives. The keystone is a search for broad solutions to some of the problems parents are facing, with the expectation that parents have the right to ask for help from outside the family (Hewlett & West, 1998). A good case can be made for additional special help to be provided to parents of deaf and hard of hearing children. Parents generally have problems with time management and the competition of work and family goals, and these strains are magnified for the parents of children with special needs. It should be possible to seek child care subsidies, broad-based tax relief, or subsidized education for parents from local, state, or federal governments, from public and private foundations, and from corporations. If society values mothers and fathers who spend more time with their children, society should expect to help make that possible.

This is by no means a small proposal. It would involve a major effort on the part of every organization involved with deaf and hard of hearing children. The needs are great, and the stakes are high. The futures of children depend on bold efforts to meet their needs—and meeting their needs begins at home.

REFERENCES

Calderon, R. (2000). Parental involvement in deaf children's education programs as a predictor of child's language, early reading, and social-emotional development. _Journal of Deaf Studies and Deaf Education, 5_(2), 140–155.

Calderon, R., & Low, S. (1998). Early social-emotional, language, and academic development in children with hearing loss: Families with and without fathers. _American Annals of the Deaf, 143,_ 225–234.

Elster, C. (1994). Patterns within preschoolers' emergent readings. _Reading Research Quarterly, 29,_ 403–416.

Erting, C.J., Thumann-Prezioso, C., & Benedict, B.S. (2000). Bilingualism in a deaf family: Fingerspelling in early childhood. In P.E. Spencer, C.J. Erting, & M. Marschark (Eds.), _The deaf child in the family and at school: Essays in honor of Kathryn P. Meadow-Orlans_ (pp. 41–54). Mahwah, NJ: Lawrence Erlbaum Associates.

Gregory, S. (1995). _Deaf children and their families._ Cambridge, England: Cambridge University Press.

Grimsley, K.D. (2000, May 3). Family a priority for young workers: Survey finds change in men's thinking. _The Washington Post,_ p. E1.

Harvey, M.A. (1989). _Psychotherapy with deaf and hard-of-hearing persons: A systemic model._ Mahwah, NJ: Lawrence Erlbaum Associates.

Harvey, M.A. (2001). "Does God have a cochlear implant?" _Journal of Deaf Studies and Deaf Education, 6,_ 70.

Hernandez, D.J. (1993). _America's children: Resources from family, government, and the economy._ New York: Russell Sage Foundation.

Hewlett, S.A., & West, C. (1998). _The war against parents: What we can do for America's beleaguered moms and dads._ Boston: Houghton Mifflin.

Hochschild, A. (1989). _The second shift._ New York: Viking.

Hochschild, A.R. (1997). _The time bind: When work becomes home and home becomes work._ New York: Henry Holt and Company.

Hofferth, S.L. (1999, Spring). Changes in American children's time, 1981–1997. _Childnews,_ 1–4.

Holden-Pitt, L., & Diaz, J.A. (1998). Thirty years of the annual survey of deaf and hard-of-hearing children & youth: A glance over the decades. _American Annals of the Deaf, 143_(2), 72–76.

Increasing prevalence of one-parent families. (1999, June 14). _USA Today,_ p. 6D.

Koester, L.S., & Meadow-Orlans, K.P. (1990). Parenting a deaf child: Stress, strength, and support. In D.F. Moores & K.P. Meadow-Orlans (Eds.), _Educational and developmental aspects of deafness_ (pp. 299–320). Washington, DC: Gallaudet University Press.

Ladd-Taylor, M., & Umansky, L. (Eds.). (1998). _"Bad" mothers: The politics of blame in twentieth-century America._ New York: New York University Press.

LaRossa, R. (1997). _The modernization of fatherhood: A social and political history._ Chicago: University of Chicago Press.

Marschark, M. (1993). _Psychological development of deaf children._ New York: Oxford University Press.

Meadow, K.P. (1980). *Deafness and child development*. Berkeley: University of California Press.

Meadow-Orlans, K.P. (1990). The impact of childhood hearing loss on the family. In D.F. Moores & K.P. Meadow-Orlans (Eds.), *Educational and developmental aspects of deafness* (pp. 321–338). Washington, DC: Gallaudet University Press.

Meadow-Orlans, K.P. (1995). Sources of stress for mothers of deaf and hard of hearing infants. *American Annals of the Deaf, 140*, 352–357.

Meadow-Orlans, K.P., Mertens, D.M., & Sass-Lehrer, M.A. (2003). *Parents and their deaf children: The early years*. Washington, DC: Gallaudet University Press.

Meadow-Orlans, K.P., & Sass-Lehrer, M. (1995). Support services for families with children who are deaf: Challenges for professionals. *Topics in Early Childhood Special Education, 15*(3), 314–334.

Meadow-Orlans, K.P., & Spencer, P.E. (1996). Maternal sensitivity and the visual attentiveness of children who are deaf. *Early Development and Parenting, 5*, 213–223.

Milkie, M.A., Bianchi, S.M., Mattingly, M.J., & Robinson, J.P. (2002). Gendered division of childrearing: Ideals, realities, and the relationship to parental well-being. *Sex Roles, 47*, 21–38.

Mohay, H. (2000). Language in sight: Mothers' strategies for making language visually accessible to deaf children. In P.E. Spencer, C.J. Erting, & M. Marschark (Eds.), *The deaf child in the family and at school: Essays in honor of Kathryn P. Meadow-Orlans* (pp. 151–166). Mahwah, NJ: Lawrence Erlbaum Associates.

Musselman, C. (2000). How do children who can't hear learn to read an alphabetic script? A review of the literature on reading and deafness. *Journal of Deaf Studies and Deaf Education, 5*(1), 9–31.

Paul, P.V. (2003). Processes and components of reading. In M. Marschark & P.E. Spencer (Eds.), *The Oxford handbook of deaf studies, language, and education* (pp. 97–109). New York: Oxford University Press.

Power, D., & Leigh, G.R. (2000). Principles and practices of literacy development for deaf learners: A historical overview. *Journal of Deaf Studies and Deaf Education, 5*(1), 3–8.

Presser, H.B. (1999). Toward a 24-hour economy. *Science, 284*, 1778–1779.

Schleper, D. (1998a, Fall–Winter). Here's how the shared reading process works. *Preview*, 1–3.

Schleper, D. (1998b, Spring–Summer). Reading together, the Shared Reading Project expands to six sites. *Preview*, 1–4.

Schleper, D. (n.d.). *Read it again and again*. [Videotape and manual]. Washington, DC: Gallaudet University, Clerc Center.

Schlesinger, H.S. (1992). Elusive X factor: Parental contributions to literacy. In M. Walworth, D.F. Moores, & T.J. O'Rourke (Eds.), *A free hand: Enfranchising the education of deaf children* (pp. 37–66). Silver Spring, MD: T.J. Publishers.

Schwartz, S. (Ed.). (1996). *Choices in deafness: A parents' guide to communication options* (2nd ed.). Bethesda, MD: Woodbine House.

Steinberg, A.G., Davila, J.R., Collazo, J., Loew, R.C., & Fischgrund, J.E. (1997). A little sign and a lot of love. . . . Attitudes, perceptions, and beliefs of Hispanic families with deaf children. *Qualitative Health Research, 7*(2), 202–222.

Sulzby, E. (1985). Children's emergent reading of favorite storybooks: A developmental study. *Reading Research Quarterly, 20*, 458–481.

Swisher, M.V. (1993). Perceptual and cognitive aspects of recognition of signs in peripheral vision. In M. Marschark & M.D. Clark (Eds.), *Psychological perspectives on deafness* (pp. 209–228). Mahwah, NJ: Lawrence Erlbaum Associates.

Swisher, M.V. (2000). Learning to converse: How deaf mothers support the development of attention and conversational skills in their young deaf children. In P.E. Spencer, C.J. Erting, & M. Marschark (Eds.), *The deaf child in the family and at school: Essays in honor of Kathryn P. Meadow-Orlans* (pp. 21–40). Mahwah, NJ: Lawrence Erlbaum Associates.

Vadasy, P.F., Fewell, R.R., Greenberg, M.T., Dermond, N.L., & Meyer, D.J. (1986). Follow-up evaluation of the effects of involvement in the fathers' program. *Topics in Early Childhood Special Education, 6*(1), 16–31.

Wells, G. (1985). Preschool literacy-related activities and success in school. In D.R. Olson, N. Torrance, & A. Hildyard (Eds.), *Literacy, language, and learning: The nature and consequences of reading and writing* (pp. 229–250). Cambridge, England: Cambridge University Press.

Wood, D., Wood, H., Griffiths, A., & Howarth, I. (1986). *Teaching and talking with deaf children.* New York: John Wiley & Sons.

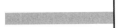

The Pennsylvania School for the Deaf

Tina Pakis and Julie Gould Marothy,
Educators at the Pennsylvania
School for the Deaf

The Pennsylvania School for the Deaf (PSD) is an urban day school serving children who are deaf and hard of hearing from infancy through high school in the Philadelphia region. PSD is our nation's third-oldest center school serving deaf children. Founded in 1820, PSD moved to its fifth campus in 1984. With that move came the change from the traditional, residential center school to a smaller, more intimate day program serving mostly urban, elementary-age deaf children. Our student demographics have changed gradually over the past 17 years (the population of African American students has gone from 20% to 58%, Caucasian students from 74% to 18%, Latino students from 5% to 17%, and Asian & other ethnic groups from 1% to 7%). Commensurate with this change has come the need for more ethnic diversity among the staff. This is a goal we continue to work toward. Among our staff who work directly with the students, 36% are deaf or hard of hearing. In addition, 85% of our families live at or below the federal poverty level, 54% of PSD households are headed by single parents/caregivers, and 50%–60% of PSD students have significant learning differences or other identified disabilities.

At PSD we have incorporated a team structure among our classes. Currently we have nine instructional teams, comprised each of two to four homeroom classes. Within this structure, we assign our staff in a manner that ensures diversity both ethnically and communicatively. Each team has a balanced staff that includes deaf or hard of hearing and African American adults. Members of other culture groups are spread throughout the school. In addition, we strive to include men on our classroom staff to serve as role models to the children. In our view, this structure not only provides the children with a staff that reflects their own culture and ethnicity but also opens the door to families, allowing them to feel more comfortable and welcome in the school, thus bridging the gap between school and home.

In keeping with the priority of diversity and reflection of the student body within the staff, our communication philosophy is designed to embrace both our students and their families. In terms of classroom instruction, we work to meet the communication needs of each child in the school. In practical terms, this could mean placing a Spanish-speaking staff member on teams with children from Spanish-speaking families. This helps link the languages of home and school and further helps families feel welcome when they can communicate directly with an adult that works with their child.

PSD places a high importance on its work with families. To meet this need we have a support team consisting of two parent-involvement coordinators, two family therapists, a home-school visitor, and several other school counselors who work with families. Further, our instructional teams host annual family and literacy events to promote family involvement and their children's literacy development. As Kathryn P. Meadow-Orlans states in her chapter, communication as the foundation of literacy cannot be emphasized strongly enough. This is the very crux of the task at hand and yet, most challenging to accomplish. Times have indeed changed for all families, including those with deaf children, and for the deaf children themselves. In this age of information, access to print is absolutely critical to success in American society. From employment to Internet access, opportunity in our American society for those with marginal literacy skills is extremely limited. In our school community it is observed that many of the mothers give a great deal of time and attention to their young deaf children. However, in many cases, when those deaf children are safely in school full time, the same parents then return to full-time work, their own schooling, or devote their attention to the younger children in the family. However, what many parents do not realize is that the need for parental involvement in helping their deaf child develop communication fluency, which is imperative to their development of print literacy, continues throughout their child's school years.

As outlined in this chapter, the challenge of helping a deaf child become literate and providing all of the components of early communication needs provides an additional strain for families. However, the benefits resulting when family members are themselves readers, enjoying their own reading materials, cannot be overlooked. That is, when family members model reading for their children, deaf or otherwise, in addition to reading children's stories to them, parents motivate their children to become readers themselves. It is very challenging to make a reader out of a child from a home with few books and magazines, in which reading is something children do not see their parents engaging in.

When a child enters our preschool program at 3 years of age, early intervention home services are usually terminated and the parents' contact with school personnel usually becomes less frequent. The parents' contact with deaf adults generally becomes less frequent as well. It has been observed in many families that as the child grows and becomes more adept with sign language communication the parents struggle to keep up with their own signing skills. The frequent result is that communication in the home begins to break down. At this point, staff members can often communicate more fluently with students than with the students' families and serve as interpreter for conversations between parents and their children. In an effort to remedy this, morning and evening sign language classes are offered free at PSD for family members of our students. Unfortunately, they are often not well attended. There are many reasons for this:

- PSD is not a neighborhood school. For parents who work, rely on public transportation, live at a distance, and have other children, coming to school functions can be a challenge, especially at night.

- Many of our families are not comfortable in a school environment.

- Their children use a language that is foreign to the families. Even if parents have been taking advantage of the sign classes we offer, it is difficult to keep up if one is not immersed in the deaf community.

All of this speaks to Meadow-Orlans's observation that parents generally respond to their deaf child's communication and developing literacy needs with either motivation and action or paralysis and inaction. It is not difficult to understand how the latter can occur, which serves as a call to action for schools.

Several adaptations by PSD make it easier for parents to be involved in evening events. The staff at PSD find that family events are better attended when the following are provided:

- Transportation

- A simple meal (e.g., pizza, hoagies)

- Babysitting services

- Interpreting services for sign language as well as other languages

Meadow-Orlans also states that involving fathers in intervention services is challenging for families. Fathers are less often available during the day, and in most families, it is the mother who attends the early intervention program and therefore becomes the person in the family who knows the most about deafness and sign language communication. Mothers also often become the interpreters in a family, which places additional stress on them. To motivate fathers to attend school functions, PSD hosted a basketball fundraiser a few years ago, and there was an amazingly good turnout of fathers, stepfathers, grandfathers, and uncles, many of whom had never been to the campus. This is now an annual event, and because of the basketball fundraiser, fathers and other male caregivers seem to be more comfortable visiting our school, attending other functions, and thus sending a positive message to their children about school involvement. Another annual event for fathers is "Bring Your Fathers to School" day in the spring. Fathers visit the classroom, eat lunch with their children, and attend a short program designed especially for them.

In an effort to address the literacy needs of our students and their families, we have become a site for the Shared Reading Project (SRP) developed by David Schleper, Jane Fernandes, and Doreen Higa. Several aspects of the SRP make it very useful for our families. For example, the sessions take place in the child's home. This makes it convenient and less intimidating for families to be involved. The visits are scheduled at a time that the family chooses, thus increasing the family's availability. The families develop a relationship with the SRP tutor, a native American Sign Language user who is most often a deaf individual. Finally, any family members and close family friends can be involved in the sessions. The SRP program has been very successful at PSD, with many families requesting to be involved with the program for additional years. To expand on this program, we have had two summers of family reading programs involving families of our emergent readers, ages 5–7. In these programs, we have provided families with the following:

- Signing storytellers in families' homes to read books and share information about literacy
- Gift books so that families can read with their children
- Ideas for literacy activities that families can do with their children, such as cooking with simple recipes, shopping with grocery lists, and labeling furniture in the house
- Information about local resources including storytelling at neighborhood libraries and how to access interpreting services for their children to participate
- Family literacy events on campus with dinner, games, professional face painters, a panel of parents with older deaf children, and workshops led by native signers on how to read the gift books to their deaf child

Helping a deaf child along the road to literacy requires a team effort. The challenge outlined in Meadow-Orlans's chapter is indeed a call to action for schools everywhere. In addition to a quality, balanced literacy program at school, the best support we can offer includes a partnership with families. That is what we have attempted at PSD. As educators, it is our experience that reaching out to families and engaging their active involvement results in the best benefits for their children.

CHAPTER THREE

Family Rights,
Legislation, and Policies

What Professionals
Need to Know to Promote
Family Involvement and Advocacy

BETH SONNENSTRAHL BENEDICT
AND BARBARA RAIMONDO

About 10 people, not including my husband and myself, at the individualized family service plan (IFSP) meeting were telling me what Scott needed. The group included sign language specialists, an audiologist, Scott's home visit teacher, a psychologist, a social worker, a local education agency representative, and others. We were so confused. We never knew we were going to have to deal with so many people. No one warned us. They never asked us if we agreed with their observations and evaluations of Scott. We never knew Scott was constantly evaluated. Was Scott their child? Was Scott that bad? Who were we to them? They were probably right that we did not have any training on raising a deaf child. Yes, we could have used a lot of information that they had to offer. But Scott lives with us, and we have found ways to interact nicely with Scott. We know what Scott enjoys and dislikes. Can we work as a team? Can we be involved in the evaluation and decision-making process as to what program Scott may benefit the best? That would be fun! (Anonymous, personal communication, March, 21, 2000)

As experts on their children, parents are their children's first and best advocates (Anderson, Chitwood, & Hayden, 1997). One of the major responsibilities of professionals is to assist parents in strengthening their ability to advocate on behalf of their child. This chapter discusses advocacy and involvement, outlines some aspects of federal law that address family involvement and advocacy, and offers advice to professionals on how to better promote involvement and advocacy of families in early intervention and education systems.

WHAT IS ADVOCACY?

What does it mean to advocate? Prominent advocates Turnbull and Turnbull defined advocacy as "taking one's own or another's perspective to obtain a result not otherwise available" (2001, p. 350). Advocacy is a strategy of taking an action to present, support, or defend a position. Three parents describe advocacy this way:

When you have a child who is "different," you start to question everything you thought you knew about child rearing. You figure you have got to give this kid more, and it's up to you, the parent, to make a home and be involved in an education for that child that is going to help him soar.

Because my deaf child's needs are different from a hearing child's needs, I have to be well informed. . . . I need to know where to gather information and how to use the information I receive.

The professionals can't know my child the way I do, and they are dealing with a caseload—I am dealing with my baby. I need to make sure they understand her needs and my needs, too.

WHAT IS FAMILY INVOLVEMENT?

To be involved is to "engage as a participant" or to "oblige to take part," "to occupy (as oneself) absorbingly," "to relate closely," or "to have an effect on" (*Webster's New Collegiate Dictionary*, 1980). Research has found that family involvement and environment strongly influence children's outcomes (Calderon, 2000; Epstein, 1987; Epstein & Dauber, 1991; Henderson & Berla, 1996; Moeller, 2000).

According to the continuum of family collaboration devised by the National Council on Disability (NCD; 1994), families who have a high participation rate in their child's education are assertive, knowledgeable, and empowered. Their time and energy have been greatly used and invested in getting the most appropriate education available for their children. However, many of these families are frustrated with the school system because they feel they are not involved in decision making. Parents want to be equal partners with the school system. Families with mid-level participation are generally satisfied with their child's educational program. They participate in the mandates of the Individuals with Disabilities Education Act (IDEA) Amendments of 1997 (PL 105-17) but usually do not have the full knowledge of the programs and outcomes. These parents are most likely to follow what is expected of them and accept whatever is suggested with some inquiries. Families with limited participation typically feel lost in the system and rarely participate in their child's education in any way. They often feel angry and intimidated by the school system, and their perception is that their child is receiving a lower quality education. "Placement" on the continuum of family collaboration is not permanent; some families and professionals move back and forth on this continuum depending on situations and times.

Family involvement—which includes advocacy—can lead to better outcomes for children. For example, Moeller (2000) examined the influence of early enrollment in an intervention program on language outcomes for children with hearing loss. She found that the children who were enrolled early and had families with a high degree of involvement fared the best. Moeller measured involvement by looking at familial adjustment, early intervention participation, effectiveness of communication with the child, and advocacy efforts. However, she also found that children who enrolled late with a high level of family involvement did better than children enrolled early with average or low family involvement. This was true regardless of the degree of hearing loss (Moeller, 2000).

Also, Calderon (2000), following a study of 28 children with hearing loss who graduated from a birth-to-three early intervention program, suggested parent involvement as a predictor in reading skills although maternal communication skills with deaf children is considered a critical factor. Mothers demonstrating better communication skills with their deaf children had children with higher language and reading scores and fewer behavior problems. Throughout the literature, family involvement is shown to be critical to the success of the child.

DIFFERENCE BETWEEN INVOLVEMENT AND ADVOCACY

All parents are involved in their children's lives and interact with their children in many ways throughout the day. For instance, being involved in their children's lives usually means that parents or caregivers feed, diaper, rock, and play with their children; they know what their children like, what they dislike, and how they might react to various situations and people. As the child enters school full time, parents typically want to be involved and have regular contact with their child's teachers. Parents expect good communication between home and school so that they can support their child's educational progress. Parents who understand and support their child's schools are most likely also to be involved with their children (Christensen & Cleary, 1990). If parents know what to expect from their child's school, such as workload and enrichment activities, they are more likely to support the school. Establishing a good relationship with school personnel can help prevent problems and can help ensure that the child and family receive appropriate services. Parents are often thoughtful consumers on behalf of their child. This is what being involved generally means.

When parents find out their infant has a hearing loss, they become keenly aware that raising their child will be different from what they expected. Typically, parents have no previous experience with hearing loss and do not know how best to enhance their child's development. In these instances, they need to learn their child's unique communication needs and determine how the family can best meet them by going beyond typical involvement and becoming advocates. Parents of children with hearing loss are usually new to the special education system, and to become advocates for their children, parents need to learn about the professionals, programs, and the variety of disciplinary fields involved; they also need to learn about the processes and procedures that they may not fully understand.

At the same time, parents may find early intervention and education systems to be imperfect. For example, skilled professionals may not be available in all geographic areas, parents may have access only to limited resources, and certain early intervention programs may not offer a wide range of options or services. Often parents discover that they must learn to navigate the school system and use the legal system to receive the right services and an appropriate education for their child. This is advocacy.

For these parents, advocacy includes elements of knowledge, how and where to obtain information, confidence in their ability to speak up for and act on behalf of their child, participation in their child's education, and the skills needed to work in the system set up to provide education to their child. Because the education system, as mandated by IDEA 1997, is premised on a high degree of family participation in decision making, it is critical that professionals provide information and support to families on behalf of their children.

Parents value this kind of support. Frequent comments from parents include the following (excerpted from Roush, 1994):

This mother and a preschool consultant were there thinking for us. It was wonderful to have their support. (p. 344)

Compliments and praise really help us parents to keep pushing on for our deaf kids. (p. 346)

Professionals should offer as much information as possible—and much of it will need to be repeated. Handouts, books, groups in the community have been extremely helpful. Frequent contact and explanations are important. (p. 346)

The people who were most helpful were the ones who took the time to find out how we were doing. They were not only interested in the children, but in how was my job, my marriage, my emotional well-being. . . . These people were always available when I needed them. Looking back these professionals helped guide me through the most difficult period of my life, I refer to them as my "dark years" and I will be forever grateful. (p. 346)

The most helpful thing our pediatrician did for us is to put us into contact with another family with a hearing impaired child. They welcomed us into their home and gently let us acclimate ourselves to the new world we were entering. They provided us names of audiologists, schools, and organizations, [and] that was valuable. (pp. 346–347)

I have also appreciated the respect I have been shown by professionals; the way they have asked for my opinions and have listened to me. I feel like parents know their children the best and professionals need to listen to what the parents are saying. (p. 347)

HISTORICAL ROLES OF FAMILY ADVOCACY

Knowledge of the history of advocacy provides a context in which to understand advocacy. Bear in mind that family advocacy approaches were altered over the past generation of families and professionals. These approaches may be as valuable to the next generation of families and professionals as early approaches appear to us now. As George Santayana stated, "Those who cannot remember the past are condemned to repeat it" (1905, p. 284).

Turnbull and Turnbull (2001) described eight major roles parents and other family members have assumed since the late 1800s. These roles may describe the environment of some parents today despite outdated perspectives. Although the roles are set in a chronological order, they may overlap somewhat. These eight roles still exist in many situations.

At the end of the 19th century, parents were considered the source of the child's disability and were to be blamed. The Eugenics movement suggested selective breeding that would improve the human race by eliminating children with disabilities. The 1930s found more parent organizations that provided parents with emotional and educational support, as well as services to develop and maintain parent networking and promote strong advocacy among parents. Until the 1950s, many children with disabilities were excluded from public schools, and services were not provided for children birth to 6 years old. Therefore, parents were viewed as service developers. Parents and charitable organizations created public awareness, raised money, operated services, and advocated for others to assume responsibility to provide services. Classes and programs for children with disabilities were held in basements, town buildings, religious institutions, and other community environments.

Due to the continuing support from communities in the 1960s, more professions were formed and more professionals became available to parents of children with disabilities. However, parents were not thought to be sophisticated enough to make decisions about educational matters, so they were expected to be the recipients of professional decisions. Because there were no laws mandating services for children with disabilities in public schools, many parents had to become their children's teachers. This caused many clashes between professionals and parents. Their roles included establishing a learning environment, setting up and maintaining a routine when teaching, and using appropriate procedures when teaching a new skill or a concept. Eventually, many parents became frustrated and dissatisfied with their children's total exclusion from the public education system.

In the early 1970s, many parents shifted to roles as political advocates, and they were an integral part of the disability rights movement. Simply being advocates of the political process was insufficient; more parents took decision-making roles and wanted to participate more fully in their child's education to more effectively support their child and improve his or her outcomes. With the passage of the Education for All Handicapped Children Act of 1975 (PL 94-142), parents became active participants in the process of educational decision making.

This eventually led to the philosophy in the early 1990s of having families as collaborators. The family works with teachers, administrators, paraprofessionals, and service providers to maximize benefits to the child. Professionals can use this team to enhance their ability to meet the child's needs. The belief was that the educational outcomes would be improved when multiple perspectives and resources exist along with shared motivation, knowledge, and skills.

Formal education for deaf children was influenced by these roles but developed somewhat differently. It began in the early 19th century when Mason Cogswell, father of a deaf girl, Alice, joined forces with Thomas Gallaudet, a local minister, to find a way to teach Alice. Cogswell sent Gallaudet to France to learn effective teaching methods, they raised funds from members of the general public and the legislature, and in

1817 in Hartford, Connecticut, Cogswell and Gallaudet founded what is now called the American School for the Deaf (Moores, 2001). In ensuing years, the number of schools for deaf children multiplied across the country. By 1907 there were 139 schools for the deaf (Lane, 1993). Changes in special education law since 1975 led to the decline in enrollment of these schools. However, the original belief remains: The desire to have his child perform on par academically with her hearing peers is what drove Mason Cogswell to advocate for his daughter, and this same desire drives parents to advocate for their children today.

FEDERAL COURT CASES LEADING TO THE PASSAGE OF SPECIAL EDUCATION LEGISLATION

In 1954, the landmark Supreme Court case *Brown v. Board of Education* struck down previously sanctioned "separate but equal" treatment for people of color. The ensuing years were a time of heightened awareness of racial discrimination and numerous attempts to eradicate this discrimination. Against this fabric of social consciousness, parents of children with disabilities also worked for fair treatment of their children.

In the early 1970s, parents brought two major federal lawsuits to obtain educational services for their children; these lawsuits are powerful examples of parents in the role of advocates. In *Pennsylvania Association for Retarded Children (PARC) v. Commonwealth of Pennsylvania* (1971) parents of children with mental retardation who were denied an education sued the Commonwealth. In *Mills v. Board of Education of the District of Columbia* (1972), parents of children with mental retardation, behavioral disorders, or emotional disturbances brought suit. The courts found that these children had a constitutional right to a free public education and an educational placement that was appropriate to their needs. The courts mandated that these and other children with disabilities be educated and drafted requirements that were to be followed in order to do so.

Although these were important victories, they only became mandates in the districts in which they were decided. In countless other school districts, denial of education or provision of inadequate education was still permitted. But these cases set the stage for the Education for All Handicapped Children Act, now renamed and reauthorized as the IDEA Amendments of 1997. (*Note:* As of 2003, the law was undergoing extensive reauthorization, which occurs every 5 years. Please consult www.ed.gov/offices/OSERS/Policy/IDEA/ for more current information.) Based on the language in the courts' opinions, the 1975 law and its regulations required, as they do today, that children with disabilities be provided with a free appropriate public education (FAPE) based on an individualized education program (IEP). These children are to be educated in the least restrictive environment (LRE) possible, alongside children without disabilities to the maximum extent appropriate. Procedural safeguards were put into place to enforce the rights of students and their parents.

Although the *PARC* and *Mills* cases were not brought on behalf of children who were deaf, the subsequent law had a profound effect on how deaf children were educated. Suddenly schools for the deaf were not considered to be appropriate placements for many children who were deaf. Because all of the students in the school were deaf, these schools were not considered to be the least restrictive environment. Local educational agencies began to mainstream these children in their local schools. As a result, enrollment in schools for the deaf began to drop, and enrollment in local schools rose. In the 21st century, professionals in all educational environments must be prepared to serve deaf and hard of hearing children and their families.

HOW IDEA AND OTHER FEDERAL LEGISLATION SUPPORT PARENT INVOLVEMENT AND ADVOCACY

IDEA 1997 emphasizes family involvement, which should occur at the individual level—that is, families supporting their own child—and at the systems level—that is, families working to provide service delivery systems for all consumers of the services. Because most professional involvement with families is at the individual level, such as working with families in the home, in classrooms, and in individual and group parent meetings, this section focuses on the individual level. This section, although not a complete summary of IDEA 1997, highlights sections of the law that support family involvement and suggests how professionals can support families within this context. Part C applies to Infant and Toddler Programs that serve children from birth to age 3, and Part B applies to children ages 3 through 21.

Part C

The implementation of Part C is based on the concept that there is an "urgent and substantial need . . . to enhance the capacity of families to meet the special needs of their infants and toddlers with disabilities" (IDEA 1997 § 631 [a]). The law recognizes that service providers have an important role in supporting parents in their use of services and in understanding and enhancing their child's development. Under the law, service providers, to the extent appropriate, are responsible for the following:

1. *Service providers must consult with parents, other service providers, and representatives of appropriate community agencies to ensure the effective provision of services in each area.*

2. *Providers must educate parents and others regarding the provision of services.* Typically parents are not familiar with the services that are available for children with disabilities, especially very young children with disabilities. Early intervention providers should explain the purposes of early intervention and the kinds of services the child and family are entitled to. This can be done in parent group meetings, one-to-one conversations, and printed materials.

3. *Service providers need to work as a multidisciplinary team to assess the child and the child's family in order to develop integrated goals and outcomes for the individualized family service plan (IFSP)* (34 C.F.R. § 303.12 [c]). (See Table 3.1 for the contents of an IFSP.) A multidisciplinary assessment is used to determine the unique strengths and needs of the infant or toddler in order to identify the services appropriate to meet such needs. A multidisciplinary assessment must include assessment of cognitive development; physical development, including vision and hearing; communication

Table 3.1. Content of the individualized family service plan

Information on the present level of functioning of the child (IDEA § 636 [d][1]).

A statement of the family's resources, priorities, and concerns related to enhancing the development of the family's infant or toddler with a disability (IDEA § 636 [d][2]).

Outcomes for the IFSP for both the child and the family (IDEA § 636 [d][3])

A statement of the specific early intervention services necessary to meet the needs of the child and the family. These could include family training, counseling, and home visits (IDEA 632 § [4][E][i]). These are services provided, as appropriate, by qualified personnel to assist the family of a child eligible under this part in understanding the special needs of the child and enhancing the child's development (34 CFR § 303.12 [d][3]).

A "justification" must be provided when services are not provided in the "natural environment" (IDEA § 636 [d][5]). There is strong encouragement to have services provided in the natural environment (IDEA § 636 [d][5] and IDEA § 635 [a][16]), which includes the home and community settings in which children without disabilities participate (IDEA § 632 [G]). However, service providers must be certain to understand that services are not *required* to be provided in the natural environment. Location of service provision should be determined by the needs of the child and family.

The identification of the service coordinator who will be responsible for the implementation of the plan and coordination with other agencies and people (IDEA § 636 [d][7]).

The steps to be taken to support the transition of the toddler to preschool or other appropriate services (IDEA § 636 [d][8]).

development; social or emotional development; and adaptive development (34 C.F.R. § 303.322[c][3][ii]).

Family-directed assessments are also perfomed. This assessment addresses the family's resources, priorities, and concerns in order to identify the supports and services necessary to improve the family's capacity to meet the developmental needs of the infant or toddler (IDEA 1997 § 636 [a][2]). Families can tell the professionals what the family can do to support the child. For example, the family may be highly motivated to learn a new mode of communication. Or perhaps the extended family lives nearby and is committed to helping support the child. The family can also let the professionals know what areas the family would like the professionals to concentrate on.

Once these assessments take place, the family and the professionals can have a dialogue about the supports and services that are necessary to address their child's needs. The family's priorities and concerns, however, may not be the same as the professionals'. In order for meaningful discussion to take place, an atmosphere of trust and respect must exist between the parents and the professional. Lacking this, parents may not be forthcoming in assessing their resources, priorities, and concerns.

The family members also need to be sure to let the professional know where they need additional support. For example, some hearing families feel comfortable serving as a spoken language model for their child but would like a native signer to serve as an American Sign Language (ASL) model. This additional support can come from outside the early intervention system, such as from a community education program. It is important to note that discussion of resources, priorities, and concerns need not be limited to what is available in the child's early intervention placement. State and local resources, such as state insurance programs, local child care centers, and parent and consumer organizations, can be tapped as well.

4. *Service providers must develop a written IFSP with the multidisciplinary team, including parents* (IDEA 1997 § 636 [a][3]). Parents must be part of this IFSP team, and they should be treated as equals. Their knowledge about and expectations for their child are as important as the information gleaned through professionals' assessments.

5. *Service providers must review the IFSP at 6-month intervals, or more often when appropriate, based on infant or toddler and family needs* (IDEA 1997 § 636 [b]). A young child changes quickly, so it is important that plans and programs for the child must be modified when appropriate. The family may observe behavior at home

that leads them to believe the IFSP should be modified. For example, the communication mode or the manner in which it is used may not be appropriate for the needs of the child. Or other factors may influence the modification of the IFSP, such as the availability of more advanced technology.

6. *Service providers must protect parents' procedural rights.* Part C includes a requirement that early intervention agencies must obtain written consent prior to the provision of early intervention services, and parents are free to decline services they do not wish to receive (IDEA 1997 § 636 [a]). In order for consent to be "informed," parents must understand what services are being offered and for what purpose. If they do not know this, it must be explained to them. Professionals must be familiar with the procedural safeguards states put into place, including procedures protecting parents' rights to examine records (§ 639 [a][4]). Because disputes can arise, states must have in place procedures to allow parents to use mediation (§ 639 [a][8]), to file an administrative complaint (§ 639 [a][1]), and to file a lawsuit (§ 639 [a][1]).

Parents have the right to receive written prior notice regarding the initiation or changing of the identification, evaluation, or placement of the infant or toddler (IDEA 1997 § 639 [a][6]). This notice must be in the parents' native language unless it clearly is not feasible to do so (§ 639 [a][7]). Professionals should be aware of these safeguards and make sure that they are followed.

Part B

Part B of IDEA 1997 provides a delivery mechanism for the provision of a "free appropriate public education" (IDEA 1997 § 612 [a][1]) for children ages 3 through 21 with disabilities. This education should be based on the child's "individualized education program" (IEP) (§ 612 [a][4]) and is to be carried out in the "least restrictive environment" (§ 612 [a][5]). As of 1997, Part B also requires that these children be provided access to the general curriculum (IDEA 1997 §614 [d][1][A][iii][II] and 34 C.F.R. § 300.347 [a][3][ii]) and included in state and districtwide assessments that are given to children without disabilities (IDEA 1997 §612 [a][17][A] and 34 C.F.R. § 300.138).

Frequently, parents find discontinuity between Part B and Part C programs. Often Part B and Part C programs are led by different agencies. Each agency may operate from a different perspective with different sources of funding and professional personnel. Also, Part B preschool programs focus most of their attention on the child, rather than the child and family as a unit, and therefore the partnership between parent and professional may decline after the switch to a Part B program.

Nevertheless, family involvement is still a cornerstone of Part B. Provisions of the law that reflect this include the following parents' rights:

1. *Parents have the right to be a part of the IEP team as equal members* (IDEA 1997 § 614 [d][1][B][i]). The U.S. Department of Education stated,

> The parents of a child with a disability are expected to be equal participants along with school personnel in developing, reviewing, and revising the IEP for their child. This is an active role in which the parents 1) provide critical information regarding the strengths of their child and express their concerns for enhancing the education of their child; 2) participate in discussions about the child's need for special education and related services and supplementary aids and services; and 3) join with the other participants in deciding how the child will be involved and progress in the general curriculum and participate in State and district-wide assessments, and what services the agency will provide to the child and in what setting. (1999, p. 12473)

Parents appreciate having professionals as equal partners when making decisions. Giving comprehensive and accurate information to families is the professional's most important task. If professionals hold back information from the parents and fail to include them when making decisions, the relationship may be damaged and trust broken. Parents may invite to be part of the IEP team individuals who have knowledge or special expertise regarding their child (IDEA 1997 § 614 [d][1][B][vi]).

2. *Parents may voice their concerns and have them documented and addressed.* In developing each child's IEP, the IEP team must consider the strengths of the child and the concerns of the parents for enhancing the education of their child (IDEA 1997 § 614 [d][3][A][i]). This information must be solicited by other members of the IEP team because many IEP forms do not include this provision on the document, and most parents do not know the law well enough to bring it up themselves. The professional chairing the meeting must ask the parents for this information. Parents' views and opinions should be documented and addressed and given the same credence as those of professionals.

3. *Parents are entitled to be a part of the team that decides their child's placement.* Each public agency is required to ensure that the parents of each child with a disability are members of any group that makes decisions on the educational placement of their child. (IDEA 1997 § 614 [f] and 34 C.F.R. § 300.501 [c]). A child with a

disability can be placed in a continuum of alternative placements including general education classes, special education classes, special schools, home instruction, and instruction in hospitals and institutions (34 C.F.R. § 300.551). The placement decision must be made by a group of people, including the parents and other people, knowledgeable about the child, the meaning of the evaluation data, and the placement options (34 C.F.R. § 300.552 [a][1]).

Because the parent is to be involved in the placement decision, the parent needs to understand the meaning of the evaluation data and the placement options, just as the professional does. Professionals administering evaluations or interpreting evaluation data must be prepared to explain those evaluations and the data to the parents. The professionals must be able to explain the purpose of the evaluation, whether it will be administered by a qualified individual, the qualifications of the evaluator, what the evaluation showed, and how the evaluation results compare with those of children without disabilities. Parents generally do not have background or any training in this area, so the professionals must be able to convey this information to the parent in plain language.

Similarly, in order for parents and other members of the IEP team to participate in an informed manner in the placement decision, they must know the capabilities for provision of special education and related services for this individual child in each environment. IDEA 1997's inferred preference for children with disabilities to be educated with children without disabilities (§612 [a][5]) is tempered by the phrase "to the maximum extent appropriate." Removal from the general education classroom is permitted if "the nature or severity of the disability is such that education in regular classes with the use of supplementary aids and services cannot be achieved satisfactorily" (34 C.F.R. § 300.550).

Parents may not be satisfied that their child's placement or proposed placement is an environment in which the child's IEP goals can be met, but they may not be aware that other placements are available. Or, if they are aware that other placements exist, they may not understand that those placements could be available to their child. Parents may have mistaken beliefs about a particular environment, such as a mistaken belief that the placement does not serve children of their child's age or that the placement does not serve children who are similar to their child in some other way. Professionals should ensure that parents receive accurate information. All of the members of the placement team should give the same legitimacy to the parents' views as they do to other members of the team. Decisions are not to be made on the basis of "majority rule"—that is, there are more members of the school district than there are parents, so the school district wins—but on the basis of shared agreement in compliance with the IEP process.

Some school systems discourage parents from investigating specialized environments for their child by not making information about the specialized environments available or by steering them away from the environments. The local or state education bureaucracy may be designed in such a way that specialized placements are difficult, if not impossible, to obtain. However, this may be in violation of U.S. Department of Education Policy Guidance. In "Deaf Students' Education Services: Policy Guidance," the Department outlined critical factors to consider for placement. That Policy Guidance states,

> The Secretary [of Education] is concerned that the least restrictive environment provisions of the IDEA and Section 504 [of the Rehabilitation Act Amendments of 1992] are being interpreted, incorrectly, to require the placement of some children who are deaf in programs that may not meet the individual student's educational needs. Meeting the unique communication and related needs of a student who is deaf is a fundamental part of providing a free appropriate public education (FAPE) to the child. Any setting, including a regular classroom, that prevents a child who is deaf from receiving an appropriate education that meets his or her needs, including communication needs, is not the LRE for that individual child.
>
> Placement decisions must be based on the child's IEP. Thus, the consideration of LRE as part of the placement decision must always be in the context of the LRE in which appropriate services can be provided. Any setting that does not meet the communication and related needs of a child who is deaf, and therefore does not allow for the provision of FAPE, cannot be considered the LRE for that child. The provision of FAPE is paramount, and the individual placement determination about the LRE is to be considered within the context of FAPE.
>
> The Secretary is concerned that some public agencies have misapplied the LRE provision by presuming that placements in or closer to the regular classroom are required for children who are deaf, without taking into consideration the range of communication and related needs that must be addressed in order to provide appropriate services. The Secretary recognizes that the regular classroom is an appropriate placement for some children who are deaf, but for others it is not. The decision as to what placement will provide FAPE for an individual deaf child—that includes a determination as to the LRE in which appropriate services can be made available to the child—must be made only after a full and complete IEP has been developed that addresses the full range of the child's needs.
>
> The Secretary recognizes that regular educational settings are appropriate and adaptable to meet the unique needs of particular children who are deaf. For others, a center or special school may

be the least restrictive environment in which the child's unique needs can be met. A full range of alternative placements as described at 34 C.F.R. § 300.551(a) and (b)(1) of the IDEA regulations must be available to the extent necessary to implement each child's IEP. (57 Fed. Reg. 49275 [October 30, 1992], citations removed)

4. *Parents may receive counseling and training when appropriate.* Parent counseling and training means "assisting parents in understanding the special needs of their child; providing parents with information about child development; and helping parents to acquire the necessary skills that will allow them to support the implementation of their child's IEP or IFSP" (IDEA 1997 § 300.24 [b][7]). This includes sign language instruction for parents, if needed.

In a letter clarifying policy, Judy Schrag, the Director of the U.S. Department of Education Office of Special Education Programs, stated,

> If a parent of a child with a hearing impairment or a school district believes that sign language instruction for the parent is needed in order for the child to benefit from the special education and related services included in the child's IEP, then the parent's need for such instruction must be considered by the participants on the IEP team. If the participants on the IEP team determine that this service is needed, sign language instruction must be provided to the parent as a related service in the form of parent counseling and training and must be included in the child's IEP. . . . In all instances, decisions as to whether a child with a disability requires a particular related service must be made on an individual basis through applicable IEP and placement procedures. (letter to Dagley, June 3, 1991, citations removed)

Other Department of Education guidance has addressed the issue of sign language instruction for families. The department has stated,

> If the IEP team determines that in order for a child who is deaf to participate in the general curriculum he or she needs sign language and materials which reflect his or her language development, those needs . . . must be addressed in the child's IEP. In addition, if the team determines that the child also needs to expand his or her vocabulary in sign language, that service must also be addressed in the applicable components of the child's IEP. The IEP team may also wish to consider whether there is a need for members of the child's family to receive training in sign language in order for the child to receive FAPE. (1999, p. 12472)

5. *Parents are entitled to protection by procedural safeguards, such as the right to examine records* (IDEA 1997 § [b][1]). Prior written

notice to the parents is necessary whenever the agency proposes to initiate or change, or refuses to initiate or change, the identification, evaluation, or educational placement of the child or the provision of a free appropriate public education to the child (§ 615 [b][3]). Written prior notice must be in the native language of the parent unless it clearly is not feasible to do so (§ 615 [b][4] and 34 C.F.R § 300.503 [c][ii]).

6. *Parents may request mediation* (IDEA 1997 § 615 [e]). The mediation process is voluntary on the part of the parent and must not be used to deny or delay a parent's right to a due process hearing. It must be conducted by a qualified and impartial mediator who is trained in effective mediation techniques. The state must maintain a list of qualified mediators who are knowledgeable about special education law. If the mediator is not selected randomly, both parties must agree with the selection of the mediator. The state is responsible for the costs of mediation. An agreement reached through mediation must be set forth in writing. Discussions that occur during the mediation process must be confidential and may not be used as evidence in any subsequent due process hearings or civil proceedings. The parties to the mediation process may be required to sign a confidentiality pledge prior to the commencement of the process (IDEA 1997 § 615 [e] and 34 C.F.R. § 300.506).

7. *Parents may file a complaint with the local and/or state education authority* (IDEA 1997 § 615 [f]). Parents may initiate a complaint regarding the identification, evaluation, educational placement, or provision of FAPE to their child. When a hearing is initiated, the public agency must inform the parents of the availability of mediation and of free or low-cost legal and other relevant services available. The hearing must be conducted by the state education authority or the public agency directly responsible for the education of the child. The parent must give notice to the public agency, including the name, address, and school of the child, a description of the nature of the problem, and a proposed resolution of the problem to the extent known and available to the parents at the time. Each state education authority must develop a model form to assist parents in filing a request for due process (34 C.F.R. § 300.507).

Any party to the hearing has the right to be accompanied and advised by an attorney and others with special knowledge with respect to children with disabilities. Parties can present evidence and confront, cross-examine, compel the attendance of witnesses, and obtain a written record of the hearing and findings of fact and decisions. Parents may obtain an electronic version of the hearing and findings. Parents also may have their child present and open the hearing to the public (IDEA 1997 § 615 [h] and 34 C.F.R. § 300.509).

Because this hearing has many elements of a formal judicial hearing, parents and their representatives must be well-versed in the facts and the law of their case before presenting it. The hearing officer's decision will stand unless it is appealed; therefore, parents should prepare thoroughly for this action.

8. *Parents have the right to file a lawsuit* (IDEA 1997 § 615 [i][2][A]). If parents are not satisfied with the decision made at the due process hearing, they may file a suit against the education agency in federal court. They may recover attorneys' fees if they prevail (IDEA 1997 § [i][3][B] and 34 C.F.R. § 513). As in a due process hearing, the court hearing the case will look at the facts, the procedures, and the law in making its decision. However, courts are reluctant to second guess individual educational decisions: they will not substitute their own judgement for the judgement of educators. Further, they will give deference to the decision made by the hearing officer. This will influence the outcome of the case.

CONSIDERATIONS WHEN DEVELOPING AN IEP FOR A DEAF OR HARD OF HEARING CHILD

In developing an IEP for a deaf or hard of hearing child, the IEP team must consider the child's language and communication needs; the child's opportunities for direct communications with peers and professionals in the child's language and communication mode; the child's academic level; and the child's full range of needs, including opportunities for direct instruction in the child's language and communication mode (IDEA 1997 § 614 [d][3][B][iv] and 34 C.F.R. § 300.346 [a][2][iv]). The following considerations should be evaluated before developing an IEP for a deaf or hard of hearing child:

Language and communication needs: Consider the language or languages used by the child; whether the child receives communication through signing, speech, or a combination of the two; whether the child expresses communication through signing, speech, or a combination of the two; whether the child experiences language or communication delays, and if so, what the needs are stemming from these delays; whether a specific acoustic environment is necessary in order for the child to be able to communicate; whether the child needs to be near the speaker or sound source in order to receive communication; and whether those around the child understand his or her words or signs.

Direct communication: Consider the opportunities for direct communications with peers and professional personnel in the child's language and communication mode and whether the child can communicate with children and adults around him or her without the intervention of an interpreter or other facilitator. (To make this possible, the children and adults in the deaf or hard of hearing child's school environment must competently be able to use the child's mode of communication.)

Academic level: Consider the child's academic level—this should be ascertained so that children are placed in a class that suits their academic level. In some programs, all of the children with hearing loss are placed in the same class regardless of the range of academic levels of the children. As a result, a class might have an academic range of first grade through fifth grade. Children with hearing loss should not be placed with other children with hearing loss just because they share a special need—their academic level must be considered as well.

Full range of needs: This provision was fashioned on the U.S. Department of Education Policy Guidance (57 Fed. Reg. 49274 [October 30, 1992]) that states that social, emotional, and cultural needs of the child also have to be considered. As the Guidance points out, "The communication nature of the disability is inherently isolating, with considerable effect on the interaction with peers and teachers that make up the educational process. This interaction, for the purpose of transmitting knowledge and developing the child's self-esteem and identity, is dependent upon direct communication" (p. 49274).

The mention of culture in the guidance, though not explicit, seems to refer to the existence of Deaf culture. Many deaf adults and parents of deaf children value interaction with the community for a deaf individual's language development, sense of identity, and community support.

Providing opportunities for direct instruction in the child's language and communication mode means that the child's teacher must be competent to transmit academic information in the child's mode of communication. The teacher must have this level of competency in the child's mode, including, for example, a visual/manual mode. If the child does not sign, the professional should use techniques to ensure that the child can understand the spoken language being used.

THE NEWBORN INFANT HEARING
SCREENING AND INTERVENTION ACT OF 2000

The Newborn Infant Hearing Screening and Intervention Act of 2000 (§ 301 of the Public Health Services Act, Title VI of the Department of Labor, Health and Human Services, and Education, and Related Agencies Appropriations Act for FY 2000, PL 106-113) envisions a high degree of parent participation in decision making about service provision for their own child as well as the policy and practice of newborn hearing screening and intervention systems. Under this law, the Health Resources and Services Administration awards grants to states to develop and monitor the efficacy of statewide newborn and infant hearing screening, evaluation, and intervention programs and systems. As of 2003, at least 38 states plus the District of Columbia have legislation pertaining to newborn hearing screening and intervention (http://professional.asha.org/resources/legislative/index.cfm). Also, the Integrated Services Branch of the Maternal and Child Health Bureau supports 53 state and territorial programs and a national technical support center (Irene Forsman, Maternal and Child Health Bureau, U.S. Department of Health and Human Services, personal communication, August 31, 2002).

As part of early intervention, PL 106-113 requires states to ensure that families are provided comprehensive, consumer-oriented information about the full range of family support, training, information services, and communication options. Further, families must be given the opportunity to consider the full range of educational and program placements and options for their child (§ [e][3]).

In order for these functions to be carried out, professionals working with families need to be aware of what resources are available, including local parent and deaf consumer organizations, state offices on deafness, and national organizations. Many of these organizations publish information specifically for parents of children newly identified as deaf or hard of hearing. Professionals should obtain publications and make contacts with representatives of these organizations so that professionals can help parents who wish to make these contacts as well.

Under PL 106-113, early intervention includes referral to schools and agencies, including community, consumer, and parent-based agencies and organizations. It also includes referral to other programs mandated by Part C of IDEA 1997 that offer services specifically designed to meet the unique language and communication needs of deaf and hard of hearing newborns, infants, toddlers, and children (§ 703 [a][1]).

Ideally, professionals will visit these programs to see for themselves what is offered and will encourage parents to visit as well. To best decide which program best meets their child's needs, parents should meet the teachers and other service providers, experience the environment, observe other children and families as they participate in the program, and talk with families in the program. Unfortunately, programs and services for children with hearing loss are virtually nonexistent in many areas. In that case, professionals should assist in exploring neighboring options or working with other professionals to develop a quality program.

In developing policy and carrying out programs under PL 106-113, the three federal agencies in charge of the law's implementation—the Centers for Disease Control and Prevention, the Health Resources and Services Administration, and the National Institutes of Health—are required to consult with consumers, families, and professionals. Such consultation should result in better policy and implementation.

OTHER FEDERAL LEGISLATION

Other laws, such as the Rehabilitation Act of 1973 (PL 93-112), as amended in 1992 as PL 102-569, and the Americans with Disabilities Act (ADA) of 1990 (PL 101-336) apply to children with disabilities, including those who are deaf or hard of hearing. Because these laws focus more on access to programs and services and less on family involvement in a child's early intervention or educational services, these laws are not addressed in depth here. Table 3.2, however, offers a brief description and comparison of these laws and IDEA 1997.

As described previously in this chapter, federal legislation supports the role of parents in the education of their children with disabilities. But, if parents are to play the active part in their child's education as envisioned by these laws, they need access to information and various supports. To ensure family involvement, professionals can advocate for families through collaboration, empowerment, and the development of alliances with families.

Collaboration

Professionals should seek to collaborate with families. Collaboration involves a partnership between the child's family and professionals. A major component in developing a positive collaboration with families is communication. What do parents know about their child that they can share with professionals? What do the professionals want to know more about? What would parents like from a professional, both for the child and for the family? It takes time to answer these questions honestly. It does not always happen in a meeting in which one person is taking notes and the other is signing papers. This kind of communication needs trust to develop—trust that is nurtured when the family and the professional spend time together, get to know each other, and form a mutual bond of respect. Therefore, the key points to develop collaboration are 1) partnership, 2) communication, 3) trust, and 4) respect.

One parent suggested that "dealing with the parents' feelings, helping them to cope and understand the tragedy first, would allow the parents and professionals to build a firm base to start a relationship" (as cited in Roush, 1994, p. 345). Every family is different, and what works in one family may not work in another (Bailey & Wolery, 1992; Calderon & Greenberg, 2000; Spencer, 2000). Collaboration is an ongoing process. The more involved the family is, the stronger the partnership between the families and professionals is likely to be. The opposite is true as well; the stronger the partnership is, the more a family is likely to be involved. This collaborative relationship may eventually build up to a strong level of advocacy.

Information sharing is one component of successful collaboration between families and professionals. Many families want more information using different approaches, not just formal training sessions on various topics. Topics of interest may range from toilet training to homework to advocacy, and may be discussed in one-to-one situations, in small groups, over the telephone, or over e-mail. Mothers are not the only family members who want to discuss questions and issues; fathers, siblings, and other extended family members may want to be more involved as well.

Individual families decide to what extent they want to be involved with their children's education. For instance, some homes have few educational resources, while others are filled with books, writing materials, educational toys, and activity centers. Although homes with more resources may be better learning environments, the amount of resources a family has does not always equal the amount of time the family actually spends with the child.

Another component of successful collaboration is responsiveness to family priorities. Most families have a lot to learn when their child has a disability. They must have information to understand child development and the effect of their child's disability on his or her development. For children with hearing loss, the most obvious area that can be affected is language and communication development (Calderon & Greenberg, 2000). Parents need to be provided with information about typical language development so that they can support their child's language and communication development and recognize delays if they occur. Parents can work with professionals to learn communication techniques and sign language, if the child will be using that. Parents also need to understand appropriate academic development so that they may help their child succeed academically and recognize delays if they occur. They need

Table 3.2. An Overview of ADA, IDEA, and Section 504

	Americans with Disabilities Act of 1990 (ADA)	Individuals with Disabilities Education Act (IDEA), amended in 1997	Section 504 of the Rehabilitation Act of 1973
Type/ Purpose	A civil rights law to prohibit discrimination solely on the basis of disability in employment, public services, and accommodations.	An education act to provide federal financial assistance to state and local education agencies to guarantee special education and related services to eligible children with disabilities.	A civil rights law to prohibit discrimination on the basis of disability in programs and activities, public and private, that receive federal financial assistance.
Who Is Eligible?	Any individual with a disability who (1) has a physical or mental impairment that substantially limits one or more life activities; or (2) has a record of such an impairment; or (3) is regarded as having such an impairment. Further, the person must be qualified for the program, service or job.	Children and youth aged 3–21 who are determined through an individualized evaluation and by a multidisciplinary team (including the parent) to be eligible in one or more of 13 categories and who need special education and related services. The categories are autism, deafblindness, deafness, emotional disturbance, hearing impairment, mental retardation, multiple disabilities, orthopedic impairment, other health impairment, specific learning disability, speech or language impairment, traumatic brain injury, and visual impairment including blindness. Children aged 3 through 9 experiencing developmental delays may also be eligible. Infants and toddlers from birth through age 2 may be eligible for early intervention services, delivered in accordance with an individualized family service plan.	Any person who (1) has a physical or mental impairment that substantially limits one or more major life activities, (2) has a record of such an impairment, or (3) is regarded as having such an impairment. Major life activities include caring for oneself, performing manual tasks, walking, seeing, hearing, speaking, breathing, learning, and working. The person must be qualified for the services or job; in the case of school services, the person must be of an age when nondisabled peers are typically served or be eligible under IDEA.

	Americans with Disabilities Act of 1990 (ADA)	Individuals with Disabilities Education Act (IDEA), amended in 1997	Section 504 of the Rehabilitation Act of 1973
Responsible to Provide a Free, Appropriate Public Education (FAPE)?	Not directly. However, ADA provides additional protection in combination with actions brought under Section 504 and IDEA. ADA protections apply to non-sectarian private schools, but not to organizations or entities controlled by religious organizations. Reasonable accommodations are required for eligible students with a disability to perform essential functions of the job. This applies to any part of the special education program that may be community-based and involve job training/placement. Although not required, an IEP under IDEA will fulfill requirements of Title II of the ADA for an appropriate education for a student with disabilities.	Yes. A FAPE is defined to mean special education and related services that are provided at no charge to parents, meet other state educational standards, and are consistent with an individualized educational program (IEP). Special education means "specially designed instruction, at no cost to the parents, to meet the unique needs of the child with a disability." Related services are those required to assist a child to benefit from special education, including speech-language pathology, physical and occupational therapy, and others. A team of professionals and parents develop and review at least annually, an IEP for each child with a disability. IDEA requires certain content in the IEP.	Yes. An "appropriate" education means an education comparable to that provided to students without disabilities. This may be regular or special education. Students can receive related services under Section 504 even if they are not provided any special education. These are to be provided at no additional cost to the child and his or her parents. Section 504 requires provision of educational and related aids and services that are designed to meet the individual educational needs of the child. The individualized educational program of IDEA may be used to meet the Section 504 requirement.
Funding to Implement Requirements?	No, but limited tax credits may be available for removing architectural or transportation barriers. Also, many federal agencies provide grants to public and private institutions to support training and technical assistance.	Yes. IDEA provides federal funds under Parts B and C to assist state and local educational agencies in meeting IDEA requirements to serve infants, toddlers, children, and youth with disabilities.	No. State and local jurisdictions have responsibility. IDEA funds may not be used to serve children found eligible only under Section 504.

(continued)

	Americans with Disabilities Act of 1990 (ADA)	Individuals with Disabilities Education Act (IDEA), amended in 1997	Section 504 of the Rehabilitation Act of 1973
Procedural Safeguards/ Due Process	The ADA does not specify procedural safeguards related to special education; it does detail the administrative requirements, complaint procedures, and consequences for noncompliance related to both services and employment. The ADA also does not delineate specific due process procedures. People with disabilities have the same remedies that are available under Title VII of the Civil Rights Act of 1964, as amended by the Civil Rights Act of 1991. Thus, individuals who are discriminated against may file a complaint with the relevant federal agency or sue in federal court. Enforcement agencies encourage informal mediation and voluntary compliance.	IDEA provides for procedural safeguards and due process rights to parents in the identification, evaluation and educational placement of their child. Prior written notice of procedural safeguards and of proposals or refusals to initiate or change identification, evaluation, or placement must be provided to parents. IDEA delineates the required components of these notices. Disputes may be resolved through mediation, impartial due process hearings, appeal of hearing decisions, and/or civil action.	Section 504 requires notice to parents regarding identification, evaluation, placement, and before a "significant change" in placement. Written notice is recommended. Following IDEA procedural safeguards is one way to meet Section 504 mandates. Local education agencies are required to provide impartial hearings for parents who disagree with the identification, evaluation, or placement of a student. Parents must have an opportunity to participate in the hearing process and to be represented by counsel. Beyond this, due process is left to the discretion of local districts. It is recommended that they develop policy guidance and procedures.

	Americans with Disabilities Act of 1990 (ADA)	Individuals with Disabilities Education Act (IDEA), amended in 1997	Section 504 of the Rehabilitation Act of 1973
Evaluation/ Placement Procedure	The ADA does not specify evaluation and placement procedures; it does specify provision of reasonable accommodations for eligible students across educational activities and settings. Reasonable accommodations may include, but are not limited to, redesigning equipment, assigning aides, providing written communication in alternative formats, modifying tests, reassigning services to accessible locations, altering existing facilities, and building new facilities.	With parental consent, an individualized evaluation must be conducted using a variety of technically sound, unbiased assessment tools. Based on the results, a team of professionals (including the parent of the child) determines eligibility for special education. Reevaluations are conducted at least every 3 years. Results are used to develop an IEP that specifies the special education, related services, and supplemental aids and services to be provided to address the child's goals. Placement in the least restrictive environment (LRE) is selected from a continuum of alternative placements, based on the child's IEP, and reviewed at least annually. IEPs must be reviewed at least annually to see whether annual goals are being met. IDEA contains specific provisions about IEP team composition, parent participation, IEP content, and consideration of special factors.	Section 504 provides for a placement evaluation that must involve multiple assessment tools tailored to assess specific areas of educational need. Placement decisions must be made by a team of persons familiar with the student who understand the evaluation information and placement options. Students with disabilities may be placed in a separate class or facility only if they cannot be educated satisfactorily in the regular education setting with the use of supplementary aids and services. Significant changes to placement must be preceded by an evaluation. Section 504 provides for periodic reevaluation. Parental consent is not required for evaluation or placement.

Reprinted from Henderson, K. (2001). An overview of ADA, IDEA, and Section 504: Update 2001. *ERIC EC Digest, #E606.* Retrieved from http://www.ericec.org/digests/e606.html

continual opportunities to practice and refine their communication skills with their child (Greenberg & Calderon, 1987). This is a lot to expect from parents; they cannot do this alone. Collaborating with professionals can help families understand and stay involved with their child's education.

Empowerment

Dunst, Trivette, and Deal (1996) defined empowerment as when a person has access and control over situations or goals, has skills in making decisions and solving problems, and uses the appropriate behavior to interact effectively with others to accomplish goals. Professionals can help families become empowered in positive ways by being empowered themselves. Many families look to professionals as role models. Actions toward building empowerment can range from making a telephone call with a question to writing letters with confidence to request a face-to-face meeting.

One way parents can be empowered is to be familiar with organizations that take an interest in their child's special needs. Many parents value organizations that are specifically geared toward parents who have children with disabilities. Although there are many organizations that focus on advocacy, empowerment, and rights in general, most organizations are categorized by disability. Getting support and participating in these types of organizations can be a healing process for parents and reassurance that they are not alone. Joining parent organizations is one of the many ways to reach out for ideas and solutions. Professionals might also want to consider joining organizations that work to improve education and quality of life for children who are deaf or hard of hearing so that they can more easily share information with parents about these organizations. Professionals can discuss these organizations on the local, regional, state, and national levels and help parents determine the level and type of participation that may benefit them most. (For a listing of various organizations, please consult the appendix at the end of the book.)

The goal of empowerment is to enable families to become competent and capable rather than having to always depend on professionals. Families who are empowered possess knowledge, or find opportunities to gain knowledge, and skills to stand on their own, and are adept at taking control of their own beliefs and goals. And when a family works toward the same goal, family ties are usually strengthened.

Turnbull and Turnbull (2001) believed that the keys to empowerment are motivation and knowledge/skills. To become motivated, families should possess self-efficacy, perceived control, great expectations, energy, and persistence. Once motivated, families and professionals can move on to the knowledge category and focus on skills that they can carry throughout their child's education. Critical skills to possess include the ability to access information (being knowledgeable), problem solving (knowing how to overcome barriers), life management skills (being skilled to handle whatever happens), and communication skills (sending and receiving expressions of needs and wants).

Empowerment is a developmental process. Because collaboration is not always a prerequisite to empowerment, and some families may know their rights before professionals come in the picture, professionals and families need to communicate their needs so they can work collaboratively. To be empowered, both professionals and families need to be motivated and have the skills/knowledge necessary to take actions that will pave the way for them and their needs.

Alliance

Professionals should also seek to form an alliance with the family. A successful collaboration between empowered professionals and families cannot happen without building a strong alliance. Developing a strong relationship is the backbone of the empowerment. Turnbull and Turnbull (2001) suggested eight major obligations by the professionals to develop the most attainable alliance with families:

1. *Know yourself.* Reexamine your beliefs, values, and biases.

2. *Know the family.* Appreciate a family's individuality. Each family has their own perceptions of and experiences with deaf people. Do not stereotype deaf people. Characteristics (cultural background, sizes, and challenges), interactions between family members, functions (responsibilities and roles), and life cycle issues should be looked at closely.

3. *Honor cultural diversity.* Cultural diversity includes race, ethnicity, religion, geographical location, education, age, income status, gender, sexual orientation, disability status, and occupation. Often, disability can influence cultural affiliations. Deaf culture is an example. Deaf people have a long history of growing up together and typically stay in close contact. Deaf adults establish relationships with others that build communities for recreation and support. Professionals need to be prepared for cultural differences. Many deaf parents, for example, are often thrilled to have deaf children. Also, different cultures have different ways of coping with disabilities. For example, some Asian/ Pacific Americans use massage, acupuncture, *cao gio* (coin rubbing), surgery, medicine, herbal medicine, *bat gio* (pinching), *giac* (placing a very hot cup on the exposed area), and other methods to heal a

disability (Cheng, 2000). Professionals also need to avoid cultural stereotyping. For instance, Hispanics represent more than 20 separate nations, so the degree of acculturation, as well as other issues, varies across families (Christensen, 2000; Turnbull & Turnbull, 2001).

4. *Affirm and build on family strengths.* Focusing on family strengths promotes family self-efficacy. Families depend on the respect they get from professionals to build alliances with others.

5. *Promote family choice.* Give families choices as to how they participate. They can decide which family member is to be involved when making collaborative decisions; how they will make decisions; which family members will work with the professionals during the service-delivery process; what the parameters of the family–professional interaction will be, such as when and where to meet; how much information to share; and what priority needs, goals, and supports they should follow up with. Families with deaf children must be informed about communication choices and education placements.

6. *Affirm great expectations.* Expectation is significant and has an impact on the child's academic achievement. Parents and professionals must have high expectations of the deaf child. Pairing children with deaf role models will definitely help; deaf adults are likely to have high expectations of deaf children, which is a strength. Professionals and families can discuss what the expectations are for the child. Professionals can share the success of other individuals with disabilities that are similar to the child's. Linking the family with other knowledgeable individuals can be helpful as well. For example, one university offers a "family matching" program, whereby the family is matched with a university student, often one who is deaf or hard of hearing, training to become a teacher. The student and family spend 30 hours together over the course of three semesters. Families benefit from the knowledge and expertise of the student, and the student learns about "real life" from the family. Often, the first person that the parents met with a disability was their own child.

7. *Communicate positively.* Often, professionals take for granted that they are skilled communicators. Communication is like an art that involves nonverbal communication skills such as physical attending and listening. People respond much better to positive, encouraging messages. Deaf children are visual learners so they watch for body language and facial expressions. Consistent communication with deaf children enhances many different aspects, emotionally, mentally, socially, and linguistically.

8. *Foster trust and respect.* Developing trust and respect between the professionals and families is of paramount importance; these qualities

are the key to a successful alliance. If trust and respect do not exist, no matter how hard professionals try or how good the ideas are, the collaboration, empowerment, and alliance fall apart. Professionals might be working with parents wishing not to have a deaf child in the family. The parents might consider giving up the child. With trust and respect when developing alliances, parents can work through some sensitive issues without feeling threatened or intimidated. Confidentiality is the key.

Parents' most important role as parents should be endorsed and advocated by professionals with no hesitation. If there is a program that parents and professionals would like to see happen, parents should not be expected to implement and maintain it. Parents of children without disabilities would not be expected to do so. Parents do not have to assume the burden to develop a program on their own since they simply would not have the time to develop and maintain a program. Most parents are treading water constantly to meet the demands of their jobs, children, and households. Parents need assurance that they are there for their own children as parents first. Therefore, parents would appreciate knowing that service development is an option and can use professional support.

Collaboration, empowerment, and alliance lead to successful partnerships between families and professionals. They are interwoven and cannot happen alone. Collaboration, empowerment, and alliance pave the way to advocacy (Turnbull & Turnbull, 2001).

FAMILY, PROFESSIONAL, AND COMMUNITY COLLABORATION

Parents may want to know how to extend what they have learned about their child and their child's disability to other family members and various members of the community (for example, members of religious groups or neighborhood groups). Parents need to know how to help their child have positive interactions with others and develop skills to use when communication breaks down. They need to know what social opportunities are available to their children, such as a playgroup for hard of hearing children. Knowledgeable and qualified professionals make information available to ensure these community and cultural connections for the families.

Unfortunately, even though parents can benefit from continual learning, many programs end parent education in the early educational years. A survey of 151 families of deaf and hard of hearing school-aged children indicated that families would like schools to initiate and support more family involvement opportunities. When their child is in first grade, for example, parents may wish to receive more information about reading and phonics. When their child is in third grade, parents may wish to know about web resources parents can recommend for their child. When their child is in fifth grade, parents may wish to understand more about the pros and cons of various placement options for middle school. When their child is in eighth grade, parents may wish to be more informed about antidiscrimination laws such as the ADA. And when their child is considering college or a vocation, parents will want to learn more about institutions that will suit the needs of their child.

Moreover, parents may want to revisit certain issues as their child gets older, such as communication options and cochlear implants. Decisions that the parents made when their child was younger may not be permanent. Responding to parents throughout the school years can help parents acquire the skills they need and help them maintain a good relationship with professionals and interest in the school. Continuing to work with parents over the years will definitely build a solid collaboration between parents and early childhood education programs. By having a solid connection with professionals and community, parents will know where to seek information as their priorities change over the years.

Education reforms and laws urge early childhood education programs to view the families and professionals in these ongoing relationships as communities of learners, where children, professionals, and parents all learn together (Sergiovanni, 1994). Parents who truly feel like they are part of the team are likely to have faith in the early childhood program and continue their involvement throughout the years. Therefore, professionals are obligated to suggest ways to involve knowledgeable parents and insights from their children and other community members (Konzal, 2001).

CREATING AN ETHNICALLY DIVERSE FAMILY CLIMATE FOR DEAF CHILDREN

The Gallaudet Research Institute survey from November 1998 indicated that 44.1% of all deaf and hard of hearing children from infancy to 18 years of age receiving services in the United States are from ethnically diverse families. There are a limited number of professionals with diverse backgrounds, however. Given the data, nearly one of two families may have views that are unfamiliar to the professionals working with them. Beginning in the 1980s, professionals began to shift their focus to meet the priorities of culturally diverse families.

More schools (Strong, 1995) have adopted a bilingual/bicultural program with the focus on ASL and English. Although the bilingual/bicultural approach was a giant step in deaf education, this approach may not be adequate to fully meet the needs of deaf children from non–English-speaking families. However, Christensen (1985) found that using ASL as a communication "bridge" between non–English-speaking parents and deaf children is a positive step toward bilingual ASL/English competence for deaf children. Nevertheless, these non–English-speaking families need extensive support services beyond what the typical bilingual/bicultural program can offer to promote academic success.

In order for professionals to better serve culturally diverse families with a deaf child, Christensen (2000) suggests that professionals become familiar with the background, language, culture, and beliefs of these families; keep variables such as child rearing, educational experiences, and values in mind; reaffirm the family's efforts to support their child; and empower families to incorporate literacy activities with their deaf children at home. More suggestions for the professional include working to gain a better understanding of how language acquisition occurs, especially when two or more languages are involved; recognizing each deaf child and his or her family as individuals; making connections with existing knowledge of the child; and understanding the reasons the families had for coming to the United States. The suggestions above are certainly not limited only to families from certain cultures.

Strategies to help improve home–school relationships and encourage greater participation from culturally diverse families include 1) providing translations of printed information for families and providing language interpreters to assure full access to school functions; 2) being specific as to what ways parents can get involved in children's education; 3) developing trusting, positive, and personal relationships with families and forming support groups; and 4) developing an advocacy system to help parents express their views without feeling intimidated (Sass-Lehrer, Gerner de Garcia, & Rovins, 1997). More strategies involve 1) arranging community meetings about school programs, resources, and services to keep lines of communication open; 2) organizing "buddy systems" to welcome new families to the school; 3) scheduling events on days and times that fit families' schedules; and 4) planning school events and programs as consulted by the individuals from the various communities associated with the school.

When parents and professionals collaborate successfully, it becomes easier for them to write an effective IFSP or IEP together and to choose a placement that is appropriate for the child. If the collaboration is to occur successfully, both parents and professionals must communicate clearly and make clear their expectations of each other.

Table 3.3.   Questions that assess professionals' skills in promoting advocacy among families

General	IEP/IFSP development
What is the atmosphere in the school or program? Are parents' views and input solicited and valued? Are their suggestions taken seriously and acted on?	Are parents involved in premeeting preparation? Are they provided an opportunity to give their views? Do they feel as though they are equal contributors?
Do professionals view families as experts on their own children?	Do parents receive adequate notice of the meeting so that they can arrange their schedule to be there? Are several times offered so that the parents can choose a time that is convenient for them? Are evening or weekend hours available if necessary?
Do professionals facilitate parents meeting other parents and deaf and hard of hearing adults?	
When there are language differences, are qualified interpreters provided in order to facilitate communication? Do staff work with interpreters to explain concepts before meetings so that the interpreter can more effectively and accurately convey meaning? Are written materials translated in the parents' native language?	Is the meeting place convenient for the family? What about families who use public transportation?
	Is sufficient time scheduled for meetings to thoroughly discuss issues? Are forms, evaluation results, and other information sent to the family well in advance for their review?
Does the family feel that their native language and culture is reflected and respected in the program?	Are parents treated as equal participants, including when differences in ethnicity, socioeconomic status, education, and disability status exist?
Is the whole family included in the early intervention and education of the child, including grandparents, siblings, non-family caregivers?	Do parents receive and understand sufficient information so that they can be equal participants?
	Do parents receive a full explanation of what is being proposed?
	Do parents receive a full explanation of the choices and options available to them and their child?
	Do parents understand the professional's responsibilities and the responsibilities of the early intervention or educational program?

CHALLENGES TO PROMOTING PARENT ADVOCACY

Early intervention and education programs are not perfect. Particularly in the case of hearing loss, which is considered a "low-incidence" disability relative to other disabilities, barriers—many that are outside the control of the professional working with the family—can keep even the most persistent advocates from obtaining the appropriate services and education for children and families.

One barrier, for example, is the lack of appropriate services or placements in certain districts. Professionals may be pressured by superiors to steer the family toward a particular choice that is convenient for the system to provide but that may not necessarily meet the developmental needs of the infant, toddler, or family. A possible solution is for the professional to work within the early intervention or education system to ensure that a broad range of services and placements are available.

Another barrier is that parent advocacy efforts may seem threatening to a professional. The professional may have been taught that he or she is the "expert" and the parent should be taking his or her advice. However, professionals who partner with families find that the family's knowledge, insights, and participation are critical to the child's success.

Lack of experience and knowledge on the part of professionals working with a child with a hearing loss can be yet another barrier. Early intervention and education for children who are deaf or hard of hearing is highly specialized and requires in-depth training and experience on the part of the professional. Professionals could advocate within the program to ensure the recruitment and hiring of qualified individuals. See Table 3.3 for questions that assess professionals' skills in promoting advocacy among families.

CONCLUSION

This chapter has provided background and ideas on parental involvement and advocacy. It is the authors' hope that professionals will use this information to support parents in making the best decisions for their child.

REFERENCES

Americans with Disabilities Act (ADA) of 1990, PL 101-336, 42 U.S.C. §§ 12101 *et seq.*

Anderson, W., Chitwood, S., & Hayden, D. (1997). *Negotiating the special education maze: A guide for parents and teachers* (3rd ed.). Bethesda, MD: Woodbine House.

Assistance to States for the Education of Children with Disabilities and the Early Intervention Program for Infants and Toddlers with Disabilities: Final Regulations, 34 C.F.R. §§ 300, 303 (1999).

Bailey, D., & Wolery, M. (1992). *Teaching infants and preschoolers with disabilities.* Upper Saddle River, NJ: Prentice Hall.

Benedict, B.S. (2003). *Perceptions of family involvement in schools among families with deaf and hard of hearing children.* Unpublished doctoral dissertation, Gallaudet University, Washington, DC.

Brown v. Board of Educ., 347 U.S. 483 (1954).

Calderon, R. (2000). Parental involvement in deaf children's education programs as a predicator of child's language: Early reading and social emotional development. *Journal of Deaf Studies and Deaf Education, 5*(2), 140–155.

Calderon, R., & Greenberg, M. (2000). Challenges to parents and professionals in promoting social-economical development in deaf children. In P. Spencer, C. Erting, & M. Marschark (Eds.), *The deaf child in the family and at school: Essays in honor of Kathryn P. Meadow-Orlans* (p. 168). Mahwah, NJ: Lawrence Erlbaum Associates.

Cheng, L.L. (2000). Deafness: An Asian/Pacific perspective. In K. Christensen (Ed.), *Deaf plus: A multicultural perspective* (p. 76). San Diego: Dawn Sign Press.

Christensen, K. (1985). Conceptual sign language as a bridge between English and Spanish. *American Annals of the Deaf, 130,* 244–249.

Christensen, K. (2000). Emergening literacy in bilingual/multicultural education of children who are deaf: A communication based perspective. In K. Christensen (Ed.), *Deaf plus: A multicultural perspective* (p. 163). San Diego: Dawn Sign Press.

Christensen, S., & Cleary, M. (1990). Consultation and the parent-education partnership: A perspective. *Journal of Education and Psychological Consultation, 1,* 219–241.

Dunst, C., Trivette, C., & Deal, A. (1996). *Enabling and empowering families: Principles and guidelines for practice.* Cambridge, MA: Brookline Books.

Education for All Handicapped Children Act of 1975, PL 94-142, 20 U.S.C. §§ 1400 *et seq.*

Epstein, J. (1987). Parent involvement: What research says to administrators. *Education and Urban Society, 19,* 119–136.

Epstein, J., & Dauber, S. (1991). School programs and teacher practices of parent involvement in inner-city elementary and middle schools. *The Elementary School Journal, 91*(3), 289–305.

Gallaudet Research Institute. (1998, November). *Regional and national summary report of data from the 1997–1998 Annual Survey of Deaf and Hard of Hearing Children and Youth.* Washington, DC: Author.

Greenberg, M., & Calderon, R. (1987). Parent education. In J. Van Cleve (Ed.), *Gallaudet encyclopedia on deaf people and deafness* (Vol. 2, pp. 264–268). New York: McGraw-Hill.

Henderson, A., & Berla, N. (1996). *A new generation of evidence: The family is critical to student achievement.* Washington, DC: Center for Law and Education.

Henderson, K. (2001). An overview of ADA, IDEA, and Section 504: Update 2001. *ERIC EC Digest, #E606.* Retrieved from http://ericec.org/digests/e606.html

Individuals with Disabilities Education Act (IDEA) Amendments of 1997, PL 105-17, 20 U.S.C. §§ 1400 *et seq.*

Konzal, J. (2001). Collaborative inquiry: A means of creating learning community. *Early Childhood Research Quarterly, 16*(1), 95–115.

Lane, H. (1993). *The mask of benevolence.* New York: Vintage Books.

Mills v. Board of Education of the District of Columbia, 348 F. Supp. 866 (1972).

Moeller, M.P. (2000). Early intervention and language development in children who are deaf and hard of hearing. *Pediatrics, 106,* 3.

Moores, D. (2001). *Educating the deaf: Psychology, principles, and practices* (5th ed.). Boston: Houghton Mifflin.

National Council on Disability. (1994). *Back to school on civil rights.* Washington, DC: Author.

Pennsylvania Association for Retarded Children (PARC) v. Commonwealth of Pennsylvania, 334 F. Supp. 1257 (1971).

Rehabilitation Act Amendments of 1992, PL 102-569, 29 U.S.C. §§ 701 *et seq.*

Rehabilitation Act of 1973, PL 93-112, 29 U.S.C. §§ 701 *et seq.*

Roush, J. (1994). Strengthening family–professional relations: Advice from parents. In J. Rousch & N. Matkins (Eds.), *Infants and toddlers with hearing loss: Family centered assessment and intervention* (pp. 344–347). Timonium, MD: York Press.

Santayana, G. (1905). *Life of reason* (Vol. 1). New York: Scribner's.

Sass-Lehrer, M., Gerner de Garcia, B., & Rovins, M. (1997). *Creating a multicultural school climate for deaf children and their families.* Washington, DC: Gallaudet University, Pre-College National Missions Programs.

Sergiovanni, T. (1994). *Building communities in schools.* San Francisco: Jossey-Bass.

Spencer, P. (2000). Every opportunity: A case study of hearing parents and their deaf child. In P. Spencer, C. Erting, & M. Marschark (Eds.), *The deaf child in the family and at school: Essays in honor of Kathryn P. Meadow-Orlans* (p. 128). Mahwah, NJ: Lawrence Earlbaum Associates.

Strong, M. (1995). A review of bilingual/bicultural programs for deaf children. *American Annals of the Deaf, 140,* 84–94.

Turnbull, A., & Turnbull, R. (2001). *Families, professionals, and exceptionality: Collaborating for empowerment* (4th ed.). Upper Saddle River, NJ: Merrill Prentice Hall.

U.S. Department of Education. (1999). Appendix A to Part 300: Notice of interpretation. *Federal Register, 64*(48), 12472–12473.

Webster's New Collegiate Dictionary. (1980). Springfield, MA: G & C Merriam Co.

A Parent's Reflection

Anonymous

It is our first year in early intervention. Everything has been over-whelming—learning about hearing loss, going to the audiologist, the different specialists . . . one tells you to do things one way, the other tells you to do it the opposite way. I guess I got pretty discouraged sometimes. But the one person I could count on was my child's early intervention teacher. She listened to us without judging, she knew where to get information, she asked me what I thought. Of course, I wanted her to make the decisions for me—it seemed easier that way. But she encouraged me to read the facts and to trust my instincts. My daughter is still young, and I have a lot to learn. But I realize that nobody knows what they're doing when they first start on this path. It's a question of trial and error. Having the teacher's support and confidence helped us get through the year—and hopefully will help us with the years to come.

SECTION TWO

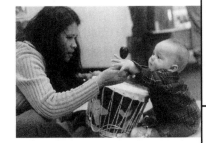

Program
Foundations

CHAPTER FOUR

Identification of Permanent Childhood Hearing Loss Through Universal Newborn Hearing Screening Programs

BRANDT CULPEPPER

M y baby girl never heard me tell her I loved her the first two years of her life. It wasn't that I didn't tell her every day, but rather that she had a hearing loss that went undetected for those two years, and was unable to hear any speech. There was no newborn hearing screening process in the hospital where she was born. (Des Georges, 1998, p. 25)

This mother's statement reflects a situation that many families who have a newborn with congenital hearing loss face and highlights the parental anguish over late identification of hearing loss and the disruption in a family's communication with unidentified hearing loss. When universal newborn hearing screening (UNHS) is not implemented, children with hearing loss are often not identified until they are toddlers. In many instances, earlier identification is possible, but the services that would detect hearing loss are not implemented as a standard of care in the hospital nursery.

Although the importance of early identification of hearing loss in infants and young children has been recognized since the mid-1900s (e.g., Ewing & Ewing, 1947), UNHS has not always been feasible (see Historical Context for Universal Newborn Hearing Screening). With the advent of new technologies in the mid-1990s, and a better understanding of the services and support necessary for infants who need follow-up, screening every infant for congenital hearing loss is now much more feasible. Professionals have worked tirelessly to develop and improve the policies, procedures, and protocols for implementing UNHS. UNHS programs now serve as the entry point to a vast array of available services for infants with hearing loss and their families. These services are commonly called the Early Hearing Detection and Intervention (EHDI) system. These advances in early identification are challenging professionals in many fields to expand and develop new service delivery systems and programming for infants and young children with hearing loss and their families (see Chapter 6).

Nationally, federal agencies, professional organizations, and state departments of health have collaborated to develop common goals regarding early identification of hearing loss. The ultimate goal of all EHDI systems is to maximize linguistic and communicative competence and literacy development for children who are deaf or hard of hearing. Through early identification and early intervention, the ultimate goal is for children with hearing loss to develop communication skills equivalent to their peers who have normal hearing, affording individuals with hearing loss the same educational, social, and vocational opportunities. Although their focus and the wording of their statements may differ somewhat, the following goals are recognized nationally by federal programs (e.g., Centers for Disease Control and Prevention's EHDI Program; Health Resources and Services Administration's [HRSA] Universal Newborn Hearing Screening and Intervention Program) and professional associations (e.g., Joint Committee on Infant Hearing, American Academy of Pediatrics, American Academy of Audiology, American Speech-Language-Hearing Association):

- All infants will be screened for hearing loss before 1 month of age.
- Audiometric assessments for all children referred from hearing screening programs will be completed before 3 months of age.
- Early intervention services for infants with hearing loss and their families will be initiated before 6 months of age.
- All children with progressive, late onset, fluctuating, or acquired hearing loss will be identified at the earliest possible time.
- All children with hearing loss will have a medical home (for more information regarding the medical home concept see Medical Care Professionals [Physicians]).
- Infant and family rights will be guaranteed through informed choice, decision making, and consent.
- Every state will have an EHDI database tracking and surveillance system that will minimize loss to follow-up.
- Every state will have a comprehensive system that monitors and evaluates progress toward EHDI goals and objectives.

Although making sure that each of the 4 million infants born annually in the United States receives hearing screening may seem daunting, it is just the first step. Ensuring that each infant who is referred for further services after hospital discharge actually receives the indicated services in a timely and appropriate manner presents a much greater challenge.

HISTORICAL CONTEXT FOR
UNIVERSAL NEWBORN HEARING SCREENING

Until 1990, relatively little national emphasis was directed toward reducing the age of identification of hearing loss, although parents and families of children who are deaf and hard of hearing and professionals working with them have long had the goal of identifying hearing loss early. With the support of then Surgeon General C. Everett Koop, the U.S. Department of Health and Human Services issued the 1990 *Healthy People 2000* report, which established goals to improve substantially the health of American citizens. Goal 17.16 of the report was to reduce the average age of identification of hearing loss to younger than 12 months (U.S. Department of Health and Human Services, 1990). Screening programs in the 1990s, however, were far from meeting this goal.

For example, in 1990 it was estimated that children with congenital hearing loss were being identified at an average age of about 24 months when programs used a predominantly high-risk registry approach. High-risk registries, as endorsed by the Joint Committee on Infant Hearing (JCIH; 1991), outlined key indicators for increased risk of having a hearing loss; infants identified as having one or more risk indicators were recommended for hearing screening. At best, however, high-risk registries identify only about half of all infants with congenital hearing loss because many children who are deaf or hard of hearing do not present any high-risk indicators (Elssmann, Matkin, & Sabo, 1987; Mauk, White, Mortensen, & Behrens, 1991; Stein, Clark, & Kraus, 1983). Even in well-established statewide programs, less than half of the infants with congenital hearing loss were identified because of loss to follow-up, missed appointments, and so forth (Mahoney & Eichwald, 1987).

The lack of resources needed to support the screening technology in the early 1990s was another challenge to meeting the *Healthy People 2000* goal. Even though audiologists had access to the auditory brainstem response (ABR) test, a powerful diagnostic test that could be used as a tool for screening infants for hearing loss, UNHS was not feasible because of cost, the time necessary to complete the measurements, and the need for highly trained professionals to interpret test results.

Fortunately, during the late 1980s, discoveries about the auditory system and advances in technology had led to the development of a new clinical tool for measuring the auditory system, the evoked otoacoustic emissions (EOAE) test (Kemp, 1988). Technological advances also facilitated the development of a computerized version of the ABR screening measurement, the automated ABR (AABR), which reduced test time and interpreted instrument data, classifying children as a "pass" or a "refer" (Hall, Kripal, & Hepp, 1988). This eliminated the need for a trained observer and drastically reduced the costs of screening newborns for hearing loss. Because screening results obtained using the AABR test were similar to those obtained from the conventional ABR test (Jacobson, Jacobson, & Spahr, 1990; Kileny, 1987), a dedicated instrument for newborn hearing screening became commercially available.

Because of the promising data collected in clinical trials using EOAE as a tool for screening newborns for hearing loss in the Rhode Island Hearing Assessment Project (Kemp & Ryan, 1993; White & Behrens, 1993; White, Vohr, & Behrens, 1993) and the potential for using AABR in newborn nurseries, the National Institutes of Health (NIH) held a Consensus Development Conference in March 1993 to review the evidence on newborn hearing screening. The statement issued from this conference, the *Early Identification of Hearing Impairment in Infants and Young Children,* concluded that

> All infants should be screened for hearing impairment. . . . This will
> be accomplished most efficiently by screening prior to discharge

from the well-baby nursery. Infants who fail . . . should have a comprehensive hearing evaluation no later than 6 months of age. (NIH, 1993, p. 1)

Endorsing UNHS was a dramatic departure from using risk indicators to target which infants should be screened. Widespread debate about the justification for screening all newborns for hearing loss was prompted by a letter to the editor in *Pediatrics* titled "Universal Screening for Infant Hearing Impairment: Not Simple, Not Risk-Free, Not Necessarily Beneficial, and Not Presently Justified" (Bess & Paradise, 1994). Although several valid points were raised in the letter, the title alone caused many proponents of earlier identification of hearing loss through universal newborn hearing screening to strongly object to the position held by the authors. Since this letter, many concerns have been addressed, technologies used as screening tools have been further defined and documented, and support has continued to grow for the earlier identification of hearing loss through UNHS programs. The number of hospital-based programs screening each newborn for hearing loss has nearly doubled every year since the 1993 NIH Consensus Statement (National Center for Hearing Assessment and Management [NCHAM], 2001). The number of professional associations, groups, and organizations endorsing the goals of screening all infants for hearing loss before 1 month of age, completing audiological diagnosis by 3 months of age, and enrolling infants with hearing loss and their families in appropriate early intervention services by 6 months of age continues to rise. Some of the more significant endorsements include those of *Healthy People 2010* (U.S. Department of Health and Human Services, 2000), the JCIH (2000), and the American Academy of Pediatrics (1999).

CURRENT STATUS OF UNIVERSAL NEWBORN HEARING SCREENING

Most professionals agree that all newborn infants should be screened for hearing loss. Before implementing UNHS, it was generally assumed that 1 infant per 1,000 was born with an educationally significant hearing loss. In most studies, the term *educationally significant* translated into at least moderate or greater bilateral sensorineural hearing loss. Since then, studies supported identification of children with milder degrees of hearing loss (Bess, Dodd-Murphy, & Parker, 1998; Blair, Peterson, & Viehweg, 1985; Davis, Elfenbein, Schum, & Bentler, 1986; Roush & Matkin, 1994; Tharpe & Bess, 1999) and unilateral hearing loss because children with any degree of hearing loss in either ear may experience

developmental difficulties (speech, language, social, or emotional) or
may fall behind in school (see Chapter 8). Infants with unilateral hearing
loss are also at risk for developing progressive or bilateral hearing loss
(Brookhouser, Worthington, & Kelly, 1994). Due to the potentially detri-
mental impact of all degrees of hearing loss, most EHDI programs in the
United States attempt to identify all infants who have any type of PCHL,
including those with mild, unilateral, or conductive hearing loss that
cannot be corrected during childhood.

Lowering the average age of identification of hearing loss through
UNHS is not only possible, it is becoming a reality. The current debate
is how to best screen for permanent childhood hearing loss (PCHL). It
is vital to ensure that families of infants who do not pass the initial hearing
screening before hospital discharge (or before 1 month of age) receive
appropriate professional referrals and are offered indicated services.

The Newborn Infant Hearing Screening and Intervention Act of 2000,
which was incorporated as Title VI of the Departments of Labor, Health
and Human Services, and Education, and Related Agencies Appropriations Act of 2000 (PL 106-113) and signed into law, provides federal
funds for competitive state grants to develop infant hearing screening
and intervention programs. In addition, through the Children's Health
Act of 2000 (PL 106-310), Congress identified specific goals to address
the problem of hearing loss in children including early hearing screening
and evaluation of all newborns, coordinated intervention and rehabilitation services, and ongoing applied research to better understand the
learning and developmental needs of children who are deaf and hard
of hearing. The number of states requiring statewide newborn hearing
screening by law or voluntary compliance increased from 11 states in
1991 to 42 states and the District of Columbia in 2003. Progress certainly
is being made in screening (see Figure 4.1), but there is still a long way
to go. For example, while 67% of infants were screened for hearing loss
before 1 month of age in 2000 (up from only 20% in 1999), more than
half of the newborns who did not pass the hearing screening were lost
to follow-up (Directors of Speech and Hearing Programs for State Health
and Welfare Agencies, 2001).

However, very encouraging data on newborn hearing screening are
emerging from Rhode Island and Hawaii, the two states with established
statewide systems (in operation for 3 years or more) that link screening
programs with follow-up services and early intervention programs. The
average ages of identification of hearing loss and intervention reported
for Rhode Island (Carty, Letourneau, & Vohr, 1998) and Hawaii (Johnson,
Kuntz, Sia, White, & Johnson, 1997) (see Figure 4.2) are substantially
lower (younger than 6 months) than the national averages (18–30
months). These statewide EHDI systems have demonstrated that it is

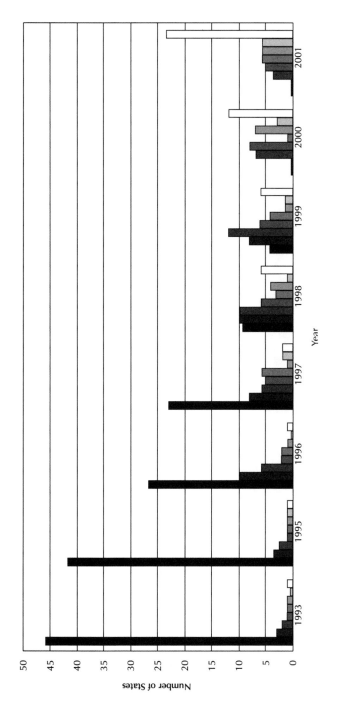

Figure 4.1.   Progression of states toward Universal Newborn Hearing Screening (UNHS) from 1993 to 2001. The number of states screening 5% or fewer of the infants born statewide is shown in black. Shading becomes progressively lighter as states screen more infants, with the number of states screening 90% or more infants shown in white. (Please note that no data were collected for 1994.)

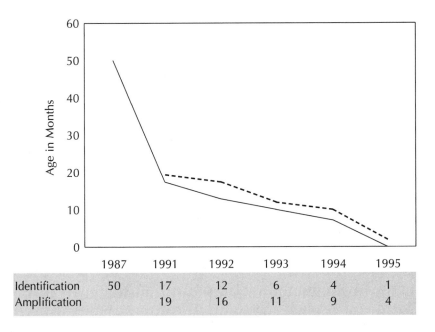

	1987	1991	1992	1993	1994	1995
Identification	50	17	12	6	4	1
Amplification		19	16	11	9	4

Figure 4.2.   Reduction in average age of identification of hearing loss and average age of amplification for children with confirmed hearing loss as newborn hearing screening programs were implemented in hospitals in Hawaii. (*Key:* solid line, identification; dashed line, amplification.)

possible to meet or exceed the goals established in *Healthy People 2010,* the *Joint Committee on Infant Hearing 2000 Position Statement,* and the *NIH Consensus Statement.*

DEFINING HEARING LOSS

Hearing loss is generally described according to three attributes: type (nature), degree, and configuration. The type or nature of hearing loss refers to where or what part of the auditory system causes the hearing loss. The degree of hearing loss refers to how severe or extensive the hearing loss is. The configuration of the hearing loss refers to the shape of hearing loss in one or both ears as hearing is plotted on the audiogram. Visual inspection of the audiogram, the most basic plot of hearing sensitivity, in association with the other information collected during a hearing evaluation provides information about the type, degree, and configuration of hearing loss.

The Audiogram

Audiologists use audiograms to plot the hearing level for each ear and create a graph of hearing. The frequency of sound (pitch) is plotted along the horizontal axis, with low frequencies on the left and high frequencies on the right. Frequency is plotted in Hertz (Hz), with higher numbers representing higher pitches. Most audiograms plot test results for pure tone frequencies between 250 to 8000 Hz. The intensity of sound (loudness) is plotted along the vertical axis. Low intensity (soft) sounds are marked on the top of the graph and high intensity (loud) sounds are marked on the bottom of the graph. Sound intensity is plotted in decibels (dB), with 0 dB being the average of the softest sounds that young adults with normal hearing can detect across the speech frequencies. Therefore, on the audiogram, soft, low-pitched sounds would be plotted in the top left corner, while loud, high-pitched sounds would be plotted in the lower right corner. The response of each ear to varied frequencies is plotted on the audiogram using red circles for right ear responses (remember "round–red–right") and blue Xs for left ear responses.

Completing an audiogram for each ear is one of the first steps in a hearing evaluation. An audiogram and other tests (e.g., tympanometry, testing with speech signals, evoked otoacoustic emissions) can be completed in a single test session, requiring only that the person being tested raise his or her hand or push a button whenever he or she hears a beep or repeat back words that he or she hears. An audiogram test is usually not a difficult task for adults and most children older than 3–4 years of age. For infants and young children, however, getting a complete audiogram may require several test sessions and may incorporate many test modifications. Infants and children are not yet capable of providing the voluntary responses such as raising a hand, pushing a button, or repeating what they have heard in response to a sound. As children age and their cognitive skills mature, obtaining results to plot on an audiogram becomes easier and can be completed more quickly. Patience and persistence are required from both families and professionals when trying to complete an audiogram for infants and young children. Families of infants and young children who are deaf and hard of hearing should be encouraged to work with audiologists with experience and expertise in pediatric testing.

For more information on hearing loss, the implications of hearing loss, or understanding an audiogram, visit the American Speech-Language-Hearing Association's public web site pages on childhood hearing loss (http://www.asha.org/hearing) or Appendix 4-D, "Relationship of degree of longterm hearing loss to psychosocial impact and educational needs," in the *Educational Audiology Handbook* (Johnson, Benson, & Seaton, 1997).

PREVALENCE OF CONGENITAL HEARING LOSS

Determining how many infants are born with hearing loss each year in the United States is not an easy task, yet estimates of the prevalence of congenital hearing loss (number of newborns with hearing loss within a specific time frame) are necessary for evaluating a program's effectiveness and estimating the professional services that will be needed to adequately serve a given population. Four major factors are known to contribute to differences in prevalence estimates: 1) the population being tested (well-baby versus special-care nurseries), 2) the definition of hearing loss (degree, type, and configuration of hearing loss targeted for identification), 3) the age of confirmation of hearing loss, and 4) the number of infants referred from the initial hearing screening who return for follow-up services. Prevalence estimates are higher for newborns needing special care than for newborns from well-baby nurseries. When newborns with milder degrees of hearing loss or unilateral hearing loss are included, prevalence will be higher.

Data from existing programs suggest that about 12,000 infants are born with congenital hearing loss every year in the United States (2–4 per 1,000 births). In addition, about one third of children with hearing loss also have vision impairment or other developmental disabilities (Gallaudet University Center for Assessment and Demographic Study, 1998; Schildroth & Hotto, 1993).

NEWBORN HEARING SCREENING TECHNOLOGIES

UNHS programs have two viable technologies: the evoked otoacoustic emissions (EOAE) test, which includes both transient-evoked otoacoustic emissions (TEOAE) and distortion product otoacoustic emissions (DPOAE), and the auditory brainstem response (ABR) test, which includes conventional ABR and screening ABR. Similarities and differences between the two technologies are presented in Table 4.1. Both EOAE and ABR instruments are commercially available from a variety of manufacturers and distributors. Both may be purchased as dedicated instruments (those that allow for performing hearing screening only) or units that may be used for a variety of purposes (e.g., screening, more comprehensive testing, data and program management). Both may be automated to provide a "pass" or "refer" result, eliminating the need for program personnel to interpret screening results. Many instruments may

Table 4.1. Comparison of EOAE and ABR

Screening tool	Response measurement	Hearing loss detection
EOAE/ABR	Objective, sensitive, physiologic measures of the auditory system that correlate with hearing status.	Do not truly test hearing status.
EOAE	Reflects energy generated by the outer hair cells within the cochlea. *Acoustic* energy is measured from a microphone in the ear canal.	May miss some reverse slope losses, some slight hearing losses. Will pass infants with auditory neuropathies.
ABR	Reflects neural response to auditory stimuli from the brainstem level activity. *Electrical* energy is measured from electrodes placed on the skin around the head and neck.	May miss some sloped, slight, and mild hearing losses. Will refer infants with auditory neuropathies.

ABR = auditory brainstem response; EOAE = evoked otoacoustic emissions.

be linked directly to computer-based data management systems designed specifically for UNHS programs. Linking hearing screening results with the data management system improves the ability of the program to ensure that infants who need follow-up services actually receive them. Many instruments also have the capability to automatically generate statistical reports and letters to parents, pediatricians, and primary care physicians.

More complete information about the technologies being used for UNHS may be found in Kurman and Spivak (1998) or at the National Center for Hearing Assessment and Management (NCHAM; 2002) web site (http://www.infanthearing.org/resources/equipment/equipmenttable .html).

APPLICATION OF NEWBORN HEARING SCREENING

As more and more EHDI programs are implemented, it is vital that the professionals who work with families understand both the big picture of the EHDI systems and the details of the system in their state or region. Although every professional cannot become an expert in PCHL, they can learn who the experts in their EHDI system are, where to make referrals, and how to link families with the appropriate people and services. The big picture is sometimes referred to as the 1-3-6 EHDI Plan, which denotes the goals for completing hearing screening, assessment, and intervention. That is, all infants should be screened for hearing loss before 1 month of age, all those who do not pass the hearing screening should receive complete audiometric and medical evaluations before 3 months of age, and all infants identified with hearing loss should be enrolled in appropriate early intervention services before 6 months of age. Although not conceptually difficult to understand, implementing fully functional EHDI systems is daunting because of the large-scale coordination of services necessary to provide a seamless system for parents from screening through intervention.

Ongoing Surveillance

Families, health care providers, and professionals who work with children must recognize that a hearing screening or a hearing test reflects the status of the child's auditory system only at the time of the test. Hearing screening results do not reflect what has happened in the past or what may happen in the future. Passing a hearing screening at birth, therefore, does not mean that hearing loss will not be a concern later in life.

Also, as reviewed in a previous section, existing technology has limitations; the two screening technologies currently available can identify hearing loss of 30 dB HL or greater. Thus, some infants with slight to mild congenital hearing loss may pass the initial hearing screening. For this reason, ongoing surveillance of each child's hearing status is necessary.

Specific indicators that place a child at risk for progressive or delayed-onset hearing loss have been identified. When an infant who has passed the hearing screening has one or more of the identified risk indicators (see Table 4.2), audiologic monitoring every 6 months is recommended until age 3 years.

Although many EHDI programs attempt to identify infants with risk indicators, some infants may not be recognized as being at risk. For instance, family history of hearing loss may not be determined before the infant is discharged from the EHDI program. Therefore, it becomes the responsibility of parents and primary care providers (PCP) to monitor infants for typical communication developmental milestones during routine medical care. Infants with frequent or persistent episodes of ear infections or otitis media with effusion (OME), will also require ongoing monitoring to address the potential adverse effects of fluctuating conductive hearing loss associated with OME (Friel-Patti & Finitzo, 1990; Friel-Patti, Finitzo-Hieber, Conti, & Brown, 1982; Gravel & Wallace, 1992; Stool et al., 1994; Wallace et al., 1988).

Table 4.2. Risk indicators for progressive or delayed-onset hearing loss

Primary or caregiver concern regarding hearing, speech, language, and or developmental delay
Family history of permanent childhood hearing loss
Stigmata or other findings associated with a syndrome known to include a sensorineural or conductive hearing loss or eustachian tube dysfunction
Postnatal infections associated with sensorineural hearing loss, including bacterial meningitis
In utero infections such as cytomegalovirus, herpes, rubella, syphilis, and toxoplasmosis
Neonatal indicators, specifically hyperbilirubinemia at a serum level requiring exchange transfusion, persistent pulmonary hypertension of the newborn associated with mechanical ventilation, and conditions requiring the use of extracorporeal membrane oxygenation (ECMO)
Syndromes associated with progressive hearing loss such as neurofibromatosis, osteopetrosis, and Usher syndrome
Neurodegenerative disorders, such as Hunter syndrome, or sensory motor neuropathies, such as Friedreich's ataxia and Charcot-Marie-Tooth syndrome
Head trauma
Recurrent or persistent otitis media with effusion for at least 3 months

These risk indicators are outlined in the JCIH 2000 Position Statement for use with infants ages 29 days to 2 years.

Roles and Responsibilities of the Family and Professionals in EHDI Systems

The success of EHDI systems depends on the family and a variety of public and private institutions, agencies, groups, professionals, and the community. The roles and responsibilities of those involved with each component of the EHDI system (that is, screening, evaluation, and intervention services) may vary among states. Regardless of which state or local agency holds the lead, provides oversight, and maintains accountability, collaborative efforts among all involved is necessary, and the roles and responsibilities of each group should be defined. In most states, an advisory committee composed of parents of children with hearing loss, professionals who work with children with hearing loss, and constituents who are deaf or hard of hearing has been developed to provide guidance and assist the lead agency in implementing and overseeing the state's EHDI program. One of the primary charges of each state EHDI program is to develop a sustainable system through public and/or private funding sources.

Funding sources vary among EHDI programs. Currently, most states and territories have received assistance to develop the infrastructures necessary for statewide EHDI programs from either (or both) the Universal Newborn Hearing Screening and Intervention program of the Maternal and Child Health Bureau of the Health Resources and Services Administration (HRSA) and/or the EHDI program of the National Center on Birth Defects and Developmental Disabilities (NCBDDD) of the Centers for

Disease Control and Prevention (CDC). Each of these federal agencies, along with the National Institute on Deafness and Other Communication Disorders (NIDCD) of the National Institutes of Health (NIH), has received funding through what is commonly referred to as the Walsh provision, in honor of Representative James T. Walsh who championed funding for the program and authored the original legislation establishing the program. Through this federal funding, HRSA is charged with helping states develop newborn and infant hearing screening and assessment and, for children who are deaf or hard of hearing, intervention systems. CDC is charged with conducting applied research and providing technical assistance to states to help them develop data management systems. NIH is charged with conducting further research in childhood hearing loss. Funding for state programs is also available through Title XIX (Medicaid) federal and state funds, Part C of the Individuals with Disabilities Education Act (IDEA) Amendments of 1997 (PL 105-17), and through reimbursement for services provided to individual children.

As outlined by the Joint Committee of the American Speech-Language-Hearing Association (ASHA) and the Council on Education of the Deaf (CED, 1994), the success of EHDI programs depends on professionals working with families on a well-coordinated team. As such, each team member must understand his or her roles and responsibilities. Although the individuals may vary for the team working with each child with a hearing loss, essential team members are families, pediatricians or primary care physicians, audiologists, otolaryngologists, speech-language pathologists, geneticists, educators of children who are deaf or hard of hearing, and other early intervention professionals involved in delivering EHDI services.

Families The families of infants and young children with hearing loss, as with the families of all children, play a vital role in the ultimate outcomes of their children. The child's best interests can only be determined within the context of the family. Therefore, families and professionals should recognize the importance of cultural, linguistic, and ethnic differences. Service provision should match the strengths and concerns of each family and their child with hearing loss. Professionals may assist families by ensuring that each family understands the importance of

- Working in partnership with professionals as part of a team
- Knowing rights regarding service provision, financial support, reimbursement, and so forth
- Talking with other parents who have children with hearing loss, both within and outside of their community. (Shared experiences and suggestions for problem solving along the way can be priceless.)

- Understanding what information should be provided at each scheduled appointment and knowing what family members want and expect to learn about their child during the appointment. Keep lists of specific questions to take to appointments.

- Keeping records of appointments, recommendations, test results, reports, and other information relevant to the child together in a folder or binder; knowing where and to whom information and reports need to be sent (names, professions, addresses, and so forth)

- Ensuring that before leaving an appointment, family members understand what the next step is, when it should happen, and who is responsible for initiating it; if possible, getting information that will allow parents to contact someone in advance, reschedule if necessary, or schedule an appointment themselves if they have not been contacted within the specified time frame

- Recognizing the importance of providing current contact information (telephone, address, e-mail, name changes, and so forth) to team members involved in the ongoing care of the child

Audiologists Audiologists serve as the experts in identification, evaluation, and auditory habilitation of infants with hearing loss. At present, becoming an audiologist requires a minimum of a college degree (about 4 years), a master's degree in audiology (typically 2 years), a clinical fellowship (about 1 year), and passing a national examination. However, by 2007, graduate programs in audiology are required to offer doctoral degrees as the minimum requirement for clinical certification in the profession. Audiologists are affiliated with two organizations, the American Academy of Audiology (AAA) and the American Speech-Language-Hearing Association (ASHA).

Audiologists are involved in each component of the EHDI process. In UNHS programs, audiologists assist in program development, implementation, management, quality assessment, and service coordination; provide education and training to hospital personnel; and develop a system for effective transitions for families among screening, evaluation, habilitation, and early intervention services. For infants referred for follow-up from UNHS programs, audiologists provide comprehensive audiologic assessment to evaluate the presence or absence of hearing loss, determine candidacy for amplification and other sensory devices and assistive technology when appropriate (see Chapter 13), and ensure prompt appropriate referrals to early intervention programs and other follow-up services (e.g., vision, genetic, speech-language therapy) as needed. In the early intervention component, audiologists provide timely fitting of personal amplification with family consent. They assist families in learning to care for the technology used by children who are deaf and hard of hearing, and monitor use, condition, and success of personal amplification. Audiologists provide family education and counseling, foster ongoing participation in the infant's individualized family service plan (IFSP), and may provide direct auditory habilitation services to infants and families.

Medical Care Professionals (Physicians)   Numerous medical care providers may be involved with the ongoing care of children who are deaf and hard of hearing, including pediatricians, neonatologists, PCPs, otolaryngologists, and family practitioners. Medical care providers work in partnership with parents, other health care providers, and nonmedical professionals serving infants and young children. The medical care professional is responsible for coordinating services for the infant's "medical home," an approach to providing health care services in which care is accessible, family-centered, continuous, comprehensive, coordinated, compassionate, and culturally competent. Using this approach that has been promoted by the American Academy of Pediatrics (1992, 2002), the infant's physician serves as the advocate for the child within the context of the medical home through identifying and accessing services that the child needs within the global plan of care for infants with hearing loss.

Pediatricians   Pediatricians, most of whom are affiliated with the American Academy of Pediatrics (AAP), are most commonly associated with providing medical care to infants and young children. Becoming a pediatrician requires the applicant to complete college (about 4 years), medical school (usually 4 years), and 3 years of intensive training in pediatrics. Board certification by the American Board of Pediatrics requires that the physician pass a rigorous written examination, which must be taken every 7 years for the physician to stay certified. Table 4.3 provides information about what may be expected at an initial evaluation by a medical care professional for a child with a hearing loss.

Otolayrngologists (Ear, Nose and Throat [ENT] Doctors)   Otolaryngologists, affiliated with the American Academy of Otolaryngology–Head and Neck Surgery, are medical doctors who specialize in the medical and surgical treatment of ear diseases and syndromes related to hearing loss. Certification from the American Board of Otolaryngology requires applicants to complete college (about 4 years), medical school (usually 4 years), and at least 5 years of specialty training. The physician must pass the American Board of Otolaryngology examination and then may choose to pursue a fellowship (1–2 years) for more extensive training in a sub-specialty area, such as pediatric otolaryngology. Parents of children who are deaf or hard of hearing may find it helpful to work with a pediatric otolaryngologist.

Table 4.3. Potential components of initial evaluation for a child who is deaf or hard of hearing by professionals

Professional	Case history	Physical/diagnostic tests
Audiologist	Takes prenatal, perinatal, and child development history; reviews risk indicators for progressive/late onset hearing loss; monitors communication development	Completes hearing evaluation, including evoked otoacoustic emissions, auditory brainstem response, tympanograms,acoustic reflexes,age-appropriate behavioral testing (e.g., visual reinforcement audiometry); determines candidacy for and selects appropriate technology (hearing aids, cochlear implants, and/or assistive listening devices) in collaboration with parents and medical care professionals
Medical care professional	Takes prenatal and perinatal history; reviews risk indicators for progressive/late onset hearing loss; reviews family history of hearing loss	Completes physical examination including blood work and/or urine sample; completes developmental/neurological examination; assists in determining candidacy for technology use; *when indicated:* orders chromosome analysis, electrocardiogram, skeletal survey, computerized tomography (CT), magnetic resonance imaging (MRI)
Geneticist	Reviews history of pregnancy, family pedigree, and developmental milestones	Completes physical examinations (or review of prior results) including a general pediatric examination, dysmorphologic examination, and a neurological/developmental evaluation; pursues specialized genetic studies, such as DNA testing (e.g., for Connexin 26)

Geneticists Three types of geneticists are becoming more involved with children with hearing loss and their families: medical geneticists (physicians), molecular geneticists (researchers), and genetic counselors. Molecular geneticists are actively involved in researching human genes that cause hearing loss. Medical geneticists are physicians who work with individuals and their families to determine what family characteristics are genetically related. And genetic counselors work with families to help them understand the science of genetics and the implications for their family. The academic preparation for geneticists varies greatly, although all geneticists hold graduate degrees in genetics. The fact that approximately 50% of all profound congenital hearing loss is genetic emphasizes the importance of referring families of infants with hearing loss for genetic services, particularly those who want to know the cause of their child's hearing loss (Marazita et al., 1993; Morton, 1991).

When a family is referred for a genetic evaluation, they may expect the geneticist to collect and interpret family history information; diagnose inherited diseases, syndromes, or conditions; perform and interpret genetic tests; and provide genetic counseling. The geneticist, with the family's permission, should communicate evaluation findings to other key team members who are working with the child with a hearing loss, particularly the parents, the PCP, the audiologist, the ENT, and other medical specialists and early intervention service providers, to promote better overall outcomes for the child with hearing loss and the family.

Early Intervention Professionals Early intervention professionals are a diverse group of professionals who are trained to provide comprehensive family-centered services. They may also have backgrounds or professional training in areas such as speech-language pathology, audiology, or the eduction of children who are hard of hearing and deaf. Early intervention professionals may also work as service coordinators or early childhood special educators. Individuals who provide services to infants with hearing loss and their families should have training and expertise in typical aspects of auditory, speech, and language development; communication approaches for infants with hearing loss and their families; and overall child development (see Chapter 6). The roles and responsibilities of early intervention personnel are many and include

- Providing information to families and associated professionals while recognizing and respecting the family's natural transitions through the grieving process at the time of initial diagnosis of hearing loss and at different intervention decision-making stages

- Periodically reviewing information (at least every 6 months) regarding the full range of intervention options in an unbiased manner and informing families about the benefit of seeking assistance from individuals and organizations for making informed decisions, such as peer models, people who are deaf and hard of hearing, and consumer and professional associations

- Assisting in service coordination among IFSP team members and service providers

- Completing a comprehensive assessment of the infant's and family's needs prior to initiating early intervention services and assisting families when making informed decisions related to those needs (Stredler-Brown & Yoshinaga-Itano, 1994) as well as providing ongoing assessments of progress to determine appropriateness of the intervention strategies. Long-term monitoring also includes continual validation of communication, social-emotional, cognitive, and later academic development to ensure that progress is commensurate with the infant's abilities.

- Monitoring participation and progress of the infant and family as well as adapting and modifying interventions as needed
- Documenting intervention approach to facilitate decision-making on program changes

THE FUTURE OF EHDI SYSTEMS

As EHDI infrastructures continue to develop all of the necessary components to ensure that newborns, infants, and young children with hearing loss are identified as early as possible and that they receive appropriate and timely follow-up services, national, state, and local EHDI systems face new opportunities and challenges. The ultimate goal of EHDI programs is for all infants and children with hearing loss to develop communication and overall developmental skills commensurate with their hearing peers. All services should be offered in the communication modality appropriate for the child and preferred by the family. The early identification of hearing loss and provision of early intervention services will try to ensure that children with hearing loss will have a good start and, as they grow, will be more likely to have access to the same educational, vocational, and social opportunities throughout their lives as those available to children without hearing loss. Meeting this goal will only be achieved by meeting challenges that are relevant at this time. As each challenge is met, opportunities will also arise.

Professional Education

Preparing preservice and in-service professionals to meet the changing needs of families who receive services for newborns and infants with hearing loss is one of the challenges being faced today (see Chapter 2). The rapid advances in technology and program implementation have created a knowledge and practice gap between those who are familiar with early intervention and the state-of-the-art methods being used in the early identification of hearing loss and those who were taught before these rapid shifts occurred. Dedicated efforts are underway in many professional organizations, including AAA, AAP, and ASHA, to provide continuing education opportunities to their members. These opportunities are beneficial not only because of the academic training they provide but also because of the resulting networking and collaborative opportunities. New avenues of communication are open among professions. More frequent, more consistent, and better exchanges of information are taking place, which is creating more coordinated care for infants who are deaf and hard of hearing and their families.

Centralized and/or Integrated
Information and Data Collection Systems

Another challenge for EHDI systems is how to centralize information and create data collection systems. EHDI programs must create tracking and surveillance systems that can be used to collect data from hospitals and UNHS programs throughout the state and that can be merged with each other or downloaded to a centralized location. Creating such systems will minimize the loss of infants referred for follow-up services and promote better coordinated child care among the growing number of agencies, systems, professionals, and constituent groups that provide services for children with special health care needs and their families. Many states are working to integrate EHDI database systems with other existing public health systems (e.g., vital statistics, live birth records, electronic birth certificate systems, immunization registries, and dry blood spot-newborn screening programs) to ensure that every infant is screened for hearing loss, to improve efficiency for follow-up services, and to coordinate services. Centralized data collection systems will allow states to monitor hospitals for quality assurance purposes, generate aggregate statistics about the EHDI system, address loss to follow-up as families move from one location to another, and promote ongoing research regarding the incidence and prevalence of PCHL. States are collaborating to standardize key data elements among programs for input into a larger, national database. Increasing the amount of information analyzed allows for improved research on topics promoting improved outcomes for children who are deaf and hard of hearing. Along with the opportunities that accompany a centralized database, there are challenges in creating systems that will allow data to be shared but that protect each individual child's and family's rights to privacy and confidentiality. Issues that must be considered include the potential impact of sharing information with insurance, educational, and vocational systems. Assurances must be established that the mechanisms for parental informed consent are in place and that they are followed according to state and/or national guidelines or laws.

Technological Advancements

Advancements in technology are yet another challenge to EHDI systems. Improvements can be expected in the AABR and EOAE technologies that are used for the initial hearing screenings, both individually and in combination. Instrumentation, procedures, and protocol improvements can be anticipated in areas of high frequency tympanometry; site of lesion testing to differentiate conductive and sensorineural hearing loss; prescriptive methods of fitting hearing aids, assistive listening devices, and cochlear implants; and perhaps techniques in telemedicine. Such advancements will bring challenges similar to those caused by current technology, that is, ensuring that professionals and children who are deaf and hard of hearing and their families are trained in the appropriate use, care, and maintenance of the advanced technologies; that families have access to computers and the Internet; and that clinical facilities have access to the software and hardware necessary for programming personal amplification devices (including hearing aids and cochlear implants).

Ongoing Research

Perhaps the greatest challenges for EHDI systems relate to ongoing research on UNHS, evaluation of PCHL, and research on outcomes for children with PCHL receiving early intervention services. Through collaborative efforts, better definition of appropriate intervention strategies and procedures will be available for children with different types, configurations, and degrees of hearing loss. Incidence and prevalence of congenital hearing loss, PCHL, auditory neuropathy, progressive or late-onset hearing loss, and others will be better understood. The role of advances in genetics relevant to PCHL will be better defined regarding hearing loss and the moral, ethical, clinical, and legal implications for incorporating genetics into ongoing practice and surveillance.

REFERENCES

American Academy of Pediatrics. (1992). Ad hoc task force on definition of the medical home. *Pediatrics, 90*(5), 774.

American Academy of Pediatrics. (2002). Policy Statement: The medical home. Medical Home Initiatives for Children with Special Needs Project Advisory Committee. *Pediatrics, 110,* 184–186.

American Academy of Pediatrics Task Force on Newborn and Infant Hearing. (1999). Newborn and infant hearing loss: Detection and intervention. *Pediatrics, 103,* 527–530.

Bess, F.H., Dodd-Murphy, J., & Parker, R.A. (1998). Children with minimal sensorineural hearing loss: Prevalence, educational performance, and functional status. *Ear and Hearing, 19,* 339–354.

Bess, F.H., & Paradise, J.L. (1994). Universal screening for infant hearing impairment: Not simple, not risk-free, not necessarily beneficial, and not presently justified. *Pediatrics, 98,* 330–334.

Blair, J.C., Peterson, M.E., & Viehweg, S.H. (1985). The effects of mild sensorineural hearing loss on academic performance of young school-age children. *The
Volta Review, 87*(2), 87–93.

Brookhouser, P., Worthington, D., & Kelly, W. (1994). Fluctuating and or progressive sensorineural hearing loss in children. *Laryngoscope, 104*, 958–964.

Carty, L.M., Letourneau, K.S., & Vohr, B.R. (1998). *RIHAP universal screening:
evolution since 1993.* Paper presented at the American Academy of Audiology
Annual Convention, Los Angeles, CA.

Children's Health Act of 2000, PL 106-310, 114 Stat. 1101, 42 U.S.C. §§ 247b *et seq.*

Davis, J., Elfenbein, J., Schum, R., & Bentler, R. (1986). Effects of mild and
moderate hearing impairment on language, educational and psychosocial
behavior of children. *Journal of Speech and Hearing Disorders, 51*, 53.

Departments of Labor, Health and Human Services, and Education, and Related
Agencies Appropriations Act of 1999, PL 105-277, 112 Stat. 2681-337.

DesGeorges, J. (1998). For the sake of Joy: A parents perspective on universal
newborn hearing screening [Special issue]. *Audiology Today, 25.*

Directors of Speech and Hearing Programs for State Health and Welfare Agencies
(DSHPSHWA). (2001). *EHDI national database.* Retrieved from http://
www.cdc.gov/ncbddd/ehdi/2000_Data/index_eval00.htm#Received

Elssmann, S.F., Matkin, N.D., & Sabo, M.P. (1987). Early identification of congenital sensorineural hearing impairment. *The Hearing Journal, 40*, 13–17.

Ewing, I.R., & Ewing, A.W.G. (1947). *Opportunity and the deaf child.* London:
University of London Press.

Friel-Patti, S., & Finitzo, T. (1990). Language learning in a prospective study of
otitis media with effusion. *Journal of Speech Hearing Research, 33*, 188–194.

Friel-Patti, S., Finitzo-Hieber, T., Conti, G., & Brown, K.C. (1982). Language
delay in infants associated with middle ear disease and mild, fluctuating hearing
impairment. *Pediatric Infectious Diseases, 1*(2), 104–109.

Gallaudet University Center for Assessment and Demographic Study. (1998).
Thirty years of the annual survey of deaf and hard of hearing children and youth:
A glance over the decades. *American Annals of the Deaf, 142*(2), 72–76.

Gravel, J.S., & Wallace, I.F. (1992). Listening and language at 4 years of age:
Effects of early otitis media. *Journal of Speech and Hearing Research,
35*, 588–595.

Hall, J.W., III, Kripal, J.P., & Hepp, T. (1988). Newborn hearing screening with
auditory brainstem response: Measurement problems and solutions. *Seminars
in Hearing, 9*, 15–33.

Jacobson, J.T., Jacobson, C.A., & Spahr, R.C. (1990). Automated and conventional
AVR screening techniques in high-risk infants. *Journal of the American
Academy of Audiology, 1*, 187–195.

Johnson, C.D., Benson, P.V., & Seaton, J.B. (1997). *Educational audiology
handbook.* San Diego, CA: Singular Publishing Group.

Johnson, J.L., Kuntz, N.L., Sia, C.C., White, K.R., & Johnson, R.L. (1997). Newborn
hearing screening in Hawaii. *Hawaii Medical Journal, 56*, 352–355.

Joint Committee of the American Speech-Language-Hearing Association and
the Council on Education of the Deaf. (1994). Service provision under the
Individuals with Disabilities Education Act-Part H, as amended (IDEA-Part
H) to children who are deaf and hard of hearing ages birth to 36 months of
age. *Asha, 36*, 117–121.

Joint Committee on Infant Hearing. (1991). 1990 position statement. *Asha*, *33*(Suppl. 5), 3–6.

Joint Committee on Infant Hearing. (2000). Year 2000 position statement: Principles and guidelines for early hearing detection and intervention programs. Retrieved from http://www.jcih.org/jcih2000.pdf

Kemp, D.T. (1988). Developments in cochlear mechanics and techniques for non-invasive evaluation. *Advances in Audiology*, *5*, 27–45.

Kemp, D.T., & Ryan, S. (1993). The use of transient evoked otoacoustic emissions in neonatal hearing screening programs. *Seminars in Hearing*, *14*, 46–56.

Kileny, P. (1987). ALGO-1 automated infant hearing screener: Preliminary results. *Seminars in Hearing*, *8*, 125–131.

Kurman, B., & Spivak, L.G. (1998). Instrumentation for newborn hearing screening. In L.G. Spivak (Ed.), *Universal newborn hearing screening* (pp. 87–119). New York: Thieme Medical Publishers.

Mahoney, T.M., & Eichwald, J.G. (1987). The ups and "Downs" of high-risk hearing screening: The Utah statewide program. *Seminars in Hearing*, *8*, 155–163.

Marazita, M.L., Ploughman, L.M., Rawlings, B., Remington, E., Arnos, K.S, & Nance, W.F. (1993). Genetic epidemiological studies of early-onset deafness in the U.S. school-age population. *American Journal of Medical Genetics*, *46*, 486–491.

Mauk, G.W., White, K.R., Mortensen, L.B., & Behrens, T.R. (1991). The effectiveness of screening programs based on high-risk characteristics in early identification of hearing impairment. *Ear and Hearing*, *12*, 312–319.

Morton, N.E. (1991). Genetic epidemiology of hearing impairment. *Annals of the New York Academy of Science*, *630*, 16–31.

National Center for Hearing Assessment and Management (NCHAM). (2001). *Annual survey of universal newborn hearing screening programs*. Logan: Utah State University.

National Center for Hearing Assessment and Management (NCHAM). (2002). *Selecting newborn hearing screening equipment*. Retrieved from http://www.infanthearing.org/resources/equipment/equipmenttable.html

National Institutes of Health. Early identification of hearing impairment in infants and young children. (1993, March 1–3). *NIH Consensus Statement*, *11*(1), 1–24.

Roush, J., & Matkin, N.D. (Eds.). (1994). *Infants and toddlers with hearing loss: Family-centered assessment and intervention*. Baltimore: York Press.

Schildroth, A.N., & Hotto, S.A. (1993). Annual survey of hearing-impaired children and youth: 1991–1992 school year. *American Annals of the Deaf*, *138*(2), 163–171.

Stein, L., Clark, S., & Kraus, N. (1983). The hearing-impaired infant: Patterns of identification and habilitation. *Ear and Hearing*, *4*, 75–87.

Stool, S.E., Berg, A.O., Berman, S., Carney, C.J., Cooley, J.R., Culpepper, L. et al. (1994). *Managing otitis media with effusion in young children. Quick reference guide for clinicians* (AHCPR Publication 94-0623). Rockville, MD: U.S. Department of Health and Human Services, Agency for Health Care Policy and Research, Public Health Service.

Stredler-Brown, A., & Yoshinaga-Itano, C. (1994). Family assessment: A multidisciplinary evaluation tool. In J. Roush & N.D. Matkin (Eds.), *Infants and toddlers with hearing loss* (pp. 133–161) Baltimore: York Press.

Tharpe, A.M., & Bess, F.H. (1999). Minimal, progressive, and fluctuating hearing losses in children: Characteristics, identification, and management. *Pediatric Clinics of North America, 46*(1), 65–78.

U.S. Department of Health and Human Services (HHS). (1990). *Healthy people 2000: National health promotion and disease prevention objectives.* Washington, DC: Public Health Service.

U.S. Department of Health and Human Services (HHS). (2000). *Healthy people 2010: National health promotion and disease prevention objectives.* Washington, DC: Public Health Service.

Wallace, I.F., Gravel, J.S., Ruben, R.J., McCarton, C.M., Stapells, D., & Bernstein, R.S. (1988). Otitis media, language outcome and auditory sensitivity. *Laryngoscope, 98*, 64–70.

White, K.R., & Behrens, T.R. (Eds.). (1993). The Rhode Island hearing assessment project: Implications for universal newborn hearing screening. *Seminars in Hearing, 14*, 1–119.

White, K.R., Vohr, B.R., & Behrens, T.R. (1993). Universal newborn hearing screening using transient evoked otoacoustic emissions: Results of the Rhode Island hearing assessment project. *Seminars in Hearing, 14*, 30–45.

Perspectives

PARENT PERSPECTIVE[1]

We are grateful for newborn hearing screening. Because of it, we found out early that our daughter, Maggie, has a severe to profound bilateral hearing loss. Early intervention worked for us because of some very dedicated and caring health care providers, but we feel that the system needs to work better. The biggest potential breakdown in the early intervention process was prevented by our exceptional pediatrician and audiologist. For the next 2 weeks [following confirmation of a severe to profound sensorineural hearing loss bilaterally] we did nothing, alternating between denial and despair. We just kept waiting for the results in the mail. We thought someone would call us and tell us what to do next. Fortunately for us, someone did. The day he got the results, Maggie's pediatrician called and asked what we were doing about Maggie's hearing loss. We told him we didn't know what to do next.

Our pediatrician gave us the phone numbers of several pediatric ear, nose, and throat (ENT) doctors. We called around to make an ENT appointment. The next available one was 3 months later! Upset about the time, we called our pediatrician back. He called the head

[1]From Meier, K. (2001). Maggie's story: A tale of early hearing detection and intervention. *ASHA Leader, 6*(8), pp. 6–7, 11. Copyright 2001 by the American Speech-Language-Hearing Association. Adapted with permission of the author.

of audiology for us to see if we could get something sooner and to discuss who would coordinate what needed to be done next.

The head of audiology (the same helpful audiologist we met at the screening in the hospital) managed to get us an ENT appointment within a month and a half. He also rush-ordered programmable hearing aids for Maggie and had her fitted with earmolds within a week. He told us that getting Maggie hearing aids as soon as was possible (ideally before 6 months) would make a tremendous difference in her speech and language development.

DEAF ADULT PERSPECTIVE[2]

Early identification in and of itself is not a problem—the "intervention" part, and parental/societal understanding and acceptance, are the concern. An ideal situation would be early identification in a natural, nonintrusive, nondisruptive, nonmedical way, with the family immediately beginning to learn sign language and becoming involved in the Deaf community. An appropriate recommendation during this process must take into consideration various factors, including culture, economic and environmental background, besides the medical and academic considerations.

The common perception and experience of the deaf community is that deafness is viewed as a medical problem, not a human difference. Because of the lack of deaf professionals [in] state planning/monitoring [bodies] and the lack of partnerships among doctors, therapists, educators, parents, and deaf adults, there is insufficient knowledge about options and understanding about deaf people and their success stories and coping strategies. The omission of sign language and deaf role models may make early intervention a problematic issue.

DEAF COMMUNITY PERSPECTIVE[3]

The National Association of the Deaf (NAD) supports 100% implementation of quality universal newborn hearing screening (UNHS) in

[2]Excerpted from Rosen, R. (2000). Perspectives of the Deaf community of early identification and intervention: A case for diversity and partnerships. *Seminars in Hearing*, *21*, 327–342.

all States. The primary concerns of the NAD relate to the quality of education and training services provided once an infant is identified with a hearing loss. The NAD urges each State to create State UNHS and/or EHDI Advisory Boards that include representatives from the deaf and hard of hearing communities as well as deaf and hard of hearing professional personnel. Such Advisory Boards should monitor protocols and outcome data progress, for the purpose of providing recommendations to hospitals, government agencies, EHDI providers, and the public regarding appropriate methodologies and guidelines for and intervention, and quality comprehensive data management systems.

EHDI should include not only newborn hearing screening, but also follow-up diagnosis and intervention services. Communication and language development in the early years are critical as a building block to excel in education for deaf and hard of hearing infants and toddlers and their families. Sign language and other visual modalities of communication must be made available to ensure the opportunity for natural language development as early as possible. Hearing aids and other amplification devices alone will often not be sufficient in providing the infant full access to the learning environment. The NAD urges all professional personnel who provide EHDI services and assess, evaluate, educate, or otherwise work with deaf and hard of hearing infants and their families [to] be proficient in American Sign Language or an appropriate visual modality, and have the specialized knowledge, skills and attributes needed to serve deaf and hard of hearing infants and toddlers and their families.

EHDI services in each State should have complete, up-to-date listings of all State resources for providers of early intervention programs and services, professional and/or consumer-based organizations serving deaf and hard of hearing communities, social services agencies, educational programs, parent resources, speech and hearing personnel, and related resources for referral purposes. States need to ensure that the parents are provided clear and comprehensive information about the full range of communication options; and

---

[3]Excerpted from National Association of the Deaf. (1997, September 2). Comments regarding EHDI presented via teleconference to the Early Hearing Detection and Intervention Ad Hoc Group of the Centers for Disease Control and Prevention; reprinted by permission.

be given the opportunity to consider the potential of various available options for their infant. Because communication access is paramount to learning and development, EHDI programs and services must above all, fully accommodate the unique communication and language needs of deaf and hard of hearing infants and toddlers, which may include sign language.

CHAPTER FIVE

Family-Centered
Developmental Assessment

JAN CHRISTIAN HAFER
AND ARLENE STREDLER-BROWN

L inda, a mother of a 3-year-old deaf child, turned, with tears in her eyes, to the early intervention team gathered around the table to discuss the results of the recent assessment. "Thank you," she said. "Kari really enjoyed herself! I learned so much being able to watch and ask questions as the assessment happened. I enjoyed playing with her, too. For the first time since we found out Kari was deaf, I feel like the assessment is accurate. I feel like you really know the little girl that we love."

What happened during the assessment that caused Linda to feel so positive about the experience? Why did Kari enjoy herself so much? Why does Linda think that this assessment yielded accurate information when other assessments never had before? Understanding what happened during Kari's assessment is at the heart of best practices in assessing young deaf and hard of hearing infants, toddlers, and preschoolers.

This chapter describes recommended practices in the developmental assessment of young deaf and hard of hearing children in order to answer three basic questions that parents ask: "What's wrong with my child?" "What will my child be like later?" and "What can be done to help my child?" (Bagnato, Neisworth, & Munson, 1997). Two assessment models, the Developmental Assessment Process for Deaf Children (DAP-D) and the FAMILY Assessment (Stredler-Brown & Yoshinaga-Itano, 1994) from the Colorado Home Intervention Program are described. Philosophies and practices common to both are highlighted, and strategies and practical suggestions for the assessment process are outlined.

THEORETICAL PERSPECTIVE

The assessment process for young children who are deaf or hard of hearing has changed over time. During the early 1970s, assessment of young children with special needs was not connected to intervention (Bagnato et al., 1997). Rather, emphasis was placed on categorizing and labeling children using traditional, norm-referenced tests for the purpose of placing students in appropriate educational settings. Testing procedures for young children with special needs were often adapted from protocols recommended for older children and children without disabilities; these highly structured practices often proved inappropriate for assessing young children. Finding assessment reports of little value in planning interventions, teachers became frustrated and often had to develop intervention plans based solely on their own observations.

Since the passage of the Education of the Handicapped Act Amendments of 1986 (PL 99-457), assessments have been structured as processes to gather information about a child to help parents answer the three questions outlined in the introduction to this chapter. Assessment sets the foundation for planning effective and supportive experiences for the child and his or her family to promote healthy development.

How do professionals help answer the three basic questions that parents ask? What tools and materials are available? What is the assessment process? Who should be a member of the assessment team? Most important, how can assessment occur in a collaborative environment with parents and professionals? The following sections provide a discussion of the information both parents and professionals need to answer these questions.

Developing a Philosophy

Before developing an assessment process for young children who are deaf and hard of hearing, professionals should examine their beliefs about working with young children and their families, by considering the following philosophies and how they intersect with their own beliefs and practices (Winton & Bailey, 1994, p. 26):

- *Family centered:* The family is a constant factor in their child's life, although services and systems may be involved only episodically.

- *Ecologically based:* Professionals need to consider how the various contexts that surround the child and family are interrelated.

- *Individualized:* Because the needs of each child and each family differ, services should be individualized to meet those unique needs.

- *Culturally sensitive:* Families come from different cultural and ethnic groups. Families reflect their diversity in their views and expectations of themselves, of their children, and of professionals. Services should be provided in ways that are sensitive to these variations and consistent with each family's values and beliefs.

- *Enabling and empowering:* Services should foster a family's independence, their unique skills, and each family member's feelings of competence and self-worth.

- *Needs based:* A "needs-based" philosophy starts with a family's expressed needs and helps families identify and obtain services commensurate with their priorities.

- *Coordinated service delivery:* Resources from a variety of informal and formal sources should be coordinated.

- *Normalized programs:* Intervention promotes the inclusion of the child and the family in their natural environments within the community.

- *Collaborative:* Early intervention services should be planned, implemented, and evaluated collaboratively, including input from parents and professionals.

Next, professionals should develop a program philosophy for working with families of young deaf and hard of hearing children. For example, a program, which should seek to serve the unique needs of each child and family (individualized), might develop a statement that incorporates the professionals' beliefs about respecting all cultures (culturally sensitive) and how it is important for parents and professionals in the child's life to work together (collaborative). The program philosophy helps to determine program goals and provides a framework for staff development. Periodic review of the philosophy will accommodate new information gathered from clinical practice and experiences.

Assessments, historically based only on a medical model to help children develop their auditory and spoken language skills, now may utilize a sociocultural model for planning and implementing education programs for deaf and hard of hearing children. Programs that employ a sociocultural perspective describe deafness as a difference, rather than a disability. The role of deaf and hard of hearing adults and the use of American Sign Language (ASL) or its various derivatives are also viewed as contributing to the child achieving academic and social success.

Inclusion of Deaf and Hard of Hearing Adults in Assessment

In addition to a commitment to working with families, a program's philosophy statement can describe the potential role of members of the Deaf community in the lives of families and how programs can include deaf and hard of hearing adults in assessment and service delivery. Deaf and hard of hearing adults can help to answer, in an authentic way, the three questions that parents usually ask. The wisdom, life experiences, and perceptions of deaf and hard of hearing adults are invaluable to a parent facing decisions regarding communication and education. Assessment programs not already employing deaf and hard of hearing adults can turn to deaf and hard of hearing people from the community to participate in the assessment process. (See Lane, Hoffmeister, & Bahan, 1996, and Padden & Humphries, 1988, for a thorough discussion of Deaf life.)

In 1913, George Veditz, President of the National Association of the Deaf, observed, "They [deaf people] are facing not a theory but a condition, for they are first, last, and all the time the people of the eye" (p. 1). Because many deaf and hard of hearing children are visual communicators and visual learners (Bodner-Johnson, Sass-Lehrer, Hafer, & Gatty, 2000; Mohay, 2000), deaf and hard of hearing adults become an essential resource in the assessment process. Deaf and hard of hearing adults are uniquely qualified to design the environment and assessment activities to support young deaf and hard of hearing children. This perspective can change in a fundamental way how assessments are conducted for deaf and hard of hearing children. Every effort should be made to professionalize the services provided by deaf and hard of hearing adults by paying a fee for their services.

Considerations for Assessment

Professionals who assess the strengths and needs of a young child who is deaf or hard of hearing can use the following best practices to ensure the assessment process yields the most accurate and helpful information. The assessment process includes a variety of measures that provide a comprehensive picture of the child's communicative abilities including verbal, nonverbal, spoken, and signed utterances. Few instruments assess this range of production; therefore, it is beneficial to use a variety of tests and tools to observe the child, and to conduct parent interviews. Consider the impact for children with limited hearing and speech when professionals score their individual test items during assessment. Do assessment protocols allow flexibility in how the questions or tasks are presented (e.g., can questions or tasks be presented using sign language, repetition, cues, and assistive listening devices)? Professionals who assess children who are deaf and hard of hearing need to communicate directly with the child. This requires having at least one professional who is skilled in the preferred method or mode of communication used by the child. These skills may include ASL and English sign systems, as well as spoken language.

Best Practices in Assessment

What are the best practices for assessing young children? Three key points are recommended by the Division for Early Childhood (DEC) (Hemmeter, Joseph, Smith, & Sandall, 2001, p. 23):

1. *Family involvement:* Professionals need to recognize and value the role parents have in the assessment process and the development of intervention plans.

2. *Developmental appropriateness of assessment:* The type and methods of the assessment must fit together with each child's unique needs and developmental stage.

3. *Team approach:* The team should include people in the child's life. Parents, caregivers, and early interventionists can participate in planning the assessment and interpreting the results.

Bagnato et al. (1997) and Hemmeter et al. (2001) expanded on these three points with the following additional recommendations. Italics are added by the authors of this chapter to indicate special considerations for children who are deaf or hard of hearing.

1. *Use of multiple perspectives:* Several informants including parents, the early interventionist, and primary care physician can make contributions regarding the strengths and needs of a child. *Whenever applicable, a deaf or hard of hearing adult can contribute his or her perspective on the child's use of visual information. The deaf or hard of hearing adult can also clarify the child's communicative attempts and recommend strategies for enhancing the child's communication skills* (Hafer, Spragins, & Hardy-Braz, 1996).

2. *Use of multiple techniques:* The assessment process includes more than one type of instrument. Observations made of the child in his or

her typical routines and natural settings yield functional information. Checklists, formal and informal testing, parent interviews, and parent questionnaires provide useful information and complement observations that are made. *The use of videotape, although beneficial for assessing all children, is particularly important for documenting the visual nature of communication with deaf and hard of hearing children. Reviewing the videotape of an assessment provides a means of examining the nuances of visual communication and how it relates to spoken communication efforts. It also can easily be made available to an outside expert for review.*

3. *Assess on multiple occasions:* To be responsive to the child, information can be collected in more than one session. This can include collecting information during multiple settings (e.g., home, child care facility, clinic), *when the child is with hearing children, or when the child is with other deaf and hard of hearing children.*

4. *Use of functional item content:* Item content may identify specific developmental milestones, functional skills, and atypical behaviors. Determining developmental milestones is useful to identify age-appropriate skills, possible delays, and challenges. *Accommodations to each item can be made when the child relies on visual communication. For example, if the item asks if a child can say his or her name, the item must be administered in the communication mode used by the child. This may include fingerspelling or signing his or her name instead of or in addition to actually saying his or her name.* Functional competence stresses unique adaptations to accomplish a skill rather than meeting a typical "standard." Documenting how a child communicates (e.g., speaking, signing) or how he or she moves across the room (e.g., scooting, walking) is fundamental to functional assessment.

5. *Making collaborative decisions:* Parents should be treated as true partners in the entire assessment process. To achieve collaboration, the professional should use clear language with limited jargon and allow family members to identify their role in the assessment process.

EXAMPLES OF EFFECTIVE DEVELOPMENTAL ASSESSMENT PROCESSES FOR YOUNG CHILDREN WHO ARE DEAF AND HARD OF HEARING

Following are two approaches to assess the developmental strengths and needs of young children who are deaf and hard of hearing. Though there are many *tools* available to practitioners that provide pieces of information about a child, an *assessment process* yields a more complete picture of the strengths and needs of a child and his or her family. The Developmental Assessment Process for Deaf Children (DAP-D) is used to train graduate students in the Family Centered Early Education Program at Gallaudet University. The Colorado Home Intervention Program, the statewide early intervention program, uses the FAMILY Assessment. Both assessment procedures incorporate the ideas discussed in this chapter, but in different ways. Both models utilize a variety of assessment tools and practices that are appropriate for use with young children who are deaf and hard of hearing.

The Developmental Assessment Process for Deaf Children Model

The Developmental Assessment Process for Deaf Children (DAP-D) model is based on the Transdisciplinary Play-Based Assessment (TPBA) created by Linder (1993). The DAP-D model makes specific adaptations to Linder's model in order to accommodate the needs of young children who are deaf and hard of hearing. The DAP-D model also makes accommodations for deaf and hard of hearing adults who participate in the assessment. The arena assessment piece is conducted in the home or in a center.

The Transdisciplinary Team—Traditional Team Members The transdisciplinary approach incorporates perspectives from multiple team members to yield a holistic, accurate assessment of the child's strengths and needs. Members of the team include professionals who have expertise in specific areas of development, including medical, psychological, motor, speech, and language. The child's parents are members of the team, providing valuable information on their child's abilities and interests. During the assessment, a parent facilitator acts as the primary contact between the parent(s) and the other team members. The parent facilitator supports the family by explaining the assessment process, answering questions, and conducting the postassessment meeting. A play facilitator interacts with the child throughout the assessment session and a video camera operator videotapes the assessment for later use.

The Transdisciplinary Team—Additional Team Members In addition to the team members already described, the DAP-D team can also include a deaf or hard of hearing adult, an interpreter for both signed and spoken languages, and a communication coach. These additional team members address the visual communication needs of the deaf or hard of hearing child and the deaf or hard of hearing adults who have joined the team.

Deaf adults have had a role in research projects assessing the communication skills of deaf toddlers and preschoolers since the advent of research on sign language in the 1970s (Klima & Bellugi, 1979; Spencer, 1993). In these research projects, analyses of videotapes that include sign language are routinely conducted by a person who is deaf in order for the analyses to be valid and reliable. Extending this role beyond the confines of research to the assessment of young children who are deaf and use sign language seems logical, especially when a child who is deaf uses ASL as a first language. The deaf or hard of hearing adult can fulfill many roles on the team. For example, the deaf or hard of hearing adult can be the play facilitator. He or she is able to use a wide range of visual communication strategies during the assessment that support the child's communicative attempts, such as bringing the object of conversation into the sign space to support visual attention. Second, deaf and hard of hearing adults may assume the role of the communication coach, helping observing team members and the play facilitator to communicate without disrupting the play process. Deaf and hard of hearing adults may also assume any role of an observing team member. Typically, they lead the evaluation of the child's communication and language skills. Sometimes this role is divided between an ASL specialist and a speech clinician.

Ten years of experience using the DAP-D model has demonstrated that the inclusion of deaf and hard of hearing adults enhances the assessment process. The assessments are generally conducted with very young children who are deaf and hard of hearing who live in different communication environments, both oral and signing. In addition to ensuring effective communication with the child, the participation of a deaf or hard of hearing adult provides an "authenticity" to the discussions about communication issues with the parents. Rather than only having hearing people making decisions about children who are deaf and hard of hearing, adults who are deaf and hard of hearing who experience the reality of being deaf offer a valuable perspective to the process. The deaf or hard of hearing adult can offer the parents an opportunity to see how an adult who is deaf or hard of hearing communicates and share their perspective on issues such as communication choices and educational options.

A sign language interpreter can also be on the transdisciplinary team. The sign language interpreter ensures that all members of the team have communication access. The interpreter may voice for some team members and sign for others. The interpreter is a valued team member in both the preassessment and postassessment meetings.

A communication coach can also be a valuable team member. It is important to create an accessible visual environment to accurately assess a child who is deaf or hard of hearing. To understand the importance of an accessible visual environment, it is necessary to consider the sequential nature of sign communication. When people who are deaf are involved in the assessment they can visually attend to only one thing at a time. The communication coach must attend to the child, the play facilitator, and the other team members in a systematic way. The coach visually scans the environment in order to check in with all team members. The observing team members make their requests to the communication coach when they want the play facilitator to elicit certain skills. The communication coach serves as a liaison between team members and the play facilitator by relaying these requests at a visually appropriate moment. The communication coach also functions as the timekeeper and alerts the team members when it is time for a transition to a new activity.

Assessment Procedure Prior to the assessment, the parent facilitator and play facilitator make a home visit. One benefit of this session is to identify parents' concerns and priorities and to establish rapport with the child. The preassessment meeting provides an opportunity to document the developmental skills of the child and to obtain an impression of the communication setting. Background information is collected at this meeting and the parent facilitator explains the assessment process and the assessment schedule. The play facilitator gets to know the child and gathers information that will be helpful in the assessment (e.g., name signs of significant people in the child's life, favorite toys, favorite activities). Taking a Polaroid picture of the play facilitator playing with the child helps in the transition to the arena assessment that is conducted at a later date.

Linder recommended a six-phase process for the assessment process that includes unstructured play, structured play, play with parent, play with peer, motor play, and snack. The order and timing of these phases are flexible. In the DAP-D model, the assessment session begins with the parent and child interacting together. This gives the team an opportunity to identify the characteristics of the communication between parent and child. The play facilitator then joins the parent–child dyad and helps the child transition to play with the play facilitator alone. At this time, the parent joins the parent facilitator to observe the remainder of the session. The child and the play facilitator then move through unstructured play in which the play facilitator follows the lead of the child. Then the child and the play facilitator move on to structured play in which the play facilitator attempts to elicit behaviors requested by the observing team members. Next, the play facilitator makes the transition to peer play. This is an opportunity to observe how the child interacts with hearing and deaf or hard of hearing children. Team members pay special attention to the communicative strategies used as the child interacts with his or her peer. Finally, the child and play facilitator participate in snack time. This activity gives the observing team members the opportunity to observe oral motor skills as well as social and functional skills.

Postassessment Meeting After the assessment session, the team meets to discuss and record their observations and to review the videotape of the assessment. During this meeting, parents have an opportunity to ask questions and contribute additional information about their child. The deaf or hard of hearing adult team member contributes their information as well, as their information may help parents to make decisions about the next steps in the intervention process.

Suggestions are made for additional assessment sessions as needed. For example, the team may determine that the child needs more in-depth assessment of his or her speech skills. If this recommendation is made, an assessment with a speech-language pathologist is scheduled. If more information is needed regarding the child's functional auditory skills, a follow-up assessment for this analysis may be scheduled. The DAP-D assessment may also indicate that the child needs further evaluation in other developmental domains. These recommendations are discussed with the family, and referrals are provided.

Formal Report   The DAP-D report, written in the style suggested by Linder (1993), is a positive narrative of the child's strengths and needs. The use of jargon is carefully monitored. The report tends to be long because supporting examples are provided. The DAP-D team looks at the preferred and optimal modes the child uses for communication. (See Table 5.1 for examples of items that are typically documented in the DAP-D report but rarely noted in assessments that are not designed for deaf and hard of hearing children.) Care is taken to record examples of both signed and spoken utterances. Educational jargon is eliminated and necessary technical terms are defined. Also, parents are given an opportunity to review and modify the report, and a copy of the report and the videotape are given to them. These two items, in addition to the postassessment meeting, provide parents with multiple ways to understand the assessment results. The videotape helps the family to explain

Table 5.1.   Examples of visual communication competencies

Makes appropriate eye contact with others

When following a conversation between two other people, shifts eye gaze from one person to another

Shifts eye gaze from a signer to an object when the signer points to an object, then shifts eye gaze back to the signer

Uses single signs or a single sign in combination with a point, facial expression, or another sign

Watches a signer and gives feedback to the signer by using facial expressions, single signs (e.g., "yes," "that," "wrong," "no"), gestures (e.g., nodding or shaking the head)

Manually babbles: uses sequences of gestures that resemble signing but are not recognizable or meaningful

Signs reflect simple, unmarked handshapes (e.g., "B" [mine], "C" [bowl], "O" [more], "A" [help], "S" [milk], "L" [mom], "5" [tree])

Signs with appropriate facial expression

Uses sign phrases such as FINISH and YOU-WANT-MORE?

the assessment to other family members and other professionals. The report and the videotape also serve as educational materials for the parents.

Supplemental Materials   The TPBA process makes provisions for the use of supplemental assessment tools. The same is true for the DAP-D process. Supplemental materials are needed to assess the visual communication skills of deaf and hard of hearing children. This area of assessment is still emerging, with few thoroughly researched tools. Many early intervention programs have developed their own checklists that include developmental items culled from the research conducted on the development of sign language. Fenson and colleagues (1992), for example, have developed the MacArthur Communicative Development Inventories and provide normative data for children who are deaf and use American Sign Language as their first language. Other tools that are used include Gallimore's American Sign Language Development Checklist (Western Oregon State College, Monmouth), the Gallaudet University Kendall Conversational Proficiency Levels (Kendall Demonstration Elementary School, the Clerc Center at Gallaudet University, Washington, D.C.), and the California School for the Deaf ASL Skills Observation Record (California School for the Deaf, Fremont, Parent Infant Preschool Kindergarten Program).

Ongoing Documentation Using Portfolios   After the initial developmental assessment is completed, ongoing observation and documentation of a child's behavior and developmental skills should continue (Katz & Swann, 1998). Observation notes, anecdotes from home, and pictures or video clips of play experiences can be collected and reviewed routinely with the family to determine progress and to establish new goals. Portfolios are an efficient and effective way to help parents and professionals document, analyze, interpret, and organize all of the important assessment data that are collected over time from multiple developmental assessments.

Summary of the DAP-D Method   The DAP-D method is a holistic, play-based, team process that is used to assess the developmental status of young children who are deaf and hard of hearing. This process recognizes the value of including deaf or hard of hearing adults in the assessment process, as their own skills contribute to an accurate determination, particularly with regard to communication, of the child's skills. The process also helps the parents understand their child's development. Use of videotape to document and analyze communication skills is an effective way to record communication. The videotape can be reviewed periodically during the intervention. Use of supplemental materials to analyze visual language, as it is used by children who are deaf and hard of hearing, is incorporated into the process. Finally, the maintenance of a portfolio for the ongoing documentation of the child's development is incorporated into the process.

The FAMILY Assessment Model

The FAMILY Assessment was started in the mid-1980s. It was developed as an assessment protocol for the Colorado Home Intervention Program (CHIP), a home-based, parent-centered early intervention program. At that time, the administration of the program was asked to prove that the intervention program was effective, cost-efficient, and valuable for children and their families. This assessment protocol was developed to obtain aggregate data to measure the progress children made over time while they were enrolled in CHIP.

As the assessment protocol was being developed, many criteria needed to be considered. First, the age of the population needed to be considered. Children in the program ranged in age from 2 months to 3 years of age. Consequently, the assessment instruments needed to be appropriate for very young children. Next, the assessment needed to portray a child's profile in a variety of developmental domains. Several tests would need to be included to obtain information about communication and language, physical development, cognitive development, motor skills, and personal-social skills. In addition to gathering information about the child's development, the assessment needed to identify the benefit parents were receiving from the program. Because CHIP used a family-centered paradigm, with the parents and/or caregivers as the primary recipients of the intervention (Winton & Bailey, 1994), it was important to measure outcomes for the family. The next consideration was the amount of time that would be needed to assess each child. How much time would it take to gather information, score the protocols, summarize the results, and review these results with the family? Another consideration was gathering reliable information. The assessment protocols needed to be sensitive to the special needs of children with hearing loss and the effects of the hearing loss on other developmental domains. And last, the assessment needed to be valid when conducted at repeated intervals.

The FAMILY Assessment (Stredler-Brown & Yoshinaga-Itano, 1994), a naturalistic assessment procedure, was launched in 1987. Although some protocols included in the assessment have changed, the aforementioned criteria and the method of collecting information have remained the same. The assessment takes place in a family's home, the most natural setting for an infant or toddler, and includes active participation by the family. The information is gathered in two ways. First, a 30-minute videotape is made of a parent and/or caregiver interacting with the child. Both the adult and the child are filmed during play or typical daily routines. The adult is instructed to select activities that will elicit typical behaviors from their child and the best language their child can use. A phonologic analysis of the child's utterances, a language sample of the child's words, and a list of communicative intentions used by the child are obtained from the videotape.

Second, the parents are asked to complete a series of parent questionnaires and protocols. Some of the questionnaires evaluate the child's skills in a variety of developmental domains. Others give the parent an opportunity to report on their own needs as parents of a child with a hearing loss. For families choosing to use sign language, parents complete an inventory of the signs they have learned. Some protocols are completed using an interview format. Using this format develops a collaborative relationship between the parents and their interventionist. The interventionist can teach the family about hierarchical development and the parents can share their observations with the interventionist. In addition, this provides an opportunity for the interventionist and the parents to converse and, subsequently, develop a trusting relationship. Mezirow (1991) and Brookfield (1987) propose that critical reflection is best achieved through dialogue with others. And, activities that engage parents in discussion about being the parent of a child with disabilities can help to make their thoughts explicit, which often increases their understanding (Bodner-Johnson, 2001).

When the videotapes, questionnaires, and protocols are complete, they are sent to the Department of Speech, Language, and Hearing Sciences (SLHS) at the University of Colorado. Through a contractual agreement supported by state funds and federal grants, the University has created a process to code and score the videotapes, protocols, and questionnaires. Undergraduate and graduate students in the department are trained to code the videotape. (Incidentally, coding the tapes has proven to be an effective way for clinicians-in-training to learn about the development of children with hearing loss). Analysis of the videotape provides information about the child, the parents, and the communicative interaction between the parent and child. Specifically, the speech skills of the child, language of both parent and child, and language strategies used by the parent are all identified when the video is coded. The information from these tools is summarized within 4 weeks. A report is generated, and this report is returned to the early interventionist working with the family. The early interventionist shares the assessment results with the family during the next home visit. The information is also used for development of the individualized family service plan (IFSP). Using these two methods to gather information, a comprehensive profile of the child is acquired, an inventory of the parents' needs is obtained, and the dynamics of the interaction between the parent and the child can be documented and analyzed. With this information, the early interventionist can obtain a baseline of the child's development, monitor changes that occur over time, and/or compare a child's skills with those of his or her hearing peers. Strategies and techniques used by the parents can be identified, and the needs identified by the family can be noted.

Uses of Videotapes   Videotapes are used for several reasons, some by design and others by chance. By design, videotape was included in order to evaluate a child's spontaneous speech, expressive communication at a preverbal level, and expressive language. After the videotape is created, a transcript is made of all oral utterances produced by the child during the assessment. The transcript includes vocalizations (referred to as non-true words) and true words. The phonologic transcript is analyzed and summarized. The summary describes the number of vowels and the vowel types that were used, the number and type of consonants and consonant blends produced, the total number of utterances, the mean number of syllables per utterance, a rating of speech intelligibility, and an evaluation of the prosodic elements of the child's speech. For true words, the Logical International Phonetics Program (1993) is used to compare the accuracy of the vowels and consonants that are produced with the target word that was intended.

Another transcript is made of all of the words produced by the child. Words produced orally and those produced in sign language are recorded using the Systematic Analysis of Language Transcripts (SALT) (Miller, 2002), a computer-assisted language sampling analysis program. SALT is capable of providing many different analyses. The FAMILY Assessment has chosen to identify the number of utterances, the percentage of utterances using spoken language and/or signed language, the types of utterances, the mean length of the utterances, the number of words, the types of words, and the type token ratio. In addition, the FAMILY Assessment evaluates the simultaneous use of voice and sign and the use of fingerspelling.

The same language sampling analysis program is used to examine the parents' language. Oral and/or signed samples of the parents' language are collected and analyzed. This information is used in several ways. First, this is a convenient way to identify the quality of the language input provided by the parent. In addition, for families learning sign language, the language sample analysis provides quantitative and qualitative measures of the number of signs used, the length of signed utterances, and the syntactical patterns that are used. From one assessment to the next, the parents can identify the improvement they make acquiring signs. When parents use both signed and spoken language, a comparison of the language produced in both modes is obtained. This is an efficient way to objectively measure the language model provided to the child.

Added Benefits of Using Videotape Although using videotapes to evaluate a child's speech and language skills continues to be valued, the use of the videotape has had another unexpected benefit. This benefit is actualized when the family and interventionist watch the tape. The videotape is viewed in the home giving the parents the opportunity to objectively observe the characteristics of their child's communication and the features of their interaction with their child. The interventionist facilitates a discussion to help families become good observers. For example, the interventionist and parent may identify specific characteristics of the child's oral language or sign language. Perhaps the child used "baby signs" that the parent did not understand or acknowledge at first. Or, the interventionist may take this opportunity to point out strategies the parent used that promoted the child's communication. And sometimes, parents will notice that they missed an opportunity to respond to their child. Over time, as parents develop their observation skills, they can regularly observe their child during typical daily routines. A good observer is able to notice what is working and feel good about it. This will help parents to determine their child's progress and to identify continued needs. Also, parents are offered a copy of the videotape, giving them an ongoing record of their child's development. The videotapes are a "baby book" of sorts, giving the family a longitudinal view of their child's development.

The early interventionists have actualized a similar benefit. During a scheduled home visit, the interventionist needs to focus on many different matters including the dynamics among family members, the behaviors of the child, the needs of the parents, and the characteristics of the parent–child interaction. Attending to all of these issues at the same time can restrict the interventionist's ability to observe particular characteristics of the child's communication and the specific strategies and techniques used by the parents. By viewing the videotape, with the parents or alone, the interventionist is able to critically analyze the appropriate issues. The interventionists laud this opportunity. Many interventionists report that, after they have viewed a videotape, they can more carefully identify strategies to teach parents during ensuing intervention sessions.

Parental Questionnaires and Protocols Early childhood programs support parents' participation in the assessment process (McWilliam & Scott, 2001). Parents are the most constant people in the child's life.

And, because parents spend countless hours with their children, they are likely to be the most familiar with their child's skills. Research has shown that parents can reliably assess the development of the child (Miller, Sedey, & Miolo, 1995; Saylor & Brandt, 1986). The FAMILY Assessment uses protocols that are designed for parent report. Some are completed through interviews and others are completed by the parents with help from their early interventionist as requested.

One protocol completed by the parent is the Minnesota Child Development Inventory (Ireton & Thwing, 1972), which provides information about the child's development in seven domains: expressive language, receptive language, gross and fine motor, personal-social, self-help, and situation comprehension. Both the Situation Comprehension Subtest and the Self Help Subtest correlate with measures of cognitive development (Yoshinaga-Itano & Snyder, 1999). Another protocol, the Play Assessment Questionnaire (Calhoun, 1987; Fewell, 1984), assesses the symbolic play skills of the child. This measure also correlates with cognitive development.

The child's vocabulary is measured using the MacArthur Communicative Development Inventories (Fenson et al., 1992). These checklists provide information about the quality of the gestures used by the child, the number of words the child understands, and/or the number of words the child produces. It describes the types of words the child has in his or her repertoire. The measure provides an easy way to track vocabulary development. Hart and Risley (1995) have identified a correlation between the rate at which vocabulary grows with rates of cognitive growth. Qualitatively, measuring vocabulary helps the interventionist to identify the categories of words that are most prevalent or occur least often.

For the child with a hearing loss, it is especially important to ensure vision skills are optimal. There are many temporary and permanent vision problems that young children may have. These vision problems can often be detected through observation. Parents and interventionists observe a child's functional visual behavior using the Observation of Vision Problems developed by Anthony (1992) to screen for problems.

Through an interview with the early interventionist, the parents complete the Functional Auditory Performance Indicators (Stredler-Brown & Johnson, 2001) to evaluate the functional auditory skills of their child (Robbins, Svirsky, Osberger, & Pisoni, 1998). While the entire scale is completed over time, the performance profile is submitted with the other assessment protocols. The profile describes the child's use of auditory stimuli in natural settings and the ability of the child to generalize these skills to different listening environments. The scoring of the protocol provides a way to objectively quantify a child's auditory development in several areas including sound awareness, identifying meaningful sound, auditory feedback, localization, auditory discrimination, short-term auditory memory, and linguistic auditory processing.

Along with considering their children's needs, parents also have the opportunity to consider their own needs and to request information. Using the Family Needs Interview (DeConde-Johnson, 1997), parents can identify information they would like their interventionist to share with them. The Rating of Parenting Events (Greenberg, 1981) asks parents to identify issues that are challenging for them in their daily routines with their child. Through this type of assessment, families gain insight about their concerns and priorities for themselves and for their child (McWilliam & Scott, 2001).

Benefits of Using Parental Involvement There is substantial research supporting use of parent-administered assessments. Moeller (2000) studied 112 children with various degrees of hearing loss. She evaluated the language development of children and rated the family's involvement in their child's intervention program. The most successful children were those with high levels of family involvement. She found that success is achieved when early identification is paired with early interventions that actively involve families. Furthermore, she found that strong levels of family involvement can buffer the effects of late enrollment to some degree. Enlisting families in the assessment process is an efficient way to promote family involvement.

Calderon (2000) studied parent–child interaction as a predictor of child outcomes. She studied 28 children with prelingual hearing loss. She measured parent involvement in the child's education program and the characteristics of maternal communication. Calderon's research showed that maternal communication skills correlate with higher language, earlier reading skills, and fewer behavior problems. Involving parents in assessing their child is a way to cultivate parent involvement. And, providing parents with an analysis of the language model they provide encourages parents to develop better communication skills.

Based on these findings, we are encouraged to look for ways to include parents in their child's early intervention program. Including parents in the assessment process is one way to encourage parent involvement. In addition, using parent-administered questionnaires and protocols, the child's behaviors are evaluated as they occur in many different situations over a period of time. This is in contrast to clinician-administered tests that assess a child's performance on specific tasks administered by a less familiar person at a specific point in time.

Sharing Assessment Results A summary of the results of the videotape analysis and the parent-completed protocols are returned to the early interventionist who shares the information with the family. The results are also used during the development of the IFSP. The information in the summary report identifies the developmental profile of the child in many developmental domains. It provides information to identify the parents' needs. Using norms for typically developing children and knowledge about child development, the interventionist can identify the unique strengths of the child and developmental areas that are delayed. The assessment information can be interpreted in three ways. Some of the information is provided in the form of developmental quotients or age equivalents, allowing a comparison of a child to his or her typically developing peers. Some tests have norms that compare a child with hearing loss to peers with similar profiles (these data obtained by Yoshinaga-Itano, Sedey, Coulter, & Mehl in 1998 at the University of Colorado can be found at www.colorado.edu/slhs/mdnc/research). These norms compare children according to the degree of hearing loss, the age of identification of the hearing loss, and the presence or absence of additional disabilities. Furthermore, the information can be used to measure a child's progress by comparing information gleaned from the first FAMILY Assessment, which is used to obtain a baseline of the child's skills, with the results of subsequent assessments. Used in this way, the information quantifies the growth that has occurred between assessments.

It can be an eye-opening experience for the parents as the strengths and needs of their child are identified. The assessment information is shared in a way that encourages parents to learn about their child, share their priorities and hopes and dreams, and develop realistic expectations. Delivering the information is not a goal in and of itself. Rather, it is part of the process by which parents discover more about their child and through which the interventionist guides the parents' learning. When subsequent tests are administered, the interventionist can explain the changes that have occurred. One goal of early intervention is to maintain a rate of development commensurate with the growing child. Hopefully, a child demonstrates 6 months of developmental gain in 6 months time.

The assessment information is also used to plan the intervention program. One caveat in choosing each assessment protocol is the availability of a developmental hierarchy. Almost all of the protocols provide a guide to help interventionists identify skills that come next in the developmental continuum. Through discussion with the parents and others involved in the child's assessment team, the child's strengths and needs can be identified, the needs of the parents can be discussed, and specific strategies and techniques for the parents to learn can be identified.

The early interventionist and the parents forge a relationship that fosters communication. The early interventionist obtains information about the child not only through observation but through the assessment process as well. Although the protocols are designed for parent report, the interventionist and the parent are encouraged to complete the assessments together. They can work collaboratively to identify the child's skills. Parents learn about child development and the sequence of activities children typically follow. This empowers parents to understand the impact of hearing loss on their child, to celebrate accomplishments, and to identify areas requiring more attention. Early interventionists in the Colorado Home Intervention Program report that the time they spend acquiring assessment information contributes to parents' understanding about the effect of hearing loss on their child's development and, subsequently, the parents' enthusiasm with the early intervention program. The interventionist learns more about the parents' expectations for their child and the parents' need for information.

An unintended benefit of the assessment is the opportunity to objectively measure the modalities a child uses to communicate and the effectiveness of the communication method. As the interventionist and the parents view the videotape and review the objective information on the summary report, they can identify the child's natural and spontaneous style of communication. Having objective information helps the intervention team and the parents to make objective decisions about communication mode and eliminates the emotional turmoil some parents have experienced.

Summary of the FAMILY Assessment Model   The FAMILY Assessment is one procedure for collecting information about child development and family needs. It can be used in its entirety, or specific protocols can be selected. It meets the requirement of Part C of the Individuals with Disabilities Act Amendments of 1997 (PL 105-17) to provide a multidisciplinary assessment for each child. It can be used to plan intervention, and it relies on parent participation that helps to empower parents. It also provides sufficient information to assist in program planning for each child. Another unintended benefit of using this assessment, which has been conducted for more than 15 years, is the extensive database that has been developed. Extensive research has been published identifying the efficacy of early identification and trends in the development of speech and language for young children who are deaf and hard of hearing (Mayne, Yoshinaga-Itano, & Sedey, 2000; Mayne, Yoshinaga-Itano, Sedey, & Carey, 2000; Obenchain, Menn, & Yoshinaga-Itano, 2000; Wallace, Menn, & Yoshinaga-Itano, 2000; Yoshinaga-Itano, 2000; Yoshinaga-Itano & Sedey, 1999, 2000; Yoshinaga-Itano et al., 1998).

PRACTICAL STRATEGIES

These following practices can help to ensure that the assessment process will be functional, comprehensive, and helpful to the family.

1. Develop a philosophy statement that will support assessment practices.
2. Incorporate deaf and hard of hearing adults in the assessment process.
3. Be aware of cultural differences, including Deaf Culture, that may influence the assessment process.
4. Establish play as the "centerpiece" in the assessment process. Supplement with additional tools.
5. Use a videotape of the assessment for parent education. Focus on the documented strengths of both parent and child.
6. Present information, both written and in person, to parents in a positive way. Emphasize the strengths of the child and family.
7. Write "jargon-free" reports that are understandable and usable for the families. If technical terms must be used, define them in the report.
8. Maintain a portfolio that includes observation notes, photos of a child's play (e.g., building towers, kitchen play) and videotape samples.
9. After the assessment, provide the family with "fridge facts": a brief list of the most important activities parents can use to support their child's development. This colorful fact sheet can be posted on the refrigerator for easy reference.
10. Use systematic observation to update skills and adjust strategies between more formalized assessments typically scheduled twice a year.

CONCLUSION

Developmental assessment of young deaf and hard of hearing children yields the most comprehensive information when a *process* is used rather than a few individual tests. The process involves parents and professionals (including deaf and hard of hearing adults) who observe the child in natural settings over time. Videotape is an essential tool in accurately documenting the communicative abilities of deaf and hard of hearing children. When professional judgment dictates, supplemental tests and checklists are used to further document the depth and range of developmental skills.

REFERENCES

Anthony, T. (1992). *Observation of vision problems.* Denver: Colorado Department of Education. (Adapted from an unpublished source)

Bagnato, S.J., Neisworth, J.T., & Munson, S.M. (1997). *LINKing assessment and early intervention: An authentic curriculum-based approach.* Baltimore: Paul H. Brookes Publishing Co.

Bodner-Johnson, B. (2001). Parents as adult learners in family-centered early education. *American Annals of the Deaf, 146*(3), 263–269.

Bodner-Johnson, B., Sass-Lehrer, M., Hafer, J., & Gatty, J. (2000, July). *Future directions in early education for deaf children and their families: Development and asessment.* Paper presented at the International Congress on Education of the Deaf, Sydney, Australia.

Brookfield, S.D. (1987). *Developing critical thinkers: Challenging adults to explore alternative ways of thinking and acting.* San Francisco: Jossey-Bass.

Calderon, R. (2000). *Parent involvement in deaf children's education programs as a predictor of child's language, early reading, and social-emotional development.* New York: Oxford University Press.

Calhoun, D. (1987). Play assessment questionnaire. In D. Calhoun, *A comparison of two methods of evaluating play in toddlers.* Unpublished master's thesis, Fort Collins, Colorado State University.

DeConde-Johnson, C. (1997). Family needs survey. In C. DeConde-Johnson, P.V. Benson, & J.B. Seaton (Eds.), *Educational audiology handbook.* San Diego: Singular Publishing Group.

Education of the Handicapped Act Amendments of 1986, PL 99-457, 20 U.S.C. §§ 1400 *et seq.*

Fenson, L., Dale, P.S., Reznick, J.S., Thal, D., Bates, E., Hartung, J.P., et al. (1992). *MacArthur Communicative Development Inventories: User's guide and technical manual.* Baltimore: Paul H. Brookes Publishing Co.

Fewell, R. (1984). *Play Assessment Scale.* Seattle: University of Washington Press.

Greenberg, M.T. (1981). *Interview rating of parenting events.* Seattle: University of Washington SEFAM Project.

Hafer, J., Spragins, H., & Hardy-Braz, S. (1996). Developmental assessment for the young set: The play is the thing. *Perspectives, 14*(4), 8–10.

Hart, B., & Risley, T.R. (1995). *Meaningful differences in the everyday experience of young American children.* Baltimore: Paul H. Brookes Publishing Co.

Hemmeter, M.L., Joseph, G., Smith, B., & Sandall, S. (2001). *DEC recommended practices, program assessment: Improving practices for young children with special needs and their families.* Longmont, CO: Sopris West.

Ireton, H., & Thwing, E. (1972). *Minnesota Child Development Inventory.* Minneapolis, MN: Behavior Science Systems.

Katz, S., & Swann, M. (1998). Portfolios and parents: An unbeatable combination, assessment with deaf and hard of hearing toddlers. *Perspectives, 17*(2), 12–13.

Klima, E.S., & Bellugi, U. (1979). *The signs of language.* Cambridge, MA: Harvard University Press.

Lane, H., Hoffmeister, R., & Bahan, B. (1996). *A journey into the deaf world.* San Diego: Dawn Sign Press.

Linder, T.W. (1993). *Transdisciplinary play-based assessment: A functional approach to working with young children* (Rev. ed.). Baltimore: Paul H. Brookes Publishing Co.

Logical International Phonetics Program (LIPP). (1993). LIPP (Version 1.40) [Computer software]. Miami, FL: Intelligent Hearing Systems.

Mayne, A., Yoshinaga-Itano, C., & Sedey, A.L. (2000). Receptive vocabulary development of infants and toddlers who are deaf and hard of hearing [Monograph]. *The Volta Review, 100*(5), 29–52.

Mayne, A., Yoshinaga-Itano, C., Sedey, A.L., & Carey, A. (2000). Expressive vocabulary development of infants and toddlers who are deaf or hard of hearing [Monograph]. *The Volta Review, 100*(5), 1–28.

McWilliam, R., & Scott, S. (2001). A support approach to early intervention: A three-part framework. *Infants and Young Children, 13*(4), 55–66.

Mezirow, J. (1991). *Transformation dimensions of adult learning.* San Francisco: Jossey-Bass.

Miller, J.F. (2002). *SALT: Systematic analysis of language transcripts.* Madison: University of Wisconsin Language Analysis Lab.

Miller, J.F., Sedey, A.L., & Miolo, G. (1995). Validity of parent report measures of vocabulary development for children with Down syndrome. *Journal of Speech and Hearing Research, 38,* 1037–1044.

Moeller, M.P. (2000). Early intervention and language development in children who are deaf and hard of hearing. *Pediatrics, 106*(3), 1–9.

Mohay, H. (2000). Language in sight: Mothers' strategies for making language visually accessible to deaf children. In P. Spencer, C. Erting, & L. Marschark (Eds.), *The deaf child in the family and at school: Essays in honor of Kathryn P. Meadow-Orlans* (pp. 151–166). Mahwah, NJ: Lawrence Erlbaum Associates.

Obenchain, P., Menn, L., & Yoshinaga-Itano, C. (2000). Can speech development at thirty-six months in children with hearing loss be predicted from information available in the second year of life? [Monograph] *The Volta Review, 100*(5), 149–180.

Padden, C., & Humphries, T. (1988). *Deaf in America: Voices from a culture.* Cambridge, MA: Howard University Press.

Robbins, A.M., Svirsky, M., Osberger, M.J., & Pisoni, D.B. (1998). Beyond the audiogram: The role of functional assessments. In F. Bess & J. Gravel (Eds.), *Children with hearing impairments: Contemporary trends* (pp. 105–116). Nashville: Vanderbilt Bill Wilkerson Center Press.

Saylor, C.F., & Brandt, B.J. (1986). The Minnesota Child Development Inventory: A valid maternal-report form for assessing development in infancy. *Developmental and Behavioral Pediatrics, 7*(5), 308–311.

Spencer, P. (1993). Communication behaviors of infants with hearing loss and their hearing mothers. *Journal of Speech and Hearing Research, 36,* 311–321.

Stredler-Brown, A., & Johnson, D.C. (2001). Functional auditory performance indicators: An integrated approach to auditory development. Retrieved from http://www.cde.state.co.us/cdesped/SpecificDisability-Hearing.htm

Stredler-Brown, A., & Yoshinaga-Itano, C. (1994). The FAMILY assessment: A multidisciplinary evaluation procedure. In J. Roush & N. Matkin (Eds.), *Infants and toddlers with hearing loss* (pp. 133–161). Timonium, MD: York Press.

Veditz, G. (1913). The genesis of the National Association. *Deaf-Mutes Journal, 62*(22), 1.

Wallace, V., Menn, L., & Yoshinaga-Itano, C. (2000). Is babble the gateway to speech for all children?: A longitudinal study of deaf or hard-of-hearing infants [Monograph]. *The Volta Review, 100*(5), 121–148.

Winton, P., & Bailey, D. (1994). Becoming family centered: Strategies for self examination. In J. Roush & N. Matkin (Eds.), *Infants and toddlers with hearing loss* (pp. 23–39). Timonium, MD: York Press.

Yoshinaga-Itano, C. (2000). Development of audition and speech: Implications for early intervention with infants who are deaf or hard of hearing [Monograph]. *The Volta Review, 100*(5), 213–234.

Yoshinaga-Itano, C., & Sedey, A.L. (1999). The relationship of language and symbolic play in deaf and hard-of-hearing children. *The Volta Review, 100*(3), 135–164.

Yoshinaga-Itano, C., & Sedey, A.L. (2000). Early speech development in children who are deaf or hard-of-hearing: Interrelationships with language and hearing [Monograph]. *The Volta Review, 100*(5), 118–211.

Yoshinaga-Itano, C., Sedey, A.L., Coulter, D.K., & Mehl, A.L. (1998). The language of early- and later-identified children with hearing loss. *Pediatrics, 102*(5), 1161–1171.

Yoshinaga-Itano, C., & Snyder, L. (1999). The relationship of language and symbolic play in deaf and hard-of-hearing children. *The Volta Review, 100*(3), 135–164.

A Parent's Perspective

Karen Ewing

As a new mother, you often gaze at your baby and wonder at the miracle of creation. A small piece of yourself and your partner lays before you, and instantly you are in love for a lifetime. As your baby grows and develops, you cannot help but conduct your own motherly assessment. Naturally, you look at other children or siblings and check that this baby is doing okay. Like every other mother, I often informally compared both my daughter and my son with not only other children but also with each other. While my son developed many health problems that doctors assured us would resolve themselves, it was shortly after he had turned 1 year old that I "felt" that something was different. I had no such feelings with my daughter, but doctors and family members assured me that once his health improved, my feelings of worry would dissipate. They did not.

I requested that my son be evaluated to determine if he did in fact have a disability. We were directed to our county's local Infants and Toddlers program. A psychologist, who served as part of a multi-disciplinary team, arrived at our house for a preassessment interview. She was warm and open. She spent time answering our questions, and she took great care and effort when interacting with our son. She clearly explained the upcoming assessment process. Our overwhelming fear concerning the unknown future for our son had been weighing heavily on our shoulders for several months. From the moment we were introduced to the education specialist and other team members, I did not feel quite as alone; rather, I felt as if I had a group of supporters behind me, making the job ahead easier in some way.

The assessment process, while hardly a carefree experience, was conducted in a positive and supportive manner. The multidisciplinary team conducted the play-based assessment as a group. I was impressed by the amount of information that the team members were able to gather in such a relaxed setting. My son was never forced; rather, he often led the various activities. The team asked and answered many of my questions. I felt like a valued member of the team, which I felt was a critical part of our successful outcome. The information gathered throughout the assessment was given to us in a constructive and clear manner. I distinctly remember feeling very appreciative of how the team focused on positive things my son was doing, rather than simply providing the laundry list of the many skill deficits that he had. Most important, the team worked with us to develop a clear road map for our son's intervention program. That road map was developed through the authentic assessment in which all of the members of the team came together in collaboration.

It has been more than 6 years since that very first assessment process, and I still depend on accurate assessments to plan and implement my son's intervention program. We have gone through many different forms of assessments since that time, and I am grateful that the first experience was so positive. My son has continued to make tremendous strides in his development into a happy, inquisitive child who is fully mainstreamed into a third-grade classroom. I continue to value the partnerships that have been established with various members of his education team. As he grows older, I still find myself conducting my own motherly assessments, and I am constantly grateful that we did take those first steps to have him assessed and receive the intervention services that were so critical for making him the amazing child he is today.

CHAPTER SIX

Programs and Services for Deaf and Hard of Hearing Children and Their Families

MARILYN SASS-LEHRER

When we discovered that our son was deaf, we cried. We didn't cry because he would never be able to hear music, hear birds sing, or hear our voices; we cried because we didn't know how we would ever be able to communicate with him. We cried because we were afraid that he would not be able to communicate with us. We cried because we wanted so desperately to have the same kind of relationship with our deaf son that we have with our hearing daughters. We were lucky in many ways. He was identified early—3 months of age, and we live in a large metropolitan area with many programs and services for families of deaf children. We got involved in the parent–infant program that provided us with home visits to help us learn about deafness and the options available for deaf children. We met other parents and their deaf children, deaf adults, and professionals who helped us realize that our son would be able to do everything that any child can do—except hear.

Few families understand how their child's hearing loss will affect their child's development and what this will mean for the child and the family. For many families, discovering that their young child has a hearing loss is just the beginning of a long journey through unexplored terrain. The key to a smooth journey is an early education program that delivers family-centered, culturally sensitive, comprehensive, developmentally and individually appropriate services. Professionals who are committed to partnerships with families, are knowledgeable about resources to tap along the way, and are sensitive to the experiences families encounter are essential guides for such a journey.

The widespread adoption of Universal Newborn Hearing Screening (UNHS) programs across the United States has resulted in the identification of hearing loss at increasingly earlier ages (see Chapter 4). Families fortunate to be referred immediately by health care professionals and audiologists to a comprehensive early education program with professionals knowledgeable about working with infants with hearing loss and their families can expect their children to achieve language and literacy abilities nearly commensurate with their hearing peers (Apuzzo & Yoshinaga-Itano, 1995; Moeller, 2000; Yoshinaga-Itano, 2003; Yoshinaga-Itano, Sedey, Coulter, & Mehl, 1998).

Even though the components of effective early education programs are no mystery, not all families have access to high quality and comprehensive services. This chapter provides an overview of the research, legislation, and professional guidelines that shape quality programming for young children who are deaf and hard of hearing and their families. Components of early education programming and models for service delivery are presented followed by program application guidelines. The chapter concludes with a discussion of future perspectives on programming for young children who are deaf and hard of hearing and their families.

RESEARCH, LEGISLATIVE, AND PROFESSIONAL PERSPECTIVES

Professionals providing services for families and their deaf and hard of hearing children find guidance for their practices from research, legislation, and professional organizations. The complex interrelationship of these three sources of knowledge informs and guides the field in the implementation of programs that support families and enhance opportunities for children who are deaf and hard of hearing.

Research Findings

Research in early intervention has encountered methodological challenges that limit the extent to which the field can accept with certainty the effectiveness of specific methods, interactions, and approaches of early intervention professionals (Guralnick, 1997). According to Calderon and Greenberg (1997), research in the early education of deaf and hard of hearing children has been complicated by the relatively low incidence of hearing loss, the heterogeneity of children and their families, the late identification of hearing loss in many children, the lack of appropriate outcome measures, the difficulty in measuring process variables (e.g., family adjustment), and the continuing controversies regarding educational and cultural issues. From a comprehensive review of the literature on the effectiveness of early intervention over the past 25 years with children with hearing losses, Calderon and Greenberg (1997) concluded that there is little scientific evidence establishing what complex array of program variables, professional characteristics, environmental conditions, or intervention approaches leads to more effective outcomes for individual children and their families.

The evidence that does exist addresses the timeliness of intervention, the importance of parental support and well-being, parent involvement, child language acquisition, social-emotional development, speech and auditory development, and communication approaches. Research suggests that the child's best chances for success depend on early identification of hearing loss followed by enrollment in a comprehensive and effective early education program (Apuzzo & Yoshinaga-Itano, 1995; Arehart & Yoshinaga-Itano, 1999; Calderon & Naidu, 2000; Moeller, 2000; Yoshinaga-Itano, 2003; Yoshinaga-Itano, Sedey, et al., 1998).

Children benefit when families feel competent and confident in their abilities to nurture and support their child's development (Carney & Moeller, 1998; MacTurk, Meadow-Orlans, Koester, & Spencer, 1993). Early intervention professionals, other parents, and adults who are deaf are important sources of social support that can strengthen and enhance the family's sense of well-being (Hintermair, 2000; Meadow-Orlans, Mertens, Sass-Lehrer, & Scott-Olson, 1997; Meadow-Orlans, Smith-Gray, & Dyssegaard, 1995).

Family involvement is essential to the child's early development and is associated with child language gains, social-emotional adjustment, and academic development, at least through the early years of school (Calderon, Bargones, & Sidman, 1998; Moeller, 2000). However, programs that involve families and also focus on enhancing family communication with their child may observe the greatest benefits in language and academic functioning (Calderon, 2000; Moeller, 2001). Parent–child communication skills not only support language and social-emotional development, but also result in enhanced parent–child relationships (Greenberg, Calderon, & Kusche, 1984; Jamieson, 1995; Spencer, Bodner-Johnson, & Gutfreund, 1992). Children need active communicative partners who are mature and fluent users in the child's preferred mode of communication for language acquisition to occur (McAnally, Rose, & Quigley, 1994).

Despite the emotional debates to the contrary, there is no evidence of the superiority of one mode of communication over another with very young children (Calderon & Greenberg, 1997; Carney & Moeller, 1998; Yoshinaga-Itano, 2000; Yoshinaga-Itano & Sedey, 2000). Speech development is strongly related to language facility and is not impeded by the use of sign language (Marschark, 1997; Wilbur, 2000). And, early hearing aid use generally results in better understanding and expression of spoken language. Parents and children who interact regularly with Deaf adults acquire better communication skills than parents and children who do not (Watkins, Pittman, & Walden, 1998). Programs that successfully establish partnerships with families and support their involvement witness effective parent–child communication and child development achievements comparable to those of hearing children with similar developmental profiles (Moeller, 2000; Yoshinaga-Itano, 2000).

In order to examine language, speech, and social-emotional development of early-identified children who are deaf or hard of hearing, the University of Colorado has conducted a series of developmental studies involving more than 400 children. Families of these children were enrolled in the Colorado Home Intervention Program (CHIP) from 6 months of age. Assessments at 3 years of age revealed that these children developed and maintained age-appropriate receptive and expressive language skills both orally and in sign language (Yoshinaga-Itano, 2000). Research conducted at The Boys Town National Medical Research Hospital in Omaha, Nebraska, with young children and families enrolled in their early intervention program by 11 months of age had similar positive outcomes. Children with the highest vocabulary and verbal reasoning skills were enrolled in early intervention earlier and had strong family involvement (Moeller, 2001). A comparison of these two successful early intervention programs reveals that they share the following characteristics: 1) they established partnerships with parents in all aspects of the program, 2) their intervention focus was on parents and caregivers with limited or no direct intervention or demonstration therapy with infants and toddlers, 3) they had strong family support and counseling components, 4) they used individualized approaches designed by parents in partnerships with professionals, and 5) they valued nonjudgmental interactions with families supporting the family's decisions (Moeller, 2000; Yoshinaga-Itano, 2000).

Guralnick (1997) called for "second-generation" research focusing on specific approaches that provided optimal outcomes and the best start for young children and their families. Calderon and Greenberg (1997) suggested that research with children who are deaf and their families should address the complex individual, family, program, and societal factors that result in successful outcomes for children with hearing loss.

Children who are deaf or hard of hearing and their families differ in many ways, and services must be adapted to fit their unique situations (Meadow-Orlans & Sass-Lehrer, 1995). Although families typically describe early intervention programs and professionals as extremely helpful, some families are frustrated by the lack of knowledge about hearing loss of some professionals, the difficulty in finding services that address their child's specific developmental needs, or the difficulty in obtaining comprehensive and unbiased information (Meadow-Orlans, Mertens, & Sass-Lehrer, 2003).

Legislative Foundations for Early Intervention

The enactment of the Education of the Handicapped Act Amendments of 1986 (PL 99-457) championed access to quality services for infants, toddlers, and preschoolers who are deaf and hard of hearing and their families. According to this law, services to young children and their families should be family-centered, culturally responsive, comprehensive, collaborative, and interdisciplinary. This legislation is currently known as Part C and Part B of the Individuals with Disabilities Education Act (IDEA) Amendments of 1997 (PL 105-17) (see Chapter 3).

At the heart of Part C of IDEA is the understanding that families, rather than the professionals, should take the lead when it comes to making decisions about their child's intervention process. The legislation recognizes families as both the consumer and the focus of early intervention efforts, and early education professionals have the responsibility of providing services that reflect this family-centered philosophy. The legislation calls for professionals and families to join together as partners to promote families' abilities to enhance the development of their young children.

According to IDEA, programs must be comprehensive and address all areas of the young child's development including cognitive, communicative, social-emotional, motor, and adaptive development. Services should be based on the infant's or toddler's needs as identified by an interdisciplinary (multidisciplinary) assessment involving family members and professionals with expertise in relevant disciplinary fields. Priorities for services should be determined by an individualized family service plan (IFSP) developed by the family in partnership with professionals (see Chapter 3 for various elements of the IFSP). Collaboration among disciplines and agencies ensures that the comprehensive needs of the child as determined by the family and professionals are met. IDEA supports the provision of services by professionals who meet the highest standards set for their specific discipline, and it suggests a system for promoting professional development.

The legislation also establishes guidelines to ensure that each family's cultural, linguistic, and ethnic diversity is respected and that their priorities, concerns, and resources are considered when implementing services. Families whose cultural or ethnic backgrounds define them as a "minority" population are overrepresented in statistical categories that may place their infants at higher risk for disabilities or developmental delays (Cohen, Fischgrund, & Redding, 1990; Iglesias & Quinn, 1997). Professionals from ethnically diverse backgrounds, however, are largely underrepresented in programs working with children who are deaf and hard of hearing (Cohen, 1993; Sass-Lehrer, Gerner de Garcia, & Rovins, 1997). Barriers imposed by language or culture often make it difficult for families to trust professionals and feel comfortable with the educational system. One parent interviewed about her experiences with early intervention programs described her feelings about professionals this way:

When you get my kid sitting there with you, don't try and tell me to leave. I want to be comfortable with who I am leaving my child with, and if I don't feel comfortable, he will not stay with you. It's that simple. I'm not going to force him to come with you; you're a stranger. (as cited in Sass-Lehrer, Mertens, & Meadow-Orlans, 2001)

In addition to IDEA, access to early education programs and services for children and families are protected by Section 504 of the Rehabilitation Act of 1973 (PL 93-112, which was amended by PL 102-569) and the Americans with Disabilities Act (ADA) of 1990 (PL 101-336). These legal provisions ensure access to programs and nondiscriminatory practices in schools, hospitals, libraries, social services agencies, nonprofit organizations, and government agencies that receive federal financial assistance (Bowe, 2000). As a result of the ADA, child development and child care programs in the community must provide "reasonable accommodations" for young children with hearing loss and their families. These accommodations may include sign language interpreters, TTYs, and other visual alerting systems (Bowe, 2000).

The Newborn Infant Hearing Screening and Intervention Act of 2000 (Title VI of the Departments of Labor, Health and Human Services, and Education, and Related Agencies Appropriations Act of 2000, PL 106-113) was passed in an effort to speed the implementation of UNHS. This legislation provides financial incentives through grants to states so they can develop early identification and early intervention systems (see Chapter 4). UNHS provides infants and their families with an early start for intervention and is changing the very nature of the programs and services provided by raising numerous questions: What are the most effective strategies for interacting with families with newborns? How should early education professionals collaborate with medical and health care professionals in newborn screening programs? What are the most effective strategies for stimulating newborns' auditory and visual channels for language acquisition? How are parents receiving and reacting to information conveyed to them about their newborn's hearing loss? How do their reactions influence the services provided and services they accept?

Professional Guidelines

Professional organizations concerned with the welfare of young children with special needs and their families have been instrumental in effecting change in early education. Professionals who work with young children who are deaf and hard of hearing can benefit from familiarizing themselves with some key guidelines and recommendations for educating typically developing young children, children with special needs, and children who are deaf or hard of hearing (see Table 6.1).

There has been remarkable consensus in research findings, legislative initiatives, and professional guidelines suggesting indicators of effectiveness for programs providing services to young children with hearing loss and their families. These findings include the following:

- Early identification and hearing screening followed by enrollment in a comprehensive, family-centered, early intervention program promotes child developmental outcomes (Moeller, 2000; Yoshinaga-Itano, 2000).

- Family-centered programming enhances a family's adaptation, decision making, and ability to promote their child's development and learning (Carney & Moeller, 1998; Moeller & Condon, 1994).

- Family support promotes family well-being and enhances quality of parent–child interaction and child developmental outcomes (MacTurk et al., 1993; Meadow-Orlans, Smith-Gray, & Dyssegaard, 1995; Meadow-Orlans & Steinberg, 1993).

- Effective programming and services to young children and their families are culturally, developmentally, and individually appropriate (Calderon & Greenberg, 1997; Meadow-Orlans et al., 2003).

- Family involvement and effective parent–child and family communication promote language acquisition and academic achievement (Calderon, 2000; Yoshinaga-Itano, 2000).

- Child and family participation in programs with well-qualified professionals supports positive developmental outcomes (Moeller, 2000; Yoshinaga-Itano, 2000).

Table 6.1. Professional guidelines and recommendations for educating deaf and hard of hearing children

Professional Organization/Report	Recommendations
Commission on the Education of the Deaf/ *Report of the Commission on the Education of the Deaf* (COED, 1988)	Recommends lowering the age of identification of hearing loss and promotes the inclusion of deaf adults as role models and facilitators in early intervention programs
National Association of the State Directors of Special Education/*Deaf and Hard of Hearing Students: Educational Service Guidelines* (Easterbrooks & Baker, 1994)	Describes program features to be considered in the design of appropriate services for deaf and hard of hearing students and families
Joint Committee of American Speech-Language-Hearing Association (ASHA) and the Council on Education of the Deaf (CED)/*Service Provision Under the Individuals with Disabilities Education Act-Part H, as Amended (IDEA-Part H) to Children Who are Deaf and Hard of Hearing Ages Birth to 36 Months of Age* (ASHA/CED, 1994)	Describes the knowledge and experiences required by professionals working with infants and toddlers birth through 36 months and their families
National Association for the Education of Young Children (NAEYC)/*Developmentally Appropriate Practice in Early Childhood Programs* (Rev. Ed.) (Bredekamp & Copple, 1997)	Offers guidelines for developmentally and individually appropriate practices for young children birth through 8 years old; practices based on child development, age appropriateness, and variations in individual abilities and needs
Division for Early Childhood (DEC)/*DEC Recommended Practices in Early Intervention/Early Childhood Special Education* (Sandall, McLean, & Smith, 2000)	Recommends practices for assessment, child-focused intervention, family-based practices, interdisciplinary models, technology applications, policies, procedures and systems change, and personnel preparation
Joint Committee on Infant Hearing/*Year 2000 Position Statement: Principles and Guidelines for Early Hearing Detection and Intervention Programs* (JCIH, 2000)	Endorses early detection of hearing loss followed by family-centered early intervention; promotes developmentally appropriate language skills, family understanding of child's strengths and needs, and family advocacy

- Deaf and hard of hearing adults are an important source of support and can facilitate families' adjustment and accommodations to a deaf child (Hintermair, 2000; Meadow-Orlans et al., 2003; Watkins et al., 1998).

EARLY EDUCATION PROGRAMS AND MODELS

Research, legislation, and professional recommendations as well as an understanding of program design are essential to the development of an effective early intervention program. Programming is comprehensive, collaborative, and interdisciplinary to address the priorities and concerns of the family related to the child's overall development. Early education program models incorporate the foundations of family centeredness and developmentally appropriate practice with an understanding of the linguistic and communication challenges for children who are deaf and hard of hearing (Sass-Lehrer & Bodner-Johnson, 2003).

Early Intervention Program Design

Early intervention programming involves the delivery of an array of services to parents, caregivers, and young children in a variety of environments by professionals using approaches, materials, and resources that are specially designed and selected to promote the child's development. A system's approach to early intervention programming provides a framework for linking the program's philosophy to assessment, goal setting, intervention, and evaluation of effectiveness (Bagnato, Neisworth, & Munson, 1997; Bricker, 1998). A linked system increases the probability that the child's abilities and needs and the family's priorities, concerns, goals, strategies, and evaluations are interrelated and anticipated outcomes are achieved (see Figure 6.1).

Philosophy Program design begins with the development of the program's philosophy and purpose, addressing the roles and relationships of families and professionals, the nature of learning in young children who are deaf and hard of hearing and their families, and the intended outcomes for both children and families.

Assessment A comprehensive child assessment covers all areas of development including cognition, communication and language, social-emotional, perceptual-fine motor, gross motor, and adaptive skills, and for preschoolers, early literacy and preacademic skills. In partnership with families, professionals from relevant disciplines identify assessment goals and protocols that will result in a complete developmental profile of the child and, if the family wishes, includes family support to strengthen their ability to promote their child's development. Support may include individual family counseling, parent support groups, communication skill development, or connecting families with resources available in their community. An effective assessment provides families and professionals with information not only on the child's developmental status and growth, but also on the developmental outcomes to be achieved. The assessment is most useful when it is linked to a developmental sequence that is both compatible with and embedded in the child's curriculum (Bagnato et al., 1997) (see Chapter 5). Suggested standards for assessment are included

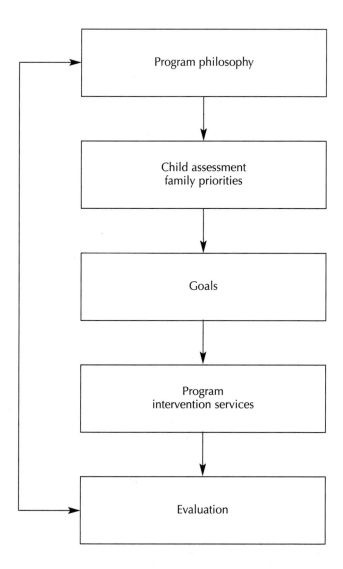

Figure 6.1. Systems approach to early intervention. (From Bricker, D., with Pretti-Frontczak, K., & McComas, N. [1998]. *An activity-based approach to early intervention* [2nd ed., p. 23]. Baltimore: Paul H. Brookes Publishing Co.; adapted by permission.)

in the Division for Early Childhood's Recommended Practices (Sandall et al., 2000, pp. 20–21).

Families are asked to provide direction to the assessment process by providing information regarding their child's development, interactions, and temperament (nature, disposition), as well as the significant people and environments that describe their child's experiences. Family aspirations for their child can be obtained over time through active listening, observing, and interviewing techniques. Several checklists and survey forms are available to stimulate discussions with families about the information, support, and skills they believe will help them promote their child's development. Often, simply asking families, "How can we help?" elicits important information that guides professionals in identifying ways to support families.

Preassessment meetings with families should focus on building a trusting, positive, and collaborative relationship. Information solicited from families, such as what they most enjoy doing with their child and their child's favorite toys, foods, people, and places, for example, help both professionals and parents focus on what the child can do rather than on his or her weaknesses or disabilities. Asking families, "How do you hope your family will benefit from early intervention services?" helps professionals understand parents' expectations as well as their thinking about the role of early education and their involvement. Families' understanding of the purpose of the assessment and their meaningful involvement in the process is essential to gathering useful information.

Goal Setting The next step in program design involves identifying outcomes or goals for the child and the family. Outcomes are broad statements that describe a desired change to occur for the child or family with the support of early intervention services. These outcomes are determined through a collaborative process between caregivers and professionals and are based on the results of the assessment process. Outcomes should address all developmental areas and be meaningful to the child and family. Families should be given the opportunity to share their priorities for their child first. Then later, professionals can add their views and suggest additional goals that may advance the child's development. After parents and professionals reach a consensus on the goals and outcomes to be achieved, professionals should work with families to identify the behaviors that will indicate that the child is making progress toward the agreed upon outcomes.

Intervention For the child who is deaf or hard of hearing, the primary focus of early intervention is usually communication and language acquisition. Because it is essential that children with hearing loss and their families communicate fluently as soon as possible, communication and language goals should not only address multiples aspects of communication and language development for the child but also emphasize communication between the child and the child's caregivers (see Chapters 11 and 12).

Implementation strategies for child and family outcomes should be based on effective practices and developmental and individual appropriateness. Options for programs and services, like other aspects of programming, require a collaborative approach by professionals with families to ensure that the family's concerns are addressed and the services the family receives reflect their beliefs and lifestyle. Flexible programming permits families to select the services and delivery approaches they feel best meet their child's and family's needs and reflects the family's choice of services. Families with infants and toddlers may select only the services that address the outcomes they believe are most important to their child's development. Families may, for example, choose not to receive services from an occupational therapist, or to delay those services, despite a recommendation that their child might benefit from those services. Preferences for where the services are provided, who provides them, and when and how often they occur should be part of a collaborative decision-making process (Moeller & Condon, 1994). Professionals have the responsibility to advocate for families and to encourage families to become self-advocates in order to receive the services that will achieve the desired expectations for their children (Mitchell & Philibert, 2002; see also Chapter 3).

Selection of communication approach and assistive technologies (e.g., hearing aids, cochlear implants) is sometimes a difficult process—one that may find professionals in disagreement with each other or the families they are working with (Meadow-Orlans et al., 2003). Moeller and Condon (1994) suggested a systematic and collaborative goal-setting approach to determine communication modality, intervention goals, and settings that offer the "best fit" for the child. The Diagnostic Early Intervention Program (DEIP) allows family members and professionals to discover the child's abilities and needs, as well as the family's preferences, using an "ecologically valid evaluation system." Using this program, families and professionals team up to discover the child's communication and language strengths through observations of parent and child interactions during play and routine interactions. Information from parent reports, interviews, and parent checklists is obtained to help determine the child's communicative strengths. Later, more formal assessments are conducted of the child's communication abilities and the progress he or she makes. This "family-guided process" places the decision making in the hands of families rather than professionals and results in satisfaction and stability in the choices made (Moeller & Condon, 1994).

Evaluation Evaluation links documentation of child progress and family satisfaction with initial and ongoing assessment, services provided, outcomes, and strategies. Families should be closely involved in the evaluation process, providing input on their children's progress as well as the effectiveness of strategies used to enhance their own abilities to promote their child's development. Several types of evaluation strategies are effective for assessing young children's progress, including parent interviews, developmental checklists, anecdotal records, videotape samples, and portfolios (see Chapter 5). Evaluations should occur at least every 6 months for children younger than 3 years of age and yearly for older children (IDEA 1997). Data obtained from evaluations should be used to update the child's individualized education program (IEP) and the IFSP by modifying outcomes for children and families and adapting program strategies to provide better services to children and their families (see Chapter 7).

Early Intervention Learning Environments

Infants are wired for learning, and they will blossom given interaction with nurturing adults and access to fluent and active communication partners and developmentally appropriate environments. Programming for infants and toddlers with hearing loss includes a variety of services and settings conducive not only to the child's growth and development but also to the family and significant others in these children's lives. Individual sessions with parents and/or caregivers, play groups, family support and information sessions, and sign language classes are the typical learning contexts for the youngest children and their families.

A traditional approach to parent–infant services is the home-based model. Although this model may have distinct advantages for some families, for others, it may be less desirable. For example, consider the Shaw family:

Both Barry and Linda Shaw work full time outside the home. Their 18-month-old daughter, Frannie, spends the day at the home of a neighbor who cares for two other young children. Both Barry and Linda are committed to providing the most effective early learning environments possible for their daughter. They understand that in addition to themselves, Frannie's care provider is a critical influence on her early development. They have requested that services be provided weekly in their neighbor's home where Barry and Linda alternate attending the sessions. In this way, Frannie's care provider can also benefit from the information and support provided by the early intervention specialist and can incorporate newly learned communication strategies into her regular routine while caring for the two other children. Barry and Linda also value their weekly parent–child playgroup sessions at the center. The center-based program gives them an opportunity to meet with the entire team of specialists and other parents with deaf and hard of hearing children and attend sign language class. They believe that this combination of settings best meets their needs.

The location of sessions should take into consideration the needs of the child and the family's preference. Many families prefer home-based services although others are more comfortable in a community setting, such as a community center or library. Others choose to travel to the program center where they may meet other families and children who are deaf and hard of hearing, or work with both deaf and hearing professionals. A family with a medically fragile child may find it too difficult to travel to a center for services and might prefer home-based services, although another family would choose a community location large enough to accommodate other family or friends who wish to participate in the sessions.

Early Intervention Program Models for Families

There is no one universally accepted model for providing services to families with very young children. The Colorado Home Intervention Program (CHIP), the SKI-HI model, and the Ready to Learn program illustrate three different early intervention program models.

The Colorado Home Intervention Program   The CHIP program, offered by the Colorado Department of Health and Environment, provides family-centered programming primarily in the family's home. A specially trained early intervention provider known as a "parent facilitator" helps family members develop techniques to promote their child's overall development including communication and language. The facilitator also promotes collaboration with agencies and services available in the family's community. A parent consultant, a consumer advisor (a deaf or hard of hearing adult), a sign language instructor, and other specialists are part of the interdisciplinary team that provides services to families. In addition to home visits by the parent facilitator and other relevant members of the team, families may participate in the Family Connections Project. This project arranges for a deaf or hard of hearing adult to visit the family on a regular basis in order to provide information, support, and sign language instruction, as well as to present a positive role model for the family.

SKI-HI Model   Another early intervention model is SKI-HI, developed at Utah State University. This model provides home-based services to families on a weekly basis that emphasize family adaptation to their child's hearing loss, understanding of hearing loss including etiology, communication, social and cognitive development, hearing aids, cochlear implants, American Sign Language (ASL), and Deaf culture. "Parent advisors" are trained to work with parents to facilitate their skills for promoting their child's communicative, language, and cognitive development. The SKI-HI family-centered, home-based programming includes curriculum, assessment materials, and resources to guide parent advisors in delivering services to families (Watkins & Clark, 1992). The goal of SKI-HI is to respond to the needs of children with hearing loss, including children who are either deaf or hard of hearing, blind or visually impaired, both deaf and blind, have multiple disabilities, or have any other special need. A revised edition of this program is expected in Fall 2003.

Ready to Learn   Another approach to programming is the Ready to Learn Parent Infant Program at the Lexington School for the Deaf in Jackson Heights, New York. This program utilizes a Mediated Learning Experience (MLE) model to engage parents, caregivers, and young children as "active participant learners" and elicit and expand their use of "cognitive actions" (Feuerstein, 1980; Kahn, 2000). The goal of a mediated learning approach is to develop efficient thinking skills that promote autonomous and independent learning (Greenberg, 1990). Professionals work in partnership with families to facilitate and support early learning and problem solving with their children. Parents and caregivers assume the role of mediator for their children's learning, acting as interpreters and guides and giving meaning and relevance to objects, events, and thoughts. The approach focuses on teaching families how to foster their children's skills of observation, thinking, reflection, and comparing. In this model, professionals are the coaches, guiding parents and caregivers through different phases of cognitive actions.

Early Childhood Program Models for Preschools

Support for a family's preparation of their child's transition from an early intervention program to preschool is essential to the child's positive adjustment. Preschool programs may be located in a variety of settings and may include individual parent–child or caregiver–child sessions, adult support and information meetings, and sign language classes in addition to center-based services for groups of children on a part-time or full-time basis. As children become more independent and developmentally able, parents and caregivers may find themselves less actively involved in their child's educational program as their child can attend programs for increasingly longer hours, and services involving the parents are typically reduced. The transition from early intervention to preschool often leaves family members without the same level of support and services that they enjoyed when their child was younger (Calderon & Greenberg, 2000). Although preschool represents a new phase of the child's development and independence, parents still need information, support, and communication instruction. Educational programming at this stage should be designed to promote family involvement, rather than discourage it, as is often the case. Consideration of the child's needs and family preferences, rather than the program structure, should determine the scope and intensity of the services provided.

Center-based programs for older toddlers and preschoolers incorporate child-centered and play-based practices that support the child's development and interests. One early education model that embeds the child's individual outcomes within an early childhood program of planned, routine, and child-initiated activities is activity-based intervention (Bricker, 1998). This approach provides a framework for incorporating individual child goals and strategies within a context of a "typical" early childhood setting. Effective early childhood programs emphasize a literature-rich environment including daily storytelling or book sharing activities (Linder, 1999). The early childhood teacher using an activity-based approach might consider how individual receptive language goals could be accomplished within a storytelling activity. Native users of American Sign Language with skills in story sharing capture the interests and attention of children with limited hearing and link the language of the story to the print in the book. For a child with limited visual attention, the teacher might use props moving them along the pages of the book at selected times to extend the child's visual attention.

Several early childhood education models developed for typically developing children are appropriate for adaptation with young children with hearing loss. Notable among these models are the Emergent Curriculum and Reggio Emilia model (Edwards, Gandini, & Forman, 1993; Gestwicki, 1999), the High/Scope Cognitively Oriented Curriculum (Hohman & Weikart, 1995), the Multiple Intelligences and Project Spectrum (Gardner, 1995; Gardner & Hatch, 1989), the Montessori Method (Goffin, 1994), and the *Read, Play, and Learn!* curriculum (Linder, 1999). Each of these models emphasizes developmentally and individually appropriate principles, stresses learning through active participation and involvement, encourages multiple avenues for learning and expression, incorporates learning across domains, and encourages learning based on child strengths and interests.

Programs for young children who are deaf and hard of hearing may also adapt educational models designed for young children with special education or linguistic needs. Inclusive education models for children with and without hearing loss have distinct advantages for some children (see Chapter 9); however, many others need complete access to language from peers and adults who communicate using sign language. Bilingual models utilize ASL as the primary language of interaction and present English primarily through print (see Chapter 12). Another approach emphasizes residual hearing to enhance spoken English and includes children who are not deaf as spoken language models for the children who are deaf.

Components of Early Intervention and Preschool Programs

Programs for young children who are deaf and hard of hearing and their families are similar in many respects to programs for children with and without special learning needs. The uniqueness lies in the knowledge and skills of the professional team, the focus on language acquisition and parent–child communication, and the nature of support and information extended to families.

Interdisciplinary Teams Professionals working with young children with hearing loss and their families may be deaf educators, speech and language pathologists, audiologists, sign language specialists, early childhood and special education professionals, occupational and physical therapists, social workers, counselors, and health care professionals. Adults who are deaf and hard of hearing and adults with other cultural and language backgrounds also have expertise and insights that make them extremely valuable team members. The composition of the professional team varies from family to family, according to the child's needs and the family's preferences and individual circumstances. Families with infants and toddlers are instrumental in selecting the professionals participating in the interdisciplinary assessment and providing services to their child and family.

The story of Michele Baum, a young mother whose infant son was born with a severe hearing loss and motor delays, illustrates an example of how an interdisciplinary team might work.

When Carey, the deaf education specialist, met Michele, she was trying hard to keep the weekly appointments with her son's audiologist to evaluate his hearing and select hearing aids. This was putting a serious strain on her time, finances, and emotions. Michele had a close relationship with a social worker who was helping her find adequate housing and child care for her infant while she attended school part time, and requested that her social worker be involved in the planning process. She also wanted her son's physical therapist to participate on the interdisciplinary team. Carey coordinated services with Michele's input, and together with her social worker, the audiologist, and the physical therapist, they discussed a plan for addressing her son's early intervention needs.

Models for interdisciplinary team collaboration vary, and Carey and Michele discussed how the team would share information, roles, and responsibilities and provide services. Due to her busy schedule, and the many people already in her infant's life, Michele selected Carey as the primary service provider. They decided that after the assessment process was completed and the IFSP developed, Michele would continue to meet regularly with her social worker but only occasionally with the physical therapist. Carey would meet weekly with the physical therapist sharing progress notes and questions and receive coaching to support Michele's interactions with her infant. Michele requested that Carey stay in close contact with the audiologist as well. This team approach enabled Michele and Carey to incorporate both auditory and physical therapy goals into the developmental and communication goals they identified. By working together in this way, they were able to simplify the service plan and minimize the number of weekly individual appointments and "therapies" so Michele could concentrate on her schoolwork.

Deaf and Hard of Hearing Adults as Team Members   Adult role models who are deaf or hard of hearing are important participants in early education programs and are beneficial to both young children and their families (Hintermair, 2000; Mohay, 2000; Watkins et al., 1998). The Deaf Mentor Project, developed by SKI-HI, provides training for adults who are deaf to meet regularly with families and their children in order to interact, model communication strategies, and share information about Deaf culture and community resources. Many programs have adopted this model. The Massachusetts State Association of the Deaf, with funding from the Massachusetts Department of Public Health, provides a 20-week Family Sign Language Program for all families in the state who are enrolled in an early intervention program. Sign language instructors who are deaf travel to the families' homes where they discuss the family's communication needs and plan an approach with the family for enhancing communication.

In early intervention and preschool classrooms, adults who are deaf and hard of hearing work side by side with other hearing professionals not only as early childhood specialists, but also as language and cultural models and integral members of the interdisciplinary team. Adults who are deaf and hard of hearing who have expertise in communication and language assessment, development, and evaluation can be invaluable in promoting communication and language goals. Deaf adults who sign often provide sign language instructional support to children (hearing, deaf, and hard of hearing) in the program, professionals, and parents.

Adults who are deaf or hard of hearing are often recruited for story-telling. Those who have been trained to use visual story-sharing techniques are very effective readers, making storybooks come alive for even the youngest children. The Shared Reading Project (described in Chapters 2 and 7) has been adapted to incorporate distance technology and brings storytelling by experienced Deaf storytellers into homes and schools in rural areas where there are few adults who are deaf (Hatfield, personal communication, 2000).

Family Support Family support is an important and yet often overlooked component of early education programs (Meadow-Orlans et al., 1997). Although information is shared with parents in many different ways (e.g., parent meetings, individual parent–child sessions, newsletters, the Internet, articles and other printed materials), counseling is often in short supply. Despite the importance of family support to the overall well-being of the family and the child's development, less than one half of parents in a national survey who have young children who are deaf and hard of hearing indicated that counseling services were available to them in early intervention programs (Meadow-Orlans et al., 1997). One program in Seattle, Washington, offers a weekly parent support group facilitated by an experienced family therapist. While parents are meeting, children and their siblings participate in a play group that facilitates interactions with other children and adults who are deaf, hard of hearing, and hearing. The parent support group encourages parents to share their experiences and concerns as they individually struggle to "do the right thing" for their child and other family members (Minkin, personal communication, 1995). One parent described the personal benefit of a parent support group:

It helps to go to a parent group, even though you don't want to talk about your problems or whatever . . . somebody there is gonna feel the same way you do. And will help you . . . because it doesn't do you or your child any good to just mope about it. (Meadow-Orlans et al., 2003)

Early Intervention and Preschool Program Settings

Center schools for deaf and hard of hearing children, local public schools, private preschools, or other centers for children with and without hearing losses may offer programs for young children and their families. Location of services, however, should be secondary to the quality and comprehensiveness of the programming provided. Part C of IDEA, which applies to children from birth to 3 years of age, requires that services be provided in the child's "natural environment," defined as the home or community settings in which children without disabilities participate (Sec. 303-18). Although some have interpreted this as a mandate from the federal government for children with hearing loss to receive services only in their homes or early childhood centers for children without hearing losses or disabilities, this should not be the case. Decisions regarding the services provided and the location of those services should be made on an individual basis by the IFSP team and include center-based services if the team agrees (NPRM, 65 Fed. Reg. 53807–53869, September 5, 2000).

Part B of IDEA applies to children from 3 years of age and older and indicates that services should be provided to the "maximum extent appropriate" in the "least restrictive environment" with children who are "not disabled." In determining placement, the IEP team must consider special communication factors for the child who is deaf or hard of hearing, including:

- Language and communication needs
- Opportunities for direct communication with peers and professional personnel in the child's language and communication mode
- Academic level and full range of needs including opportunities for direct instruction in the child's language and communication mode
- Assistive technology devices and services (IDEA 1997)

Programs that address communication needs of deaf and hard of hearing children may be found in a variety of settings. Location of the program is often an important consideration; however, many parents believe that communication modality is even more important (Meadow-Orlans et al., 2003). Whether the program is public or private or includes children with or without hearing losses or other special needs is less important than whether the environment is appropriate for meeting the individual communication and language needs of the child (Solit & Bednarczyk, 1999).

Professional Understandings and Practices

Regardless of the physical setting or model, programs should be staffed by professionals with knowledge and expertise in general education, education of individuals with hearing loss, early childhood education and development, families, and the impact of deafness on development (Joint Committee of ASHA/CED, 1994; Bodner-Johnson, 1994; Easterbrooks & Baker, 1994; JCIH, 2000; Sandall et al., 2000).

Professionals working with young children with hearing loss and their families should be proficient in the language and communication modes that provide the child with full access to communication. Professionals must be able to adapt and modify their communication to match the cognitive and linguistic abilities of the young child and provide appropriate scaffolding to support the child's development. Scaffolding techniques are especially effective with children whose home language or culture is different from others in the classroom and can be used to create a language learning environment that reduces frustration and increases motivation to take "safe risks" (Christensen, 2000). Although young children who are hearing acquire language naturally from parents and caregivers, children who are deaf and hard of hearing often depend on teachers and other professionals in addition to their parents and caregivers to acquire language (see Chapter 12). As experts in the area of communication, early education professionals not only provide support, information, and skill development to parents and caregivers, but they are also language models for young children.

Early Education Program Application Guidelines

Guidelines for early education programming for young children who are deaf and hard of hearing and their families have their roots in early intervention research, legislation, and professional guidelines and practices. Although individual and family characteristics vary and program and community resources differ, there are many aspects of programming that appear to be essential for advancing the best interests of young children who are deaf and hard of hearing and their families.

Family-Centered Programming Enhances Family Adaptation, Decision-Making, and Ability to Promote Child Development and Learning Family-centered programming begins with establishing relationships with families that recognize families as the primary caregivers and the natural, most effective agents for facilitating their child's development (Bodner-Johnson, Sass-Lehrer, Hafer, & Howell, 1992). Professionals should embrace an ecological and family system's perspective that promotes the strengthening of each family (Bodner-Johnson & Sass-Lehrer, 1999), and a collaborative decision making model that promotes family confidence and competence (Moeller & Condon, 1994).

Knowledge and Support Enhance Family Adaptation and Ability to Promote Child Development and Learning Professionals should provide comprehensive and unbiased information to families through a variety of formats (e.g., guest speakers, panel of "experts," informal discussion groups, observations, videotapes, workshops, Internet sites) compatible with adult learning perspectives, family preferences, and resources. Social support from a variety of sources including professionals, other parents with deaf children, family members, and friends promotes parental well-being and positively affects parent–child interaction, responsiveness, and child development (Calderon & Naidu, 2000; Dunst, 1999; MacTurk et al., 1993; Meadow-Orlans & Steinberg, 1993). Children benefit when parents and other caregivers feel supported.

Early Education Programs Should Promote Parent–Child and Family Communication and Early Language Acquisition   Enhancing communication among family members may be the most significant factor influencing positive outcomes in early intervention (Calderon, 2000; Moeller, 2001). Families need information and communication skills to ensure their children have consistent access to communication and the language models they need to support their acquisition of language. Adults who are deaf and hard of hearing in professional and paraprofessional roles can enhance the understanding of what it means to be deaf, promote positive expectations, and enhance the quality of communication within the family (Hintermair, 2000; Watkins et al., 1998).

Early Education Programming Must Incorporate Recommended Practices from Research, Legislation, and Professional Guidelines Early intervention and preschool programs are organized around sound early childhood developmental principles and adult learning theories and strategies. Programming is flexible and services reflect the unique strengths and needs of the child, along with the family's priorities, resources, and concerns. Professionals provide programming that is holistic, addressing all areas of development, while ensuring that the unique communication needs of the child and family are met (Sass-Lehrer & Bodner-Johnson, 2003). Expectations for development for children and families enrolled early in comprehensive early intervention programs are realistically high.

Early Education Programming and Services Are Based on Assessment and Outcome and Linked to the Curriculum   The identification of appropriate outcomes for children and families is enhanced when a family-centered and individualized assessment and evaluation approach is employed (Sandall et al., 2000). Assessments should be culturally sensitive and linguistically appropriate. Outcomes generated from these assessments are part of a linked system that informs the selection of goals and services and guides the evaluation of the child's progress. Progress is monitored closely and adaptations are incorporated to effect positive change in all areas of development.

Collaboration Supports Appropriate Early Intervention Programming   Collaboration among medical agencies, Part C coordinators, community service providers, and other professionals is critical to the provision of quality services to families and their children. Collaboration with medical and health care professionals ensures timely referrals to appropriate early intervention programs. Working collaboratively with community-based agencies and professionals from different disciplinary backgrounds provides families and their children with the expertise and support they need to address their individual, and often complex, needs.

Early Intervention Programs Must Support Professional Development to Provide the Highest Quality of Services to Families and Young Children Families with young children who are deaf or hard of hearing are best served by professionals who not only understand how to provide family-centered services, but who also understand deaf and hard of hearing children and their families' unique communication, social, and developmental challenges. Professionals include adults who are deaf and hard of hearing and other language and cultural models. Families should expect professionals to communicate fluently using the communication modality(ies) that provide their child with the best access to language. Professional development should be provided to ensure that professionals employ practices that are most likely to result in positive outcomes in all areas of development for children and their families (Sass-Lehrer, 2002).

FUTURE DIRECTIONS

The opportunities for young children with hearing loss and families are expanding rapidly due to the nearly universal realization of universal newborn hearing screening. Early intervention programs are scrambling to meet the increased demand for services. Research suggests that the power of early identification and intervention may go beyond the expectations of even the most ardent pioneers of newborn hearing screening. By channeling input to newborns with limited hearing through vision and touch and providing hearing aids or cochlear implants that maximize infants' potential to receive auditory information, young children with hearing loss may be expected to achieve language and other developmental milestones similar to their peers without hearing losses.

Programs and services for infants and toddlers with hearing losses and their families are strained by the increase in the number of newborns identified. Still, many children are left behind without access to screening programs, lack of follow-up, or limited access to quality early intervention (see Chapter 4). Professionals in early education programs who have become accustomed to working with toddlers are challenged to learn more about the infancy period in order to provide the most effective services. Professionals enter the lives of many families shortly after the birth of their child and need a heightened sensitivity and understanding of this very personal, and often challenging, time for families. Programs that primarily served families of young children with profound hearing losses are now serving many more young children with less severe hearing losses. This "new population" demands the development and evaluation of different strategies that are appropriate for these children and their families.

Families of young children who are transitioning into early education and school programs may be better communicators and advocates for their children than those families whose children were not identified until well after their first or even second birthdays. Longer stays in early intervention provide increased opportunities for families to develop an in-depth understanding of the issues and options for children and adults with hearing losses. This new generation of parents will challenge educators and the educational system, unaccustomed to families who are highly involved, and expect to continue as partners in the educational planning of their children.

Most significant will be the realized potential of children with hearing losses. With comprehensive and quality early intervention programs, educators will witness growing numbers of children with hearing losses with language and cognitive potentials approaching those of children without hearing losses. School programs will be expected to provide services that continue to promote development for these children and their families. Programs for children who are deaf and hard of hearing often struggle to make up critical time lost in the early years of life due to late identification and limited early intervention. The challenge of the future is to maintain the early advantages achieved through early identification and intervention by providing continued specialized services to children and support for their families throughout the school years.

REFERENCES

Apuzzo, M.L., & Yoshinaga-Itano, C. (1995). Early identification of infants with significant hearing loss and the Minnesota Child Development Inventory. *Seminars in Hearing, 16,* 124–139.

Arehart, K., & Yoshinaga-Itano, C. (1999). The role of educators of the deaf in the early identification of hearing loss. *American Annals of the Deaf, 144,* 19–23.

Bagnato, S., Neisworth, J.T., & Munson, S.M. (1997). *LINKing assessment and early intervention: An authentic curriculum-based approach.* Baltimore: Paul H. Brookes Publishing Co.

Bodner-Johnson, B. (1994). Preparation of early intervention personnel. In J. Roush & N. Matkin (Eds.), *Infants and toddlers with hearing loss: Family centered assessment and intervention* (pp. 319–336). Baltimore: York Press.

Bodner-Johnson, B., & Sass-Lehrer, M. (1999). Family-school relationships: Concepts and premises. In *Sharing ideas: A series of occasional papers.* Washington, DC: Laurent Clerc National Deaf Education Center. Available in print or on the web: http://clerccenter.gallaudet.edu/Products/Sharing-Ideas/family-school/family-school.html

Bodner-Johnson, B., Sass-Lehrer, M., Hafer, J., & Howell, R. (1992). *Family centered early intervention for deaf children: Guidelines for best practice.* Unpublished manuscript.

Bowe, F. (2000). *Birth to five: Early childhood special education* (2nd ed.). Albany, NY: Delmar.

Bredekamp, S., & Copple, C. (Eds.). (1997). *Developmentally appropriate practice in early childhood programs* (Rev. ed.). Washington, DC: National Association for the Education of Young Children.

Bricker, D. (with Pretti-Frontczak, K., & McComas, N.). (1998). *An activity-based approach to early intervention* (2nd ed.). Baltimore: Paul H. Brookes Publishing Co.

Calderon, R. (2000). Parent involvement in deaf children's education programs as a predictor of child's language, early reading, and social-emotional development. *Journal of Deaf Studies and Deaf Education, 5,* 140–155.

Calderon, R., Bargones, J., & Sidman, S. (1998). Characteristics of hearing families and their young deaf and hard of hearing children: Early intervention follow up. *American Annals of the Deaf, 143,* 347–362.

Calderon, R., & Greenberg, M. (1997). The effectiveness of early intervention for deaf children and children with hearing loss. In M.J. Guralnick (Ed.), *The effectiveness of early intervention* (pp. 445–482). Baltimore: Paul H. Brookes Publishing Co.

Calderon, R., & Greenberg, M. (2000). Challenges to parents and professionals in promoting socioemotional development in deaf children. In P. Spencer, C. Erting, & M. Marschark (Eds.), *The Deaf child in the family and at school: Essays in honor of Kathryn P. Meadow-Orlans* (pp. 167–185). Mahwah, NJ: Lawrence Erlbaum Associates.

Calderon, R., & Naidu, S. (2000). Further support for the benefits of early identification and intervention for children with hearing loss [Monograph]. In C. Yoshinaga-Itano & A. Sedey (Eds.), Language, speech, and social-emotional development of children who are deaf or hard of hearing: The early years. *The Volta Review, 100*(5), 53–84.

Carney, E.A., & Moeller, M.P. (1998). Treatment efficacy: Hearing loss in children. *Journal of Speech, Language and Hearing Research, 41,* 561–584.

Christensen, K. (2000). *Deaf plus: A multicultural perspective.* San Diego: Dawn Sign Press.

Cohen, O.P. (1993). Educational needs of African American and Hispanic deaf children and youth. In K. Christensen & G. Delgado (Eds.), *Multicultural issues in deafness* (pp. 45–67). White Plains, NY: Longman.

Cohen, O.P., Fischgrund, J., & Redding, R. (1990). Deaf children from ethnic, linguistic, and racial minority backgrounds: An overview. *American Annals of the Deaf, 135,* 69–78.

Commission on Education of the Deaf (1988). *Toward equality: Education of the deaf.* Washington, DC: U.S. Government Printing Office.

Departments of Labor, Health and Human Services, and Education, and Related Agencies Appropriations Act of 1999, PL 105-277, 112 Stat. 2681-337.

Dunst, C. (1999). Placing parent education in conceptual and empirical context. *Topics in Early Childhood Special Education, 19*(3), 141–147.

Easterbrooks, S., & Baker, S. (Eds.). (1994). *Deaf and hard of hearing students: Educational service guidelines.* Alexandria, VA: National Association of State Directors of Special Education.

Edwards, C., Gandini, L., & Forman, G. (Eds.). (1993). *The hundred languages of children: The Reggio Emilia approach to early childhood education.* Norwood, NJ: Ablex.

Education of the Handicapped Act Amendments of 1986, PL 99-457, 20 U.S.C. §§ 1400 *et seq.*

Feuerstein, R. (1980). *Instrumental enrichment: An intervention program for cognitive modifiability.* Baltimore: University Park Press.

Gardner, H. (1995). Reflections on multiple intelligences: Myths and messages. *Phi Delta Kappan, 77,* 200–209.

Gardner, H., & Hatch, T. (1989). Multiple intelligences go to school: Educational implications of the theory of multiple intelligences. *Educational Researcher, 18*(8), 4–10.

Gestwicki, C. (1999). *Developmentally appropriate practice: Curriculum and development in early education* (2nd ed.). Albany, NY: Delmar.

Goffin, S. (1994). *Curriculum models and early childhood education: Appraising the relationship.* New York: Merrill/Macmillan.

Greenberg, K.H. (1990). Mediated learning in the classroom. *Journal of Cognitive Education and Mediated Learning, 1,* 33–44.

Greenberg, M.T., Calderon, R., & Kusche, C. (1984). Early intervention using simultaneous communication with deaf infants: The effect on communication development. *Child Development, 55,* 607–616.

Guralnick, M.J. (1997). Second-generation research in the field of early intervention. In M.J. Guralnick (Ed.), *The effectiveness of early intervention* (pp. 3–20). Baltimore: Paul H. Brookes Publishing Co.

Hintermair, M. (2000). Hearing impairment, social networks, and coping: The need for families with hearing-impaired children to relate to other parents and to hearing-impaired adults. *American Annals of the Deaf, 145,* 41–51.

Hohmann, M., & Weikart, D.P. (1995). *Educating young children: Active learning practices for preschool and child care programs.* Ypsilanti, MI: High/Scope Press.

Iglesias, A., & Quinn, R. (1997). Culture as a context for early intervention. In S.K. Thurman, J.R. Cornwell, & S.R. Gottwald (Eds.), *Contexts of early intervention: Systems and settings* (pp. 55–71). Baltimore: Paul H. Brookes Publishing Co.

Individuals with Disabilities Education Act (IDEA) Amendments of 1997, PL 105-17, 20 U.S.C. §§ 1400 *et seq.*

Jamieson, J. (1995). Interactions between mothers and children who are deaf. *Journal of Early Intervention, 19,* 108–117.

Joint Committee of the American Speech-Language-Hearing Association and the Council on Education of the Deaf. (1994, August). Service provision under the Individuals with Disabilities Education Act-Part H, as amended (IDEA-Part H) to children who are deaf and hard of hearing ages birth to 36 months of age. *Asha, 36,* 117–121.

Joint Committee on Infant Hearing. (2000). Year 2000 position statement: Principles and guidelines for early hearing detection and intervention programs. *American Journal of Audiology, 9,* 9–29.

Kahn, R.J. (2000). Dynamic assessment of infants and toddlers. In J. Carlson (Series Ed.), C.S. Lidz, & J.G. Elliott (Vol. Eds.), *Advances in cognition and educational practice: Vol. 6. Dynamic assessment: Prevailing models and applications* (1st ed., pp. 325–373). New York: JAI Elsevier Science.

Linder, T.W. (1999). *Read, play, and learn!: Storybook activities for young children.* Baltimore: Paul H. Brookes Publishing Co.

MacTurk, R.H., Meadow-Orlans, K.P., Koester, L.S., & Spencer, P.E. (1993). Social support, motivation, language, and interaction: A longitudinal study of mothers and deaf infants. *American Annals of the Deaf, 138,* 19–25.

Marschark, M. (1997). *Raising and educating a deaf child.* New York: Oxford University Press.

McAnally, P.L., Rose, S., & Quigley, S.P. (1994). *Language learning practices with deaf children* (2nd ed.). Austin, TX: PRO-ED.

Meadow-Orlans, K., Mertens, D., & Sass-Lehrer, M. (2003). *Parents and their deaf children: The early years.* Washington, DC: Gallaudet University Press.

Meadow-Orlans, K., Mertens, D., Sass-Lehrer, M., & Scott-Olson, K. (1997). Support services for parents and their children who are deaf and hard of hearing: A national survey. *American Annals of the Deaf, 142*(4), 278–293.

Meadow-Orlans, K., & Sass-Lehrer, M. (1995). Support services for families of children who are deaf: Challenges for professionals. *Topics in Early Childhood Special Education, 15*(3), 314–334.

Meadow-Orlans, K., Smith-Gray, S., & Dyssegaard, B. (1995). Infants who are deaf or hard of hearing with and without physical/cognitive disabilities. *American Annals of the Deaf, 140,* 279–286.

Meadow-Orlans, K., & Steinberg, A., (1993). Effects of infant hearing loss and maternal support on mother-infant interactions at 18 months. *Journal of Applied Developmental Psychology, 14,* 407–426.

Mitchell, L., & Philibert, D.B. (2002). Family, professional, and political advocacy: Rights and responsibilities. *Young Exceptional Children, 5*(4), 11–18.

Moeller, M.P. (2000). Early intervention and language development in children who are deaf and hard of hearing. *Pediatrics, 106*(3), E43.

Moeller, M.P. (2001). Intervention and outcomes for young children who are deaf and hard of hearing and their families. In E. Kurtzer-White & D. Luterman (Eds.), *Early childhood deafness* (pp. 111–138). Baltimore: York Press.

Moeller, M.P., & Condon, M. (1994). D.E.I.P. A collaborative problem-solving approach to early intervention. In J. Roush & N. Matkin (Eds.), *Infants and toddlers with hearing loss: Family-centered assessment and intervention* (pp. 163–192). Baltimore: York Press.

Mohay, H. (2000). Language in sight: Mothers' strategies for making language visually accessible to deaf children. In P. Spencer, C. Erting, & M. Marschark (Eds.), *The deaf child in the family and at school: Essays in honor of Kathryn P. Meadow-Orlans* (pp. 151–166). Mahwah, NJ: Lawrence Erlbaum Associates.

Notice of Proposed Rulemaking (NPRM) on the Early Intervention Program for Infants and Toddlers with Disabilities, 65 Fed. Reg. 53807–53869, September 5, 2000.

Sandall, S., McLean, M., & Smith, B. (2000). *DEC recommended practices in early intervention/early childhood special education.* Longmont, CO: Sopris West.

Sass-Lehrer, M. (2002). Early beginnings for families with deaf and hard of hearing children: Myths and facts of early intervention and guidelines for effective services. Washington, DC: Laurent Clerc National Deaf Education Center, Kids World Deaf Net. Retrieved February 10, 2003 from http://clerc center2.gallaudet.edu/KidsWorldDeafNet/e-docs/EI/index.html

Sass-Lehrer, M., & Bodner-Johnson, B. (2003). Early intervention: Current approaches to family-centered programming. In M. Marschark & P. Spencer (Eds.), *Handbook of deaf studies, language and education* (pp. 65–81). New York: Oxford University Press.

Sass-Lehrer, M., Gerner de Garcia, B., & Rovins, M. (1997). Creating a multicultural school climate for deaf children and their families. In *Sharing ideas: A series of occasional papers*. Washington, DC: Laurent Clerc National Deaf Education Center. Available in print or on the web: http://clerccenter.gal laudet.edu/Products/Sharing-Ideas/creating/

Sass-Lehrer, M., Mertens, D.M., & Meadow-Orlans, K. (2001). *Experiences of families with young children who are deaf and hard of hearing: Implications for professional preparation.* San Diego: Association of College Educators-Deaf/Hard of Hearing.

Solit, G., & Bednarczyk, A. (1999). *Issues in access: Creating effective preschools for deaf, hard of hearing, and hearing children.* Washington, DC: Gallaudet University Press.

Spencer, P., Bodner-Johnson, B., & Gutfreund, M. (1992). Interacting with infants with a hearing loss: What can we learn from mothers who are deaf? *Journal of Early Intervention, 16,* 64–78.

Watkins, S., & Clark, T. (1992). *The SKI-HI model: A resource manual for family-centered, home-based programming for infants, toddler, and preschool-aged children with hearing impairment* (2nd ed.). Logan, UT: HOPE.

Watkins, S., Pittman, P., & Walden, B. (1998). The deaf mentor experimental project for young children who are deaf and their families. *American Annals of the Deaf, 143*(1), 29–34.

Wilbur, R.B. (2000). The use of ASL to support the development of English literacy. *Journal of Deaf Studies and Deaf Education, 5*(1), 81–104.

Yoshinaga-Itano, C. (2000). Successful outcomes for deaf and hard of hearing children. *Seminars in Hearing, 21,* 309–325.

Yoshinaga-Itano, C. (2003). From screening to early identification and intervention: Discovering predictors to successful outcomes for children with significant hearing loss. *Journal of Deaf Studies and Deaf Education, 8*(11), 11–30.

Yoshinaga-Itano, C., & Sedey, A. (2000). Early speech development in children who are deaf or hard of hearing: Interrelationships with language and hearing [Monograph]. In C. Yoshinaga-Itano & A. Sedey (Eds.), Language, speech, and social-emotional development of children who are deaf or hard of hearing: The early years. *The Volta Review, 100*(5), 181–211.

Yoshinaga-Itano, C., Sedey, A.L., Coulter, D.K., & Mehl, A.L. (1998). The language of early- and later-identified children with hearing loss. *Pediatrics, 102,* 1161–1171.

Reflections on an Interview with Debra Cushner and Helen Sweetney

Marilyn Sass-Lehrer

Parents, caregivers, grandparents, aunts, uncles, infants, and toddlers are on the floor playing at the bi-weekly parent–infant program play-group at the Kendall Demonstration Elementary School (KDES). Adults are playing with their own children, sometimes they are play-ing with another child, often they are just chatting with each other. This is a diverse group that includes families from different countries, many of whom are using languages other than English. The families are rich, poor, hearing, deaf, and hard of hearing. It's often difficult to distinguish the parents from the professionals.

In the room is the parent–infant teacher, Debbie; the assistant teacher, Helen; a sign language interpreter; and Spanish, Russian, or Bengali language interpreters, depending on the families present. Sometime during the morning, the audiologist, the speech/communi-cation specialist, the occupational therapist, and the sign language specialist join the group.

The professionals move around the room complimenting the parents on their interactions or new signs or techniques they are using with their children. They applaud the children's newly acquired skills and progress and share personal comments or pass on an observation. To an outsider, the activity seems a bit chaotic. But, after a few minutes, the experienced observer recognizes that the apparent chaos is actually well-orchestrated with careful attention to many details.

The playgroup is only one part of the KDES Parent–Infant Program's comprehensive services for families with children who are deaf and hard of hearing. The program includes twice weekly parent–child play groups, including bi-monthly parent "open-discussion" sessions or presentations by specialists. Families may receive visits at home, visits at their child care centers, or visits at the parents or caregivers' places of work at a time and frequency that works well for the family.

Debbie describes the program philosophy as family centered, evolving over time with input from families. Parents understand that they are truly partners and share ownership of the program. The overall goal of the program is simple: to develop families' confidence and competence in providing for their child. Everything is directed toward this purpose.

Debbie says the program is about relationships and understanding where families are coming from. She tries to put herself in each parent or caregiver's shoes and imagine how she might feel if she had an infant with a special need. "I'm shy," she says. "If it were me, I might be sitting in the parking lot crying. After gathering up enough nerve to come in, how would it feel to walk into this room full of strangers, with different languages being spoken and hands flying?" She tries to imagine how she might feel if she were a recent immigrant from Bangladesh with a newborn who has a hearing loss. How would she feel if she were a grandmother who "inherited" primary responsibility for her deaf granddaughter? What would she want from early intervention if she were an attorney with a very busy practice and three children, one of whom is a toddler who is hard of hearing and has a visual impairment? Or, what might it be like for a Deaf parent with an infant whose hearing loss seems to fluctuate from moderate to profound? Imagining how each family feels helps her respond empathetically.

Debbie says that hearing parents often think they are already behind. They worry that they will never be able to learn to sign, that they won't be able to catch up. Her first goal is to make families feel comfortable. Debbie describes herself as a good listener. She says it's important to give parents time. Beginning an early intervention program can be very overwhelming, and many parents need time to adjust. She wants to get to know every family and let them get to know her. The relationship, Debbie says, must go both ways. She also wants to help parents get to know each other, make connections, and feel supported. One of her favorite expressions is, "How can we work together?"

Central to accomplishing this goal is a strong, competent, and supportive interdisciplinary team who enjoys working with adults and young children. The team is diverse in hearing status, ethnicity, and age. Helen, for example, is an African American hearing mother who has a son who is deaf, and now a grandmother of eight including one grandson who is deaf. Together, the team provides an environment that is welcoming, comfortable, and nurturing. A key to the success of the program is the team's flexibility. Despite a well-planned schedule, it is impossible to predict what issues will pop up on any given day. The team is always prepared to alter their schedules to accommodate the families and children. For example, from time to time a parent arrives with a suspicion that his or her child has an ear infection, and Debbie or Helen will go with the parent to see the audiologist. Parents also "pitch in." Debbie recalls a time when the sign language specialist was unavailable and a parent who is deaf quickly volunteered to take over story time.

The room is set up with several play areas, each designed to encourage adult–child interaction, and all activities and materials are developmentally appropriate for young children. There are books strategically positioned all over the room so no one is ever far from one. The room has a comfortable couch, rocking chair, and other soft, cozy areas for the tired or difficult-to-console child. There are books, catalogs, videos, and notices about upcoming events for parents. There is always at least one pet in the room—most recently, tropical fish. The room is cheery, brightly lit, and colorful with pictures and posters on the walls and mobiles hanging from the ceiling. Toys and furniture are thoughtfully arranged to allow easy movement from one area of the room to another. Visibility to all parts of the room is a priority in the room arrangement.

Open and accessible communication is essential to the success of this program. Sign and spoken language interpreters are always available to facilitate communication between deaf and hearing adults. Parents are encouraged to sign, and sign language interpreters are there to be sure that nobody's message is ever lost. Spoken language interpreters do more than interpret the spoken language, they often double as cultural mediators, helping both parents and professionals understand each other's traditions and views. One mother from Bangladesh explained through an interpreter that body language and gestures were not viewed positively by her culture. Using her hands to communicate felt awkward to her. However, as time went on, and she developed a special relationship with one of the deaf parents in the program, she began signing with more comfort, even in front of the group.

Debbie says that she feels like she is throwing a party every Tuesday and Thursday as she prepares for the play group. Food is an important ingredient that encourages conversation and makes everyone feel comfortable. There is always a pot of coffee and tea ready, and parents take turns bringing snacks for the adults to share. Parents begin arriving around 9:30 in the morning. From 9:30 until about 10:15, parents and children play in all areas of the room while professionals circulate and visit with each family. Debbie makes a point of talking individually with every parent during this time. Around 10:15, the lights flash and everyone knows that it's time for the "surprise box." Every week, a special toy or activity is presented in the "surprise box." This activity is followed by time to wash up before snack, then, weather permitting, everyone goes outside to play.

Twice a month, parents leave the room for an adult "open discussion" session or presentation on a topic of their choosing. The sessions function as a support group with parents sharing concerns as well as triumphs and receiving guidance and encouragement from the others. Debbie regularly shares information about upcoming events at school and in the community. Parents also make announcements or share information with the group, for example, the announcement of a new infant, a child's first steps, an upcoming birthday, or the discovery of a great toy or helpful book or video.

American Sign Language (ASL) story time is at 11:30. The story is told as much for the parents as it is for the children so that parents may develop the skills they need to retell the story at home. A video of each story is made, and parents take turns taking the video home to watch and re-watch so they can learn to sign the story themselves. By noon, most parents are on their way home; however, it's not unusual to see parents stay past noon. Some parents even bring lunch and stay to chat with Debbie and Helen.

On the surface, there are elements of this program that are commonplace: play time, group activity, snack, and story time. However, there is a sense of community in this program that is unusual. The team often develops close relationships with families, and it is not unusual to see professionals show up at birthday parties, baby showers, or other family events.

Debbie believes it is important that every parent leaves the playgroup feeling their needs were met. Whether it was time to speak to the audiologist about their child's hearing aid or meet with the ASL specialist to review a few signs, parents and caregivers leave with something. Debbie and Helen check in with each parent or caregiver before they leave to say something positive that they noticed about their child over the course of the morning. The good-bye is as important in this program as the welcome. Helen talks about the "power of the hug." She says, "We don't just say hello or good-bye here, we give everyone a big hug."

CHAPTER SEVEN

Evaluation of Early Intervention Programs

DONNA M. MERTENS, LINDA DELK, AND LISA WEIDEKAMP

I n 1973, my Head Start project that included children with disabilities was located in a small preschool 50 miles into the swamps of Florida. In the second year of the project, we were informed that we would be evaluated. I had no idea what the evaluation questions would be. I dutifully prepared everything I could think of, including a list of the places where letters and materials had been sent. I thought they might ask why we spent so much on postage. At least it seemed like a lot to me. My preparation efforts resulted in three boxes of materials and controlled anxiety on my part. The evaluation results were "fine," and our funding continued. But I really wanted to know how to improve our services and how to reach families that did not participate in the program. (Margaret Hallau, Director of the National Outreach, Research, and Evaluation Network [NOREN], Laurent Clerc National Deaf Education Center, Gallaudet University)

The 1997 amendments to the Individuals with Disabilities Education Act (IDEA; PL 105-17) contain provisions that ensure services for infants and young children with disabilities; these amendments emphasize families and fostering parent–professional partnerships in early intervention programs. As the early intervention field has begun to adapt to this emphasis on family involvement, so too have program evaluation efforts.

Evaluation of early intervention programs involves systematic inquiry to determine the effectiveness of those programs. Program evaluations may examine what works and what does not work in various settings, under various conditions, and with various people. These questions can be asked at different stages in the planning, development, and implementation of early intervention programs. For example, during the planning stage of a program, parents and professionals might ask what type of assessment is needed. When the program is operational and established, parents and professionals might ask what outcomes the program actually achieves with children and their families.

This chapter is intended to assist program decision makers, practitioners, and other stakeholders in early childhood education in planning, implementing, and using the results of program evaluations. This chapter also outlines the steps involved in planning and conducting an inclusive evaluation. Emphasis is placed on the importance of generating a comprehensive list of stakeholders, with special efforts to include those who have been traditionally under-represented. Throughout this chapter, the evaluation of the Shared Reading Project is used to illustrate many of the principles and strategies involved in an inclusive evaluation (Delk & Weidekamp, 2001).[1] This chapter includes options for developing or selecting performance indicators, data collection strategies, standards for assessing the quality of the evaluation, and guidelines for making ethical choices in the planning and conducting of an evaluation. Finally, future developments in evaluation are explored.

DESCRIPTION OF THE SHARED READING PROJECT

The Shared Reading Project is designed to provide hearing parents and caregivers with visually based strategies to read books to their children who are deaf and hard of hearing, age birth through age 8. David Schleper, Jane Fernandes, and Doreen Higa first began the Shared Reading Project

---

[1]This project of the Laurent Clerc National Deaf Education Center at Gallaudet University in Washington, D.C., was evaluated by a team of six internal evaluators, including Linda Delk and Lisa Weidekamp, two co-authors of this chapter.

at the Hawaii Center for the Deaf and the Blind in 1993. Subsequently, the program was implemented at the Kendall Demonstration Elementary School (KDES) on the Gallaudet University campus in Washington, D.C., where it has been in operation ever since. In 1997–1998, other schools and organizations began receiving training and setting up their own Shared Reading Projects.

The Project is based on 15 book-sharing principles derived from research about how adults who are deaf read books to young children who are deaf (Schleper, 1997). The project's developers intend the Shared Reading Project to be implemented as follows: A trained Shared Reading tutor (most of the tutors are deaf) visits the family once a week with a book bag. Each book bag includes a storybook, a videotape of the story in American Sign Language, an activity guide, and a bookmark printed with book-sharing tips. The tutor coaches the parents or caregivers on how to sign the books to their young children who are deaf or hard of hearing. The family keeps the book bag and practices reading the book to their children between tutor visits. Each week for 20 weeks the tutor brings a new book bag to the family.

The short-term goals for families participating in the Shared Reading Project are improving parent–child communication and increasing the children's interest in sharing books, as well as increasing the time parents spend reading to their children who are deaf and hard of hearing, and family enjoyment of shared books. The long-term goals are for the children to become better readers in school and to improve their academic achievement.

Programs that implement the Shared Reading Project experience costs related to administrative support; hiring, training, and supervision of tutors; recruitment and orientation of traditionally underserved families; purchase, maintenance, and distribution of book bag components; interpreting and translation services; and program evaluation. Programs seeking external start-up funds must consider the requirements of funding agencies as well as expectations of internal program administrators.

PROGRAM EVALUATION

Professionals, parents, advocates, and policy makers are in general agreement as to principles and values that underlie the provision of early intervention services to children who are deaf or hard of hearing and their families (Guralnick, 1997). Because the early years constitute a unique opportunity for influencing child development and supporting families, Guralnick described an emerging consensus among these groups regarding society's responsibility to provide needed early intervention programs for children with disabilities. Guralnick also described a set of broad principles that can be used to guide early intervention programs, such as placing importance on the needs of the family, basing the intervention program in the local community, and coordinating services from numerous agencies. However, this awareness of societal responsibility does not give practitioners or the families they serve specific information about developing and providing effective programs, nor does it give specific information about how to best match the characteristics of the program to those of the children and families in order to yield optimal development outcomes. The only way to acquire this information is through a program evaluation.

Program evaluation has long been defined as a systematic method of investigating the merit or worth of a program or system for the purpose of reducing uncertainty in decision making (Mertens, 1998; Scriven, 1995). Historically, evaluation has focused on the information needs of the top level of decision makers, such as funders and program administration. However, many leaders in the field recognize that this top-down approach to evaluation leaves the voices of important constituencies unheard or inaccurately represented (Chelimsky, 1998; Mertens, 1998, 1999; Weiss, 1998). Effective program evaluation incorporates the perspectives and voices of all the people who are involved in or affected by the program, including those who have been traditionally excluded from decisions about the program evaluation itself, such as parents, individuals with disabilities, and local program staff. This recognition spurred the development of the inclusive approach to evaluation.

The inclusive approach to evaluation emphasizes the accurate and credible representation of marginalized groups in and through the process of systematic inquiry (Mertens, 1999). The goal of inclusive evaluation shifts from that of presenting credible data to decision makers, to that of providing such data to enhance the possibility of social change for the least advantaged. It involves a shift in power from the program administration to include those served by the program and sometimes those who are denied access to it. From the perspective of social transformation, knowledge is not neutral but is influenced by human interests. All knowledge reflects the power and social relationships within society. An important purpose of knowledge construction, including the information generated by program evaluation, is to help people transform and improve society (Banks, 1995).[2]

Inclusive evaluation is particularly appropriate for use in the context of family-centered early intervention programs for infants and toddlers who are deaf and hard of hearing. The National Association for the Education of Young Children (NAEYC) supports active participation of all "stakeholders" in the evaluation process. NAEYC's accreditation criteria (1998) require annual program and staff evaluations of early intervention programs that involve all interested parties, including children where appropriate.

STEPS IN CONDUCTING AN INCLUSIVE EVALUATION

Six steps are generally useful in planning an evaluation (Mertens, 1998). These steps should not be viewed as a linear process, but rather as a cyclical, iterative framework in which each step is revisited throughout the planning process. This allows the evaluation to be more responsive to various information needs as they are revealed through the planning process. Early intervention program staff need to decide whether they will hire an external evaluator to plan and implement the evaluation or have someone on the staff undertake the responsibility (an internal evaluator). Larger programs may even utilize a team of evaluators, made up of both internal and external evaluators. The following six steps are relevant to both internal and external evaluators, although different issues arise depending on the relationship between the program staff and the evaluator.

---

[2]The following references are provided to readers interested in pursuing the theoretical and philosophical assumptions of the transformative paradigm of research and that underlie the practice of inclusive evaluation. The transformative paradigm's central tenet is that evaluation and research should be conducted with the goal of transforming for the better the lives of those who experience discrimination and oppression. Inclusive evaluation shares the same theoretical underpinnings as research and evaluation perspectives termed emancipatory (Clough & Barton, 1998; Lather, 1992; Mertens 1998), anti-discriminatory (Humphries & Truman, 1994; Truman, Mertens, & Humphries, 2000), participatory (DeKoning & Martin, 1996; Reason, 1994; Whitmore, 1998), and Freirian approaches (McLaren & Lankshear, 1994). It is exemplified in the writings of feminists (Alcoff & Potter, 1993; Fine, 1992; Hill-Collins, 2000; Reinharz, 1992), racial/ethnic minorities (Madison, 1992; Stanfield, 1999; Stanfield & Dennis, 1993), people with disabilities (Clough & Barton, 1998; Gill, 1999; Mertens & McLaughlin, 2003; Oliver, 1992), and people who work on behalf of marginalized groups. The common characteristic of these approaches is their emphasis on the importance of seeking out the social constructions of reality as expressed by members of oppressed groups. The approaches are differentiated based on the aspects of oppression that are most central (i.e., class, sex, race/ethnicity, disability, or sexual orientation).

STEP 1: FOCUSING THE EVALUATION

Focusing the evaluation involves describing the program to be evaluated, identifying the stakeholders to be included in the evaluation, describing the purpose of the evaluation, and determining the resources needed and the constraints within which the evaluation will take place.

Describing the Program

The evaluator needs to determine what it is that is being evaluated—usually it is a program or part of a program—and develop a description of the program's characteristics and how the program being evaluated is intended to work. The evaluator gathers information about the nature, status, and scope of the program to be evaluated. Is it a new or well-established program? Or, is it just an idea that has not yet been implemented? Does the entire program or just selected components need to be evaluated? Other aspects that might be considered in the evaluation of early intervention programs include child or family functioning, staff performance, educational materials, transition practices, center-based environments, parent participation, curriculum, program expenditures, and community programming needs (Sandall, McLean, & Smith, 2000).

Describing the program to be evaluated can be challenging. The following questions can guide the process of program description (Mertens, 1998):

1. Is there a written description of the program (e.g., program descriptions in brochures or reports)?

2. What is the status of the program? Is the program relatively stable and mature, new, or developing? How long has the program been providing services (This information can come from program reports or legislative directives.)?

3. In what context will (or does) the program function (e.g., public school, social services agency, hospital)?

4. Who is the program designed to serve (e.g., families, deaf and hard of hearing children, children of a certain age range)?

5. How does the program work? How is it supposed to work (e.g., early intervention visits to homes, materials given to families)?

6. What is the program supposed to do (e.g., increase hearing aid use, stimulate language development)?

7. What resources are being put into the program (e.g., funding, time, staff, materials)?

8. What outcomes are expected? How can these outcomes be evaluated? What outcomes actually occur (e.g., language development, social-emotional growth)?

9. Why is the program being evaluated (e.g., to initiate a new service, to improve an existing one)?

10. Whose description of the program is needed to get a full understanding of the program to be evaluated (e.g., program staff, families served or not served)?

One way to depict the program description is through the use of a program logic model. The logic model provides a roadmap of the program that highlights how it is expected to work, what activities need to come before others, and how desired outcomes are achieved (W.K. Kellogg Foundation, 1998). Early childhood programs typically involve many different activities and intended outcomes. A program logic model helps to describe a program by portraying the theory or rationale and assumptions that underlie the program, as well as linking program outcomes (short- or long-term, real or intended) with program activities and processes.

The logic model is developed by reviewing relevant program documents and related literature, observing the program in action, and discussing the program with relevant stakeholders (Mertens, 1998). Different individuals with different relationships to the program may view the program in various ways. It is important to share these differences in order to develop a shared understanding among stakeholders of what the program is intended to do and how it works; this increases the chances that the program depicted in the logic model accurately describes the functioning program.

A sample logic model for the Shared Reading Project is presented in Figure 7.1. The project evaluators developed the logic model based on conversations with the project developers, reviewing published articles about the project, and project documentation. The logic model illustrates the complex sequence of activities that are expected to lead to improved literacy skills among children who are deaf. The interactive process used to develop the model was useful in raising questions concerning the appropriate focus of different phases of the evaluation and selection of process indicators and outcome measures.

The iterative nature of the planning process becomes apparent when describing a program. At first, program description might seem like a simple task; however, the description of the program will evolve as different sources are consulted, including program documentation, literature related to the program, developers' views of the program, observations of the program in action, and perceptions of representatives of different stakeholder groups.

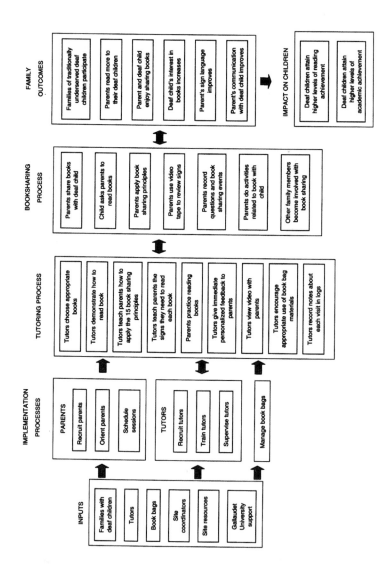
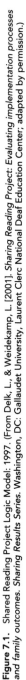

Figure 7.1. Shared Reading Project Logic Model: 1997. (From Delk, L., & Weidekamp, L. [2001]. *Sharing Reading Project: Evaluating implementation processes and family outcomes. Sharing Results Series.* Washington, DC: Gallaudet University, Laurent Clerc National Deaf Education Center; adapted by permission.)

Identifying Stakeholders

As mentioned previously, the development of the logic model requires conversations with key stakeholder groups. However, once the logic model has reached at least a preliminary state of stability, it is important to generate a complete list of the stakeholders who will be involved in or affected by the evaluation. A stakeholder is any person who has a stake in the outcomes of the evaluation. Because the philosophy of the early intervention initiative supports active participation of all stakeholders in the evaluation, it is important that an inclusive list of stakeholders is generated, with special efforts to include those who have been traditionally underrepresented.

The following questions help ensure that the list of stakeholders is inclusive (Mertens, 1998):

1. Who is involved in the administration and implementation of the program?
2. Who are the intended beneficiaries?
3. Who has been excluded as being eligible for participation in the program?
4. Who stands to gain or lose from the evaluation results?
5. Which individuals and groups have power in this setting? Which do not?
6. Did the program planning and evaluation planning involve those with marginalized lives?
7. Who is representative of the people with the least power?
8. What opportunities exist for mutual sharing between the evaluators and those without power?
9. What opportunities exist for the people without power to criticize the evaluation and influence future directions?
10. Is there appropriate representation on the basis of gender, ethnicity, disability, and income levels?

Some stakeholder groups to consider include sponsors and funders, governing and advisory boards, state and federal level agency representatives, policymakers, administrators (at various levels), staff members, children, parents and other caregivers of children, grassroots organization representatives in the community, and public community representatives. The primary stakeholders for the Shared Reading Project, for example, included the administrators and Shared Reading Project staff of the Clerc Center, external oversight groups for the Clerc Center, program administrators at new project sites, tutors, and deaf and hard of hearing children and their families. Because the Shared Reading Project was targeted at traditionally underserved groups, important stakeholders at each project site included hearing families with deaf and hard of hearing

children who were members of diverse ethnocultural groups, had secondary disabilities, lived in rural areas, or used a language other than English
in the home.

Deciding on the Purpose of the Evaluation

Description of the program, including development of a logic model, can
help to focus the purpose of the evaluation. With program ideas that are
just beginning to be developed, the evaluation may take the form of a
needs assessment: What are the goals that need to be addressed? What
resources are required to accomplish the goals? With new programs,
one might be interested in evaluating what areas need to be improved
(formative evaluation). Or, with more established programs, the focus
might be on whether the intended outcomes of the program are being
achieved.

Consider alternative interests of key stakeholders when deciding on
the purpose of the evaluation. Who are the audiences for information
generated by the evaluation? How will they access and use the evaluation
information? How can evaluation activities be designed to facilitate the
discussion and intended use of the evaluation results? In early intervention programs, evaluations might be used to make decisions about an
individual program; formalize policy; determine the viability of implementing a new program; determine who is and is not benefiting from the
program; modify and improve program practices; determine how funds
should be allocated; support the continuation, expansion, or discontinua-
tion of a program; or demonstrate accountability or cost-effectiveness.

Evaluators talk about a multiplicity of possible purposes of evaluations. Three possible types of purposes include context, implementation,
and outcome evaluation. *Context evaluation* examines the influence of
the context within which the program functions, such as the project
setting and the economic, social, cultural, and political environment of
the surrounding community. In planning a new program or planning an
expansion or a revision of an existing program, the purpose of the evaluation might be viewed as a needs assessment. A needs assessment reviews
the needs, assets, and resources of target families in order to plan relevant
and effective interventions within the context of their community. If the
program has been running for a year or so and it is encountering difficulties in continuing to serve the target population, then the purpose of
the evaluation might be an organizational assessment. An organizational
assessment focuses on identifying the political, social, and administrative
strengths and weaknesses of both the community and the project.

Implementation evaluation examines the processes of the program, including planning, setting up, carrying out, and evolution of a
program. An implementation evaluation is designed to provide information about how the program is actually operating compared with how

it is intended to operate and why certain goals are or are not being accomplished. Implementation evaluations also help program leaders make decisions about the allocation of resources within the program.

Outcome evaluation examines the short- and long-term results of the program. Outcomes can be reviewed at the child, family, program, organization, or community level. Although certain types of evaluations receive greater emphasis at different stages of the program, most evaluation plans include some attention to program context, implementation issues, and outcomes. The following questions can be used among stakeholders to discuss the purpose of their evaluation (Mertens, 1998):

1. What is the purpose of the evaluation?
2. What events triggered the need for the evaluation?
3. What is the intended use of the evaluation findings?
4. Who will use the findings and for what purpose?
5. Whose views should be represented in the statement of evaluation purpose?

THE PURPOSE OF THE SHARED READING PROJECT PROGRAM EVALUATION

The Shared Reading Project was evaluated at five program sites to determine if anticipated short-term results with families were achieved and how the project was actually implemented in diverse types of settings serving different target populations. This information was needed by the Clerc Center project staff to assist in developing a site coordinator training course, which would enable other schools and organizations to start their own Shared Reading Projects. Information about how Shared Reading was implemented was also needed for the planning of later evaluation of the long-term impact of the project on the academic reading skills of students who are deaf and hard of hearing. Therefore, this evaluation was an inquiry into 1) the different contexts in which the Shared Reading Project was implemented, 2) how the project was actually being implemented compared with the program logic model, and 3) the achievement of short-term family book sharing outcomes.

Resources and Constraints of an Evaluation

The final step in the initial focusing of the evaluation plan is to identify resources that are available and constraints that may affect how the evaluation is conducted. Types of resources and constraints can be identified by considering the following issues (Mertens, 1998):

- Money: How much money is budgeted for the evaluation?
- Family: What cultural or language issues must be addressed? How will confidentiality of information be assured?
- Time: When do the results of the evaluation have to be ready for decisions that need to be made?
- Personnel: How much time can stakeholders give to the evaluation activities?
- Existing data: What data are already collected that could be used for the evaluation?
- Politics: Who would benefit if this program were eliminated?
- Legislation: What does the legislation require the program to do?

Evaluations are always conducted in a political environment. For example, many political issues are well documented in the deaf community related to communication choices and educational placement decisions (Meadow-Orlans, 2000). Sensitivity to political issues is important throughout the process of planning and implementing the evaluation. Therefore, establishing acceptable lines of communication among project staff, decision makers, project participants, evaluators, and other key stakeholders is important at the beginning of the evaluation.

RESOURCES AND CONSTRAINTS IN THE SHARED READING PROJECT

The 1992 Amendments to the Education of the Deaf Act (PL 102-421) charged the Clerc Center with developing and evaluating programs and strategies that meet the educational needs of five groups of traditionally underserved deaf and hard of hearing students, including members of diverse ethnocultural groups, students who have secondary disabilities, students who live in rural areas, students who come from homes in which a spoken language other than English is used, and students who are lower achieving academically. Following this legislative mandate, the Shared Reading Project was designed to meet the needs of these target populations. The evaluation inquired into the extent to which programs were successful in recruiting families of traditionally underserved children who are deaf and hard of hearing to participate in the Shared Reading Project.

Describing the program (logic model), compiling an inclusive stakeholder list, deciding on a purpose, and determining resources and constraints are important components of the first step in the evaluation planning process. Before moving to Step 2, it is important for the evaluator to share the focused part of the plan in a synthesized form with the stakeholder groups and ask for feedback.

STEP 2: CLARIFYING THE EVALUATION QUESTIONS

The statement of purpose for the evaluation can provide a guide for the development of the evaluation questions. Developing the evaluation questions can involve holding brainstorming sessions with stakeholder groups, borrowing questions from previous evaluation studies, or generating questions through a theoretical framework that is relevant to the study. The *W.K. Kellogg Foundation Handbook* (W.K. Kellogg Foundation, 1998) suggests possible evaluation questions that correspond to the three components of evaluation: context, implementation, and outcome evaluation. The following list of questions may be helpful in developing evaluation questions. They are adapted from sample questions from the *W.K. Kellogg Foundation Handbook,* the U.S. General Accounting Office (Shipman, MacColl, Vaurio, & Chennareddy, 1995), and Mertens's textbook on research and evaluation methods (1998).

Sample Context Questions

Context questions ask about factors in the program content that relate to identifying needs for a new, expanded, or revised program (needs assessment) or identifying strengths or weaknesses in the community or program (organizational assessment). Examples of needs assessment questions include

- What are the needs and gaps in services in the community?
- What strengths and opportunities exist in the community?
- What are the differences in perceptions of diverse groups regarding the needs and gaps in services and the strengths and opportunities in the community?

Examples of organizational assessment questions include

- What financial, physical space, and other cooperative or administrative relationships influence the program functioning? Are these adequate?
- How does the leadership and organizational structure of the project influence its effectiveness? What are the characteristics of the project staff and leadership? What resources (e.g., funding, staffing, organizational and/or institutional support, expertise, educational opportunities) are available to the project?

- To what extent are opportunities available for diverse stakeholders to participate in the evaluation?

Sample Implementation Questions

Implementation questions tell how and to what extent activities have been implemented as intended and whether they are targeted to appropriate populations or problems. Examples of implementation questions include

- What strategies or activities for the program are being implemented? Which are not? Why or why not?
- Which project operations work well? Which aren't working? Why or why not? Is the program reaching its intended audience? Why or why not? What changes must be made to reach intended audiences more effectively?
- Does the program conform to the intended program model or to professional standards of practice?

Sample Outcome Questions

Outcome questions address the program effects. Examples at various levels of outcomes and impact include

Individual Family- or Child-Level Outcomes

- What changes occurred in family communication, circumstances, status, quality of life or functioning, attitude or behavior, knowledge, and skills as a result of participating in this program? How did the impact or outcomes vary across participants and approaches? What changes occurred in the families' perceptions of the early intervention program?
- What other important effects relate to the program (side effects)? What unforeseen effects came from the program (either positive or negative) on problems or individuals it was designed to address?
- How does the program compare with an alternative strategy for achieving the same ends?

Program- and System-Level Outcomes

- How has the program had an impact on shared decision-making processes among relevant stakeholders?
- How has the program had an impact on the efficiency of provision of services to deaf and hard of hearing children and their families?

Broader Family and Community Outcomes

• How has the program affected increased parent–child–program interactions (e.g., kept children safe from neglect or abuse)?

• How has the program affected community involvement and participation, shifted authority and responsibility to community-based agencies and community resident groups, or provided more intensive collaboration among community agencies and institutions?

Impacts on Organizations

• How have the lives and career directions of project staff been affected by the program? What new skills have the staff acquired?

• Are collaborations among agencies strengthened?

EVALUATION QUESTIONS
FOR THE SHARED READING PROJECT

1. How was the Shared Reading Project implemented at each site? How did the unique contexts and resources at each site facilitate or impede implementation of the Project?

2. To what extent did families of traditionally underserved children who are deaf or hard of hearing participate in the Project?
   a. Why did families choose to participate or not participate?
   b. What factors seem to be related to family persistence in the Project?

3. Did participating families read more to their children?
   a. How did families change as a result of participating in Shared Reading?
   b. Did parents and children enjoy reading together?

STEP 3: DATA COLLECTION PLANS

The data collection planning process is tied directly to the purpose of the evaluation and the intended outcomes of the program. The program logic model can be used to identify important program characteristics, processes, and outcomes that need to be assessed, along with ways to measure them.

Before determining which data collection plans to use, evaluators must determine which performance indicators are appropriate. Performance indicators are statements that define the critical level of performance needed in order to judge if a program has successfully achieved its goals. The performance indicators lead directly to discussions concerning ways to measure the intended program characteristics, activities, and outcomes. The evaluator must align the performance indicators and sampling plans with the evaluation purpose, questions, and intended program outcomes until they have a good fit with each other. Reference to the program logic model, which depicts what is needed to implement the program, how the program is intended to work, and the intended outcomes of the program, can guide the identification and selection of relevant performance indicators.

When the U.S. Congress passed legislation that was intended to improve the efficiency and effectiveness of federal programs, they recognized the importance of identifying performance indicators to monitor programs' progress toward achieving their determined results (U.S. General Accounting Office, 1997). The Government Performance and Results Act (GPRA) of 1993 (PL 103-62) requires agencies, including those who fund early intervention programs, to focus on the results of their programs and to document their effectiveness. Many state and local governments, as well as private foundations, have also taken up the practice of requiring performance indicators for projects that they fund.

The importance of performance indicators in evaluation is also supported by the activities of private funding organizations, professional associations, and accrediting bodies in early intervention. Three very valuable resources that list performance indicators are available to service providers and other stakeholders in the area of early intervention. These include the NAEYC Accreditation Criteria and Procedures, the Division for Early Childhood (DEC) of the Council for Exceptional Children (CEC) recommendations, and a technical report issued by the Joint Committee of the American Speech-Language-Hearing Association and the Council on Education of the Deaf.

PERFORMANCE INDICATORS AND THE SHARED READING PROJECT

The Shared Reading Project evaluation used its logic model to help identify appropriate performance indicators for its evaluation questions. For example, the five sites included in the evaluation were selected because they served high proportions of children who are deaf and hard of hearing who belonged to traditionally underserved groups. The expectation was that each site would focus their recruitment efforts on the families of these children. The performance indicators related to this expectation were that a high proportion of the participating families would have children who belonged to traditionally underserved groups, and that the proportion of such families participating at each site would be representative of the pool of eligible families of traditionally underserved children. Existing documentation of children's educational and demographic characteristics served as the data sources for these performance indicators.

Another expected outcome of the project was that participating families would share books more often with their children than they did before they joined the Shared Reading Project. The performance indicator for this outcome was that families would report a greater number of book sharing events after they participated in the Shared Reading Project than they did before the Shared Reading Project. Data were collected using at least three measures for this indicator: the frequency of book sharing parents reported on pre- and postparticipation surveys, the number of book sharing events parents recorded per week on log forms, and interviews with parents about how book sharing in the family changed during their participation in the project (Delk & Weidekamp, 2001).

NAEYC (1998) developed Accreditation Criteria and Procedures. NAEYC's accreditation system is designed to engage early childhood program personnel in a process that improves the quality of the programs that serve young children. Although the accreditation system does not specifically focus on programs for young children who are deaf and hard of hearing and their families, it does provide an inclusive set of overall criteria for high-quality early childhood programs that covers the physical, social, emotional, and cognitive development of the children and adults (parents, staff, and administrators) who are involved in the programs. The criteria are divided into 10 goals—interactions among teachers and children, curriculum, relationships among teachers and families, staff qualifications and professional development, administration, staffing, physical environment, health and safety, nutrition and food service, and evaluation—each with a brief goal statement and rationale, and criteria that indicate that the goal is being achieved (see Table 7.1 for examples of three goals and criteria).

The Division for Early Childhood of the Council for Exceptional Children developed recommended practices in early intervention programs for infants and young children with special needs and their families (Sandall et al., 2000). Recommendations were developed for seven areas:

Table 7.1. Sample goals and criteria from the National Association for the Education of Young Children Accreditation Criteria (1998)

Goal A: Interactions among teachers and children	Criteria A-4: Teachers treat children of all races, religions, family backgrounds, and cultures with equal respect and consideration. Teachers provide children of both sexes with equal opportunities to take part in all activities. Teachers make it a firm rule that a person's identity (age, race, ethnicity, language, or disability) is never an acceptable reason for teasing or rejecting. Teachers initiate activities and discussions to build positive self-identity in each child and also teach the value of difference. Teachers talk positively about each child's physical characteristics and cultural heritage (p. 18).
Goal B: Curriculum	Criteria 3b: The program is designed to be inclusive of all children, including children with identified disabilities and special learning and developmental needs. Staff are aware of the identified/diagnosed special needs of individual children and are trained to follow through on specific intervention plans, Individualized Education Plans (IEPs) or Individualized Family Service Plans (IFSPs) ... Staff work in collaboration with appropriate professionals (such as early childhood special educators, therapists) and/or make appropriate professional referrals where necessary. Therapy is developed appropriately and incorporated within classroom activities as much as possible, rather than removing the child from the classroom. Family members are involved in development and use of individual education plans. Staff address the priorities and concern of families of children with special needs (pp. 23–24).
Goal C: Relationships among teachers and families	Criteria C-1: Information about the program is given to new and prospective families, including written descriptions of the program's philosophy and operating procedures. Families have opportunities to have input regarding policies and procedures, and plans for meeting children's individual needs. Programs with non-English-speaking families provide materials in the parents' native language or arrange for translation (p. 30).

assessment; child-focused interventions; family-based practices; interdisciplinary models; technology applications; policies, procedures, and systems change; and personnel preparation. For example, DEC recommended that families and professionals working under an interdisciplinary model, including regular caregivers, work as team members in planning, delivering, and evaluating early intervention/early childhood special education (EI/ECSE) services. DEC, with regard to the use of technology, also recommended that professionals use and select assistive technology that is based on families' preferences within assessment, implementation, and evaluation activities. Recommendations such as these could be used as a basis to develop indicators of quality for a program's evaluation planning process.

A Joint Committee of the American Speech-Language-Hearing Association (ASHA) and the Council on Education of the Deaf (CED) issued a technical report (1994) regarding service provision for children who are deaf and hard of hearing from birth to 36 months of age. The provision of services listing can be used for developing performance indicators. For example, the Joint Committee recommended that early identification, assessment, and management should include the family in an active, collaborative role with professionals in the planning and provision of early intervention services. As an indicator, this could mean, for example, that 90% of parents agree that they were placed in a central role in the evaluation of their infant or young child. The report outlines a number of areas in early intervention programs that can guide the development of performance indicators. ASHA and CED continue to review and revise their recommendations related to early intervention indicators.

Once appropriate performance indicators have been identified, data collection methods and instruments can be determined based on the data collection's ability to provide evidence concerning the degree to which the performance indicator has been achieved. Data collection methods can involve the review of documents, use of tests and assessment tools, portfolios, interviews (individual or group, e.g., focus groups), surveys (in-person, mail, telephone, Internet; structured or unstructured), and observations. A more complete picture can be obtained if both quantitative (numbers) and qualitative (words/pictures) data are collected. When constructing the data collection plan, the following questions may be useful:

- What data are already collected that could be used for the evaluation study (e.g., individual assessment, project files, portfolios)?
- What kind of data will the stakeholders (e.g., parents, staff) find credible?
- What kind of methods and instruments can detect the kind of issues, changes, and outcomes that are important to the evaluation?

Sample tools for data collection include

1. The four instruments NAEYC uses in their accreditation self-studies: The Early Childhood Classroom Observation Scale, the Administrator Report, the Teaching-Staff Questionnaire, and the Family Questionnaire (National Association for the Education of Young Children, 1998). Please note, however, that these forms are only available to those who have applied and paid a fee for participation in an accreditation assessment by NAEYC.

2. A self-evaluation checklist Project DAKOTA developed to measure family involvement and family perceptions of their involvement (Kjerland, Mendenhall, Perez, Wilkins, & Corrigan, 1998).

3. The standardized SKI-HI Data Sheet, completed by parents and parent advisors, that the SKI-HI program in Utah developed to measure

progress and outcomes (Strong et al., 1994). The Data Sheet includes demographic information such as hearing aid use and language development. Parents record data on steps achieved in auditory, cognitive, and communication skills. The SKI-HI Language Development Scale is used to measure receptive and expressive language for deaf and hard of hearing children, ages birth to 5 years. The sheet also provides data on how well parents are managing their child's hearing disability.

When implementing the data collection strategies, the evaluator must be sensitive to issues that might influence the quality of the data. For example, in the Shared Reading Project, the evaluators originally intended to conduct end-of-the-year interviews with tutors by telephone using a telecommunications device for the deaf. This strategy was based on the assumption that all the tutors hired by the expansion sites would be fluent in English as well as ASL, so an English-based interview would not be an impediment to clear communication. Several of the site coordinators reported, however, that some of the tutors they hired were strong ASL users and had excellent interpersonal skills with parents but were less fluent in English. One of the deaf site coordinators strongly recommended that the tutor interviews be conducted face-to-face using sign language. The Shared Reading Project staff concurred and also recommended that these interviews be conducted by a deaf interviewer and that they be videotaped because the evaluators wanted to have a verbatim record of the interviews for analysis. On-site videotaping, however, would be difficult to arrange and expensive to analyze. After much discussion, the Shared Reading Project staff and evaluators decided on a different strategy for the tutor interviews. A deaf interviewer fluent in ASL was trained and traveled to each of the sites with an interpreter to interview the sample of tutors, as recommended by the site coordinators. Each interview was audiotaped, using an interpreter to voice into the tape recorder for both the interviewer and interviewee. In this way, the interview was conducted in a manner conducive to clear, direct communication, and a verbal record of the interview was obtained for analysis.

A sample data collection plan for the Shared Reading Project is displayed in Figure 7.2. The components of the Shared Reading Project are listed in the first column. The various data collection strategies used in the project appear across the top row. The checks in the figure indicate which data collection strategies were used to evaluate the different parts of the logic model.

Another part of the data collection plan, known as sampling, determines from whom data will be collected and when the data will be collected. In many evaluation studies, the sample includes funders, staff,

Data Collection Instruments

INPUTS, PROCESSES, & OUTCOMES	Family/Child master list	Family master list	Parent pre/post survey	Tutor information	Family reading record	Tutor log	Parent interview	Tutor survey	Tutor interview	Site Coordinator interview
SRP INPUTS										
Environmental/Site characteristics	✓	✓	✓	✓			✓	✓	✓	✓
Family and child characteristics	✓	✓	✓				✓	✓	✓	✓
Tutor characteristics				✓			✓		✓	✓
SRP PROCESSES	✓	✓	✓	✓	✓	✓	✓	✓	✓	✓
Site coordinator training					✓					✓
Family and tutor recruitment		✓								✓
Tutor training								✓	✓	✓
Selection and use of materials						✓	✓	✓	✓	
In-home tutoring					✓	✓	✓	✓	✓	
Book sharing within the family			✓		✓		✓	✓	✓	
SRP OUTCOMES	✓	✓	✓		✓	✓	✓		✓	✓
Underserved families participate		✓			✓		✓			✓
Families share books more often			✓		✓		✓			✓
Parents' communication with child improves							✓	✓	✓	✓
Parents use book sharing strategies			✓			✓	✓	✓	✓	
Child's interest in book increases						✓	✓		✓	

Figure 7.2. Some sources of data for evaluating Shared Reading Project (SRP) inputs, processes, and outcomes. (From Delk, L. [1998, March 16]. *Evaluation of the Shared Reading Project: FY 98* [Unpublished document]. Washington, DC: Gallaudet University, Pre-College National Mission Programs; adapted by permission.)

parents, and kids, and sometimes nonparticipants and community members as well. However, an issue that is somewhat controversial involves the use of control groups. The U.S. General Accounting Office (USGAO) recognizes that early intervention programs have documented improvement of skills for participating children; however, the USGAO concluded that the results on effectiveness were not definitive because they were not based on random assignment of children to programs or control groups (Shaul, 2000). Yet, the USGAO also recognizes the ethical challenges in randomly assigning children to an unserved control group in order to assess effectiveness. Therefore, many programs choose to look at growth scores rather than deny services to eligible children (Calderon & Greenberg, 1997).

SAMPLING IN THE SHARED READING PROJECT

In the evaluation of the Shared Reading Project, data were collected from the major stakeholders at the five expansion sites. This included site coordinators, parents and caregivers, and tutors. The ethics of using a control group of interested families who would not participate in the Shared Reading Project was discussed by the project staff and evaluators. It was finally decided that this evaluation would track changes in book sharing for participating families only. The evaluators collected data from parents using pre- and postparticipation surveys of family book sharing and by asking parents to record how many times they read to their child each week during the tutoring period. Although a no-treatment group was not used, book sharing rates of Shared Reading families were compared with rates of a national sample of families from the general population, using the U.S. Department of Education's National Household Education Survey.

STEP 4: DATA ANALYSIS AND INTERPRETATION

The data analysis and interpretation plan should be directly related to the data collection plan. Only data that are needed for the planned analysis should be collected. Data that may be interesting but that are not tied to the program logic model and plans for analysis can place an undue burden on programs and participants.

Make a plan to analyze all of the data that need to be collected and determine how to involve key stakeholders in the interpretation process. With quantitative data, determine the extent to which statistical analysis is appropriate. Is it sufficient to present descriptive statistics, such as means or frequencies, or is it necessary to do group comparisons that call for inferential statistics? If the data are qualitative, would it be appropriate to use a computer-based qualitative analysis program to assist in the search for emerging themes that are relevant to the evaluation questions or to use more traditional content analysis (Berg, 1998; Creswell, 1998; Fielding & Raymond, 1998)? To complete the data analysis plan, refer to a statistics or research methods book or an evaluation or statistics consultant for guidance (Mertens, 1998; Miles & Huberman, 1994; Moore & McCabe, 1993).

In the Shared Reading Project, both quantitative and qualitative data were collected. Qualitative data came from open-ended questions on parent and tutor surveys and from interviews with site coordinators, parents, and tutors. The responses to open-ended survey questions were analyzed using traditional content analysis in which the number of occurrences of different types of responses were coded and tabulated, such as the different types of problems parents encountered when they tried to share books with their children before participating in the Shared Reading Project. In contrast, the interviews were analyzed using a different approach. Rather than counting the number of occurrences, researchers reviewed the interview transcripts for broad organizing themes and patterns. For example, two themes that were discovered from qualitative analysis of the interviews were "the tutor as catalyst" and "reasons parents wanted to participate in the Shared Reading Project." This analysis sought to increase understanding of the nature of Shared Reading relationships from the parents' perspective rather than counting how many times particular responses occurred.

Remember to include opportunities for stakeholders to provide feedback on the interpretation of the results throughout the evaluation process. This can improve the accuracy and add to the stakeholder comfort with the evaluation results, and may lead to a greater likelihood that the results will be viewed as credible and useful.

DATA ANALYSIS AND THE SHARED READING PROJECT

The Shared Reading Project evaluation resulted in a complex, multilevel data set, representing sites, families, and individual children. Before any analysis could be done, the quantitative data were entered and organized in a relational database. This permitted data at the child level to be aggregated to the family level for families that had more than one child who was deaf or hard of hearing, or to the site level. Descriptive statistics, repeated measures analysis of variance, and multiple regression were used to analyze the data and answer the evaluation questions. The qualitative data, which consisted of about 50 interviews with site coordinators, parents, and their tutors, were transcribed, double checked against tape recordings and notes, and formatted for analysis by a qualitative data analysis program. The major themes explored were how the Shared Reading Project was implemented at different sites and the nature of the parent–tutor–child relationship. As the different data sources were processed, the analysis began to address each of the evaluation questions.

The Shared Reading Project collected both quantitative and qualitative data—a mixed method approach—to address its evaluation questions. The questions that call for a quantitative analysis included words like "to what extent . . . " and "did they read more?" For these questions, descriptive and inferential statistics were calculated using the Statistical Package for the Social Sciences (SPSS). The characteristics of the children, families, and tutors were tabulated and reported as numbers and percentages to describe the different groups of stakeholders participating in the evaluation.

Data on the number of times families shared books were analyzed using a repeated measures analysis of variance to determine if there was a statistically significant increase in the number of book sharing events during the project. Surprisingly, this analysis showed that most families read to their children a consistent number of times per week from the beginning until the end of the tutoring sessions. This analysis did not tell anything, however, about how the families changed in the way they shared books.

Here is where the qualitative data collected through in-person, on-site interviews helped explain what was happening. Parents described how they began to improve their sign language, how they gained confidence, how they began to understand better the questions their children were asking about the books, and how they learned to use more facial and body expression to make the stories more interesting to their children. The interviews with the parents, tutors, and site coordinators also revealed that, although many of the parents increased their book sharing abilities during the 20-week intervention, they still had more to learn and still struggled with different aspects of the story-reading process. Many of the parents asked their tutors and site coordinators if they could continue with the Shared Reading Project the following year.

STEP 5: MANAGEMENT OF THE EVALUATION

The management plan for the evaluation should include a personnel plan with a time line and a budget. The personnel plan specifies the evaluation tasks and how, when, and by whom they will be done. The evaluation tasks are determined by the purpose of the evaluation, the evaluation questions asked, and the data collection and analysis plan. A very important part of the personnel plan is the selection of dates and mechanisms for periodically communicating progress and results of the evaluation to the other stakeholders. Therefore, milestones should be included for sharing interim reports of the evaluation in various formats with diverse groups. Connected to these reports should be plans for how the results will be used at that point in the project (e.g., will the results be used to modify curricular materials or revise staff training?). A second part of the management plan is the cost plan or budget that specifies anticipated expenses of the evaluation in categories such as personnel, travel, supplies, communication, and consultants. Together, these two parts of the management plan can be used as a basis for a formal contract between the evaluator and the sponsoring agency.

STEP 6: PLANNING FOR META-EVALUATION

The meta-evaluation plan specifies how the quality of the evaluation itself will be evaluated. Typically, the meta-evaluation specifies when reviews of the evaluation will be conducted, who will conduct them, and to what standards the evaluation will be held. Evaluation in the United States of America functions with a set of standards and a set of guiding principles that can be used to assess the quality of the evaluation plan and implementation. The Joint Committee on Standards for Educational Evaluation (1994) developed *The Program Evaluation Standards: How to Assess Evaluations of Educational Programs. The Standards* guides the evaluation of educational and training programs, projects, and materials in a variety of settings; they provide one comprehensive (albeit not all-encompassing) framework for examining the quality of an evaluation.

The standards outlined by the Joint Committee on Standards for Educational Evaluation are explained through guidelines and illustrative cases and are organized according to four main attributes of evaluations:

1. *Utility:* These standards are intended to ensure that an evaluation will serve the information needs of intended users.

2. *Feasibility:* These standards are intended to ensure than an evaluation will be realistic, prudent, diplomatic, and frugal.

3. *Propriety:* These standards are intended to ensure that an evaluation will be conducted legally, ethically, and with due regard for the welfare of those involved in the evaluation, as well as those affected by its results.

4. *Accuracy:* These standards are intended to ensure than an evaluation will reveal and convey technically adequate information about the features that determine worth or merit of the program being evaluated.

The Standards have been criticized for insufficiently addressing the complexities of conducting interpretive-constructivist evaluations (Lincoln, 1995) and for inadequately addressing the concerns about diversity and multiculturalism (Kirkhart, 1995; Mertens, 1995, 1998). Kirkhart (1995) proposed consideration of multicultural diversity in evaluation as an additional attribute for *The Standards* that would address more specifically concerns about pluralism and diversity in evaluation.

The *Guiding Principles for Evaluators* (Shadish, Newman, Scheirer, & Wye, 1995), developed by the American Evaluation Association, outlines principles intended to guide professional practice of evaluators and inform evaluation individuals and the general public about the principles they can expect to be upheld by professional evaluators. The five major principles include

1. *Systematic inquiry:* Evaluators conduct systematic, data-based inquiries about whatever is being evaluated.

2. *Competence:* Evaluators provide competent performance to stakeholders.

3. *Integrity/honesty:* Evaluators ensure the honesty and integrity of the entire evaluation process.

4. *Respect for people:* Evaluators respect the security, dignity, and self-worth of the respondents, program participants, individuals, and other stakeholders with whom they interact.

5. *Responsibilities for general and public welfare:* Evaluators articulate and take into account the diversity of interests and values that may be related to the general and public welfare.

The Standards and *Guiding Principles* can be used as indicators in the assessment of the quality of the evaluation plan. Meta-evaluation is typically scheduled at three points during the evaluation: after the preliminary plan is finished, during the implementation of the evaluation, and after the evaluation is completed. The meta-evaluation can be accomplished by asking a person outside of the setting to review the evaluation planning documents, the progress reports, and the final report. It can also involve feedback from the stakeholder groups.

META-EVALUATION AND
THE SHARED READING PROJECT

The Shared Reading Project evaluation addressed meta-evaluation issues at several points. An external group of researchers and evaluators reviewed the initial evaluation plans and direction while the evaluation was still in its planning stages. Before the evaluation plan was finalized, the new site coordinators for the expansion sites reviewed the proposed data collection procedures and were invited to comment and make recommendations about them. The University's Institutional Review Board for the Protection of Human Subjects reviewed the evaluation plan to ensure that the data collection, analysis, and reporting plan adhered to ethical guidelines. During the expansion year, the Shared Reading Project developers, trainers, and evaluators met regularly to monitor the progress and needs of the five sites and discuss training and evaluation issues. Ongoing Shared Reading Project oversight and direction are provided by the Clerc Center's Vice President's administrative team.

The National Mission Advisory Panel for the Clerc Center reviewed the initial findings of the evaluation and made recommendations concerning future steps for the project and its evaluation. This panel represents educators and administrators of programs serving students who are deaf and hard of hearing in different educational settings, parents, members of the deaf community, and alumni of the Clerc Center's demonstration school programs. The site coordinators and their program administrators received draft copies of the Shared Reading Project final evaluation report and were invited to give the evaluators their reactions and feedback before the report was finalized.

In conclusion, program evaluation is a complex process that provides a means to address the need for unbiased information related to a program's goals, processes, and outcomes. The six-step process explained in the chapter can provide general guidance. However, the implementation of the evaluation planning process must be responsive to the specific information needs of the program and its stakeholders.

FUTURE PERSPECTIVES IN EVALUATION

Emerging trends present many opportunities and challenges to the evaluation of early intervention programs for children who are deaf and hard of hearing and their parents. Trends such as the provision of services from infancy and the use of cochlear implant technology bring more issues to the evaluation table (Calderon & Greenberg, 1997). Given the increased demand for family involvement and the need to focus on child outcomes, as well as the new technologies that are available, it is becoming more important to find out not only what the outcomes of a program are but also how programs work and why expected outcomes did or did not occur (Horsch, 1998).

Along with understanding how programs work, there is an increasing need to build more evaluation capacity in local programs, particularly if participatory, empowerment, and inclusive evaluation approaches are to be used. Coffman (1997) stated that building organizational capacity and becoming a "learning organization" that constantly evaluates and improves itself go hand in hand. Local program providers, staff, and parents have much to contribute to the design, conduct, interpretation, and reporting of evaluations if those evaluations are to be relevant and useful to them. Local programs tend to use evaluations to assess needs, improve programs, and advocate for the program. Achieving a balance between evaluating to determine program effectiveness and evaluating for advocacy can be precarious if the results of the evaluation are to be viewed as credible. Most evaluators and project funders reject the advocacy role as biased and lacking in needed objectivity (Chelimsky, 1998). Yet, if key stakeholders who have traditionally lacked power in determining the course of evaluations are included in the planning, conduct, and dissemination of evaluation results, then the purpose of evaluations and the use of evaluation results will undoubtedly address the issue of advocating for the program.

One of the challenges of evaluating early childhood programs from an inclusive framework is how to conduct credible evaluations that are useful for internal improvement purposes and may be used to support policy and funding initiatives, as well as provide an unbiased assessment of the program. For this reason, it is important for local programs to identify and work with experienced program evaluators when evaluating their early childhood programs. The American Evaluation Association maintains a web site (http://www.eval.org) that can provide access to trained evaluators with the necessary background in early intervention and disabilities. Trained evaluators can guide program evaluation efforts and help the local program staff build basic capacities for self-evaluation.

TOOLS FOR EVALUATION
TRAINING: SHARED READING PROJECT

The Shared Reading Project offers a week-long training course for people who want to become Shared Reading Project site coordinators. One module in this training course deals with program evaluation. Participants are guided through the basics of deciding on goals and outcomes for their local adoption and adaptation of the Shared Reading Project. They are also provided with an evaluation tool kit that includes modified data collection instruments that were developed as part of the Shared Reading Project evaluation. Site coordinators who successfully complete the training course have access to Clerc Center evaluators with whom they can talk and receive advice about designing evaluation needs specific to their site.

At the same time that local programs are searching for ways to evaluate their programs, the movement at the state and national level toward performance-based assessment challenges funders to find ways to evaluate projects that are funded at multiple sites. Local sites often have a great deal of latitude in designing and implementing federally and state-funded programs to meet local needs and objectives. Funders and local programs alike are learning to work together to find ways of appropriately evaluating multisite projects so that the evaluation information needs of both funders and local programs are met.

Because many early intervention programs address the needs of the whole child and the family, projects often require the collaboration of multiple agencies to design and provide the array of needed services. Funders often require that grant applicants establish collaborations with parent groups, service agencies, or school programs for early intervention projects. In these cases, the project evaluation plan may address not only the merit and worth of the project at the child and family level, but also the success of the agency level collaboration. How to assess collaborative efforts, or determine if a collaboration is the best approach to take, is an emerging aspect of more and more program evaluations. Here again, an inclusive, participatory, process approach to evaluation is essential.

REFERENCES

Alcoff, L., & Potter, E. (Eds.). (1993). *Feminist epistemologies.* New York: Routledge.

Banks, J.A. (1995). The historical reconstruction of knowledge about race: Implications for transformative teaching. *Educational Researcher, 24*(2), 15–25.

Berg, B.L. (1998). *Qualitative research methods for the social sciences* (3rd ed.). Needham Heights, MA: Allyn & Bacon.

Calderon, R., & Greenberg, M. (1997). The effectiveness of early intervention for deaf children and children with hearing loss. In M.J. Guralnick (Ed.), *The effectiveness of early intervention* (pp. 455–482). Baltimore: Paul H. Brookes Publishing Co.

Chelimsky, E. (1998). The role of experience in formulating theories of evaluation practice. *American Journal of Evaluation, 19*(1), 35–56.

Clough, P., & Barton, L. (Eds.). (1998). *Articulating with difficulty: Research voices in inclusive education.* Thousand Oaks, CA: Sage Publications.

Coffman, J. (1997). Building the capacity to build capacity. *The Evaluation Exchange, III*(1), 5–6.

Creswell, J.W. (1998). *Qualitative inquiry and research design: Choosing among five traditions.* Thousand Oaks, CA: Sage Publications.

DeKoning, K., & Martin, M. (Eds.). (1996). *Participatory research in health.* London: Zed Books.

Delk, L. (1998, March 16). *Evaluation of the Shared Reading Project: FY 98* (Unpublished document). Washington, DC: Gallaudet University, Pre-College National Mission Programs.

Delk, L., & Weidekamp, L. (2001). *Sharing Reading Project: Evaluating implementation processes and family outcomes. Sharing Results Series.* Washington, DC: Gallaudet University, Laurent Clerc National Deaf Education Center.

Education of the Deaf Act Amendments of 1992, PL 102-421, 20 U.S.C. §§4301 *et seq.*

Fielding, N.G., & Raymond, M.L. (1998). *Computer analysis and qualitative research.* London: Sage Publications.

Fine, M. (Ed.). (1992). *Disruptive voices.* Ann Arbor: University of Michigan Press.

Gill, C. (1999). Invisible ubiquity: The surprising relevance of disability issues in evaluation. *American Journal of Evaluation, 20*(2), 279–288.

Government Performance and Results Act of 1993, PL 103-62, 31 U.S.C. §§ 1115 *et seq.*

Guralnick, M.J. (1997). Second-generation research in the field of early intervention. In M.J. Guralnick (Ed.), *The effectiveness of early intervention* (pp. 3–22). Baltimore: Paul H. Brookes Publishing Co.

Hill-Collins, P. (2000). *Black feminist thought: Knowledge, consciousness, and the politics of empowerment.* New York: Routledge.

Horsch, K. (1998). Interview with Carol H. Weiss. *The Evaluation Exchange, IV*(2), 5–6.

Humphries, B., & Truman, C. (Eds.). (1994). *Re-thinking social research.* Aldershot, UK: Avebury.

Individuals with Disabilities Education Act Amendments of 1997, PL 105-17, 20 U.S.C. §§ 1400 *et seq.*

Joint Committee of the American Speech-Language-Hearing Association and the Council on Education of the Deaf. (1994). Service provision under the Individuals with Disabilities Education Act-Part H, as amended (IDEA-Part H) to children who are deaf and hard of hearing ages birth to 36 months of age. *Asha, 36,* 117–121.

Joint Committee on Standards for Educational Evaluation. (1994). *The program evaluation standards: How to assess evaluations of educational programs.* Thousand Oaks, CA: Sage Publications.

Kirkhart, K.E. (1995). Seeking multicultural validity: A postcard from the road. *Evaluation Practice, 16*(1), 1–12.

Kjerland, L., Mendenhall, J., Perez, A.M., Wilkins, R., & Corrigan, K. (1998). *Project DAKOTA outreach.* Eagan, MN: Project Dakota.

Lather, P. (1992). Critical frames in educational research: Feminist and post-structural perspectives. *Theory into Practice, 31*(2), 1–13.

Lincoln, Y.S. (1995). *Standards for qualitative research.* Paper presented at the annual meeting of the American Educational Research Association, San Francisco.

Madison, A.M. (1992). Minority issues in program evaluation. *New directions for program evaluation* (Vol. 53). San Francisco: Jossey-Bass.

McLaren, P.L., & Lankshear, C. (Eds.). (1994). *Politics of liberation.* New York: Routledge.

Meadow-Orlans, K. (2000). Social change and conflict: Context for research on deafness. In M.D. Clark, M.J. Marschark, & M. Karchmer (Eds.), *Context, cognition, and deafness* (pp. 161–178). Washington, DC: Gallaudet University Press.

Mertens, D.M. (1995). Identify and respect differences among participants in evaluation studies. In W.R. Shadish, D. Newman, M.A. Scheirer, & C. Wye (Eds.), *The American Evaluation Association's Guiding Principles* (pp. 91–98). San Francisco: Jossey-Bass.

Mertens, D.M. (1998). *Research methods in education and psychology: Integrating diversity with quantitative and qualitative approaches.* Thousand Oaks, CA: Sage Publications.

Mertens, D.M. (1999). Inclusive evaluation: Implications of transformative theory for evaluation. *American Journal of Evaluation, 20*(1), 1–14.

Mertens, D.M., Farley, J., Madison, A.M., & Singleton, P. (1994). Diverse voices in evaluation practice: Feminists, minorities, and persons with disabilities. *Evaluation Practice, 15*(2), 123–129.

Mertens, D.M., & McLaughlin, J. (2003). *Research and evaluation methods in special education.* Thousand Oaks, CA: Sage Publications.

Miles, M.B., & Huberman, A.M. (1994). *Qualitative data analysis* (2nd ed.). Thousand Oaks, CA: Corwin Press.

Moore, D., & McCabe, D. (1993). *Introduction to the practice of statistics.* New York: Freeman.

National Association for the Education of Young Children. (1998). *Accreditation criteria & procedures of the National Association for the Education of Young Children.* Washington, DC: Author.

Oliver, M. (1992). Changing the social relations of research production? *Disability, Handicap, & Society, 7*(2), 101–114.

Reason, P. (Ed.). (1994). *Participation in human inquiry.* London: Sage Publications.

Reinharz, S. (1992). *Feminist methods in social research.* New York: Oxford University Press.

Sandall, S., McLean, M.E., & Smith, B.J. (2000). *DEC recommended practices in early intervention/early childhood special education.* Denver, CO: Division for Early Childhood Education of the Council for Exceptional Children.

Schleper, D.R. (1997). *Reading to deaf children: Learning from deaf adults.* Washington, DC: Gallaudet University, PreCollege National Mission Programs.

Scriven, M. (1995). *Evaluation thesaurus* (4th ed.). Thousand Oaks, CA: Sage Publications.

Shadish, W.R., Newman, D., Scheirer, M.A., & Wye, C. (Eds.). (1995). *The American Evaluation Association's guiding principles.* San Francisco: Jossey-Bass.

Shaul, M. (2000). *Preschool education: Federal investment for low-income children significant but effectiveness unclear* (GAO/T-HEHS-00-83). Washington, DC: U.S. General Accounting Office.

Shipman, S., MacColl, G.S., Vaurio, E., & Chennareddy, V. (1995). *Program evaluation: Improving the flow of information to the Congress: Report to the ranking minority members, Committee on Labor and Human Resources, U.S. Senate.* Washington, DC: U.S. General Accounting Office.

Stanfield, J.H., II. (1999). Social action research as vehicles of empowered social change in multiethnic and ethnically different communities. *American Journal of Evaluation, 20*(3), 415–432.

Stanfield, J.H., II, & Dennis, R. (Eds.). (1993). *Race and ethnicity in research methods.* Thousand Oaks, CA: Sage Publications.

Strong, C.J., Clark, T.C., Johnson, D., Watkins, S., Barringer, D.G., & Walden, B.E. (1994). SKI-HI home-based programming for children who are deaf or hard of hearing: Recent research findings. *Infant-Toddler Interventions: The Transdisciplinary Journal, 4,* 25–36.

Truman, C., Mertens, D., & Humphries, B. (Eds.). (2000). *Research and inequality.* London: Taylor & Francis.

U.S. General Accounting Office. (1997). *The Government Performance and Results Act: Government-wide implementation will be uneven* (Chapter Report, 06/02/97, GAO/GGD-97-109). Washington, DC: Author.

Weiss, C. (1998). Have we learned anything new about the use of evaluation? *American Journal of Evaluation, 19*(1), 21–34.

Whitmore, B. (Ed.). (1998). Understanding and practicing participatory evaluation. *New directions in evaluation* (Vol. 80). San Francisco, CA: Jossey-Bass.

W.K. Kellogg Foundation. (1998). *W.K. Kellogg Foundation evaluation handbook.* Battle Creek, MI: Author.

Determining
Program Effectiveness

Margaret Hallau, Director,
National Outreach, Research,
and Evaluation Network (NOREN)

When I read this chapter, my first reaction was, "I wish this informa-tion had been available in 1973." At that time, I was the training coordinator of a federally funded early childhood project, 1 of 14 that were part of a national network developing ways to include chil-dren with disabilities in Head Start programs.

Of course, in those days determining program effectiveness was in its infancy. The concept of including the perspectives and voices of all of the people involved or affected by the program had not yet emerged. The valuable resources provided by national groups and legislation to delineate performance indicators had not yet been developed. Although there was a focus on outcomes, I am not sure that those outcomes focused on what actually made a difference in the lives of the families we served. But because no one asked them, we didn't really know.

Almost 25 years later, I have had the privilege of watching the Shared Reading Project blossom. It began in Hawaii when hearing parents expressed their concern about knowing how to read to their deaf children. While they knew it was important to read to their chil-dren, they were not sure how to go about it. When Jane Fernandes and David Schleper brought the Shared Reading Project to

Kendall Demonstration Elementary School, which is a part of the Laurent Clerc National Deaf Education Center at Gallaudet University, they expanded some of the principles and began to work with other members of the Clerc Center to implement the Shared Reading Project at other sites. The long-range goal was to develop a training package that could be implemented in their schools and programs. In order to develop this training package, the Clerc Center needed to evaluate how the project was implemented at each site, the extent to which families of traditionally underserved children participated in the Project, and whether the participating families read more to their deaf or hard of hearing children.

This chapter provides the reader with guidelines for evaluating early intervention programs, using the Shared Reading Project as an example of how some of the guidelines were implemented for one project. By incorporating this comprehensive framework for planning and conducting an inclusive evaluation, early intervention programs will be taking a step toward developing the capacity to constantly evaluate and improve. They will not only find out about the outcomes of their programs but also understand better how their programs work and why expected outcomes did or did not occur. The authors also identify challenges in conducting inclusive evaluations for multiple purposes and discuss how an inclusive, participatory, process approach can be used for evaluating projects at multiple sites and those that incorporate collaborations.

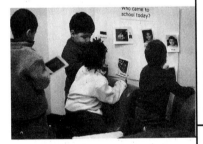

Challenges
in Early
Education

CHAPTER EIGHT

The Hard of Hearing Child

The Importance of Appropriate Programming

NANCY RUSHMER

I watch my daughter, Julie, as she maneuvers the vehicle around the high school parking lot. I watch with pride as she learns another essential skill in her life. She is no longer a child, yet not an adult. She is somewhere in the middle. In other aspects of her life, in terms of social interaction and communication, Julie is also in the middle. She is not deaf and she is not hearing; she is hard of hearing.

It is a unique position to be not deaf and not hearing, to be able to be understood, but often not able to understand, a place where frustration and patience go hand in hand. Julie chooses to talk more than she signs, yet she has more in common with Deaf people. She is somewhere in the middle. It is imperative that both parents and professionals understand the particular needs of the hard of hearing child. Being hard of hearing is a unique state, not without its own struggles, but the hard of hearing child can thrive, provided she is given the best communication tools, beginning in infancy, to utilize this special place.

We continue the driving lesson. I watch my daughter as she perfects a turn, and know deep within my heart that the skills she has learned will carry her for a lifetime—right down the middle. (Mason, 2000)

With appreciation to Nancy Hatfield, Ph.D., for her thoughtful contributions to this work.

223

Children who are considered hard of hearing have varying degrees of hearing loss. This extensive group includes a boy about to turn 5 and enter kindergarten who is deaf in one ear but has "only" a mild loss in the other ear—and neither is diagnosed until late in his fourth year because of his near-typical speech and language development. It includes a 3-year-old girl with a permanent conductive hearing loss who signs in fluent American Sign Language (ASL) with her Deaf parents, then talks intelligibly to her preschool classmate. And it also includes a 6-month-old infant with a mild hearing loss who (unaided) turns and reaches for his musical toy, activated from behind by his grandpa, convincing disbelieving grandparents that the tests were wrong and that he hears just fine. This group may well include deaf children with cochlear implants that bring their aided responses into the normal range.

Generally, the term *hard of hearing* is applied to individuals with mild, moderate, and severe sensorineural or permanent conductive hearing loss, either unilateral or bilateral, who have sufficient hearing to develop speech through audition, typically with the benefit of hearing aids. This includes infants identified at birth and those with onset during early childhood. A more precise definition of the term is difficult because the auditory characteristics of individuals with hearing loss are complex and use of the term often reflects the perspective, professional training, and/or goals of the individual using the term. A Position Statement of the Joint Committee of the American Speech-Language-Hearing Association (ASHA) and the Council on Education of the Deaf (CED) recommends that "terminology to describe individuals with hearing loss reflect respect for personal and family/caregiver preference(s) and the complexity of the communication interchange, as well as facilitate opportunities for personal, educational, social and vocational development" (Joint Committee of ASHA/CED, 1998).

When a child's hearing loss is identified, professionals provide his or her family with the audiological definition of their child's hearing loss, and the family uses this to understand and describe the loss. (Audiological classifications of degree of hearing loss can be found in Northern & Downs, 1991, pp. 13–14.) As children reach adolescence, many begin to identify themselves independently of audiological descriptions and more in accordance with social and/or cultural definitions that they find more acceptable. Some individuals audiologically classified as hard of hearing function more as if they were deaf and refer to themselves as deaf. Conversely, some profoundly deaf individuals function as if they were hard of hearing and choose to identify themselves as such.

The term *hard of hearing* can be extended to infants and toddlers with otitis media who concurrently experience temporary hearing loss. In fact, the most common cause of hearing difficulties in children from birth to 5 years is middle ear problems, such as serous otitis media, either chronic or intermittent, that can cause fluctuating hearing loss and may even lead to permanent hearing loss. Although chronic serous otitis media can be difficult to treat, it usually resolves during the preschool years. The timing of these hearing problems, however—during the prime years for acquisition of language and preacademic skills—amplifies their seriousness. A large body of research documents the long-term effects of hearing loss resulting from middle ear problems, including its impact on development of reading skills (Shriberg, Friel-Patti, Flipsen, & Brown, 2000).

And what about deaf children who have cochlear implants—where do they figure into this description of children with hearing loss? Are they considered normally hearing? Some deaf children with cochlear implants receive minimal benefit and function as if they were deaf. Others function very much like hard of hearing children, and some hear better than many hard of hearing children. The issues discussed here regarding hard of hearing children will apply to many deaf children who have cochlear implants.

JULIE

Remember Julie? Her family typifies the challenges faced by families with children who are hard of hearing. Because Julie babbled and sang as a toddler, doctors had difficulty taking seriously her parents' concerns about her hearing. Julie sometimes responded to voices and environmental sounds, making it hard for her family to trust their perceptions that she was not hearing them at times. Her moderate sloping to profound sensorineural hearing loss was finally diagnosed when Julie was 2 years old. Her family had already begun using ASL with her (they had learned it in college) and continued to sign after her hearing loss was "officially" confirmed. Julie attended a parent–infant program for children with hearing loss as well as a neighborhood preschool until she was 4 years old, at which time she was enrolled in a preschool for deaf and hard of hearing children that used simultaneous communication (signed and spoken English). Her mother believes that the early support Julie received from having concepts presented unambiguously through sign language and speech helped her speech and language fluency improve. In third grade, Julie began attending her neighborhood public school with a full-time interpreter who provided only instructional information, and used speech for class participation and peer interaction. Julie was fortunate. Her mother advocated effectively for her, making sure that each new teacher and set of classmates understood the educational implications of Julie's hearing loss and lobbying for the assistive listening devices and classroom modifications that Julie needed to ensure full participation in her neighborhood school. Julie is now bilingual—fluent in ASL and spoken English—with both hearing and deaf friends, code-switching with ease. An avid reader from an early age, she has excelled academically, taking honors and advanced placement classes in high school and reading at college level by age 16. Julie's outcomes could have been very different had her family and school programs not provided the specific supports she needed.

Children who are hard of hearing pose challenges for educators as well as for families. With hearing loss now being identified in the first weeks of life as a result of universal newborn hearing screening (UNHS), there is an assumption in the field that these children will be able to function with ease in a hearing world. Does this mean that they will not require special supports and accommodations at home and in school? What happens when ASL or signed English is introduced early to help establish a language base? Will listening and speech skills suffer as a result? Will these early-identified hard of hearing children perform best in a classroom with hearing peers, or in a classroom with deaf and hard of hearing peers? How will their social skills, identity, and self-esteem be affected by the early decisions made for them? These are the kinds of questions that families continue to face. They must be answered for each hard of hearing child individually with programming decisions reevaluated periodically.

This chapter discusses the importance of appropriate programming for hard of hearing infants and toddlers and their families. The potential obstacles facing hard of hearing children between the ages of birth and 5 years and their families are reviewed, and suggestions are offered concerning early programming to remove or minimize those obstacles. In particular, it is emphasized that the benefits of early identification and early intervention must be supported by continual improvement in programming for hard of hearing children throughout all stages of development. Professionals and parents can draw from the experiences of school-age children and young adults who are hard of hearing to inform the decisions they make on behalf of children during the first years of life. Late-identified children who are hard of hearing, even those for whom amplification can raise hearing thresholds to normal or near-normal levels, currently face serious challenges in language development, academic achievement, and social inclusion (Davis, 1990; Ross, 1990). Children identified at birth as hard of hearing will have to face many of these same challenges unless clinical and educational professionals, families, and the children themselves recognize and understand the special needs of hard of hearing children. Early identification of hearing loss in itself will not solve many of the later challenges faced by the hard of hearing child, but it certainly provides hope of moderating them.

DEMOGRAPHICS

Clearly, the ways in which individuals with hearing loss are defined will determine how many and which individuals receive appropriate professional and public services. Currently, there are no *complete* national survey statistics or incidence figures on numbers of hard of hearing children. States that mandate UNHS are asked to submit yearly data on numbers of infants identified as having hearing loss, including degree and type of loss, to the United States Centers for Disease Control and Prevention (CDC). Most states, however, do not have systems in place that allow them to provide complete information (J. Holstrum, personal communication, November, 2001). The data do show that the majority of newborns identified through these programs are hard of hearing (K. White, personal communication, January, 2000; Directors of Speech and Hearing Programs in State Health and Welfare Agencies Data Forms, 2000), which necessitates a change in practice for birth to 3 providers who, prior to UNHS, saw few infants and toddlers with mild or unilateral hearing loss.

The figures for children who are hard of hearing receiving services increase considerably as those late onset or progressive losses occurring during the early years are added to the count. According to Noel Matkin (personal communication, August 22, 2000), pulling from a number of studies we can conservatively estimate that at least 10 children per 1,000 are hard of hearing, with 2 or 3 of these having permanent unilateral hearing loss. He added, "With these numbers of children identified as hard of hearing, in addition to those with severe and profound losses, we should not continue to refer to hearing loss as a 'low incidence' disability."

HARD OF HEARING CHILDREN WITH ADDITIONAL DISABILITIES

One of three families with children who are hard of hearing surveyed by Meadow-Orlans, Mertens, and Sass-Lehrer (2003) indicated that their children had special developmental needs in addition to hearing loss. Families and early intervention personnel must monitor all areas of development, especially vision. The incidence of vision problems in children with hearing loss is higher than in the general population. Of the 501 parents of deaf and hard of hearing children surveyed by Robards (1991), 31% reported that their children also had vision problems. Among those diseases and conditions with a high probability of vision impairment in addition to hearing loss are maternal rubella, CHARGE association, prematurity, neurofibromatosis, Usher syndrome, cytomegalovirus (CMV) and Stickler syndrome.

Children with Down syndrome also are at risk for hearing loss; it occurs in 40%–60% of affected children (Kosma, 1995), most of them falling within the mild to severe range. Generally, these hearing losses are conductive and caused by fluid buildup in the middle ear or by abnormal or fixed middle ear bones (Kavanaugh, 1995). Children with Down syndrome can also have sensorineural hearing loss (about 10%) or mixed sensorineural and conductive loss, with the conductive component masking the sensorineural loss. The hearing loss may not be present at birth, but it can develop over time. Even so, every child should be tested for hearing at birth, with follow-up testing at least once a year.

CULTURAL AND ETHNIC CONSIDERATIONS

According to the Gallaudet Research Institute (2001), 45% of children who are deaf and hard of hearing in educational programs in the United States are from minority backgrounds. In 2001, it was estimated that 20.8% of deaf and hard of hearing children were from Spanish-speaking backgrounds, 16.3% were African American, 4% were Asian/Pacific Islander, and 9% were Native American. These cultural differences have implications for the provision of services. Some of these children may be identified late, in particular those who come from regions of the country in which early identification and intervention services are not available. There also may be differences in the kinds of services these families are likely to choose and accept, based on their cultural values and beliefs (Christensen, 2000; Meadow-Orlans et al., 2003). For example, the family and specialist will need to agree on a language of instruction for the hard of hearing toddler when the family does not speak English. Specialists will also need to modify their approach and expectations for families who, initially, may not be comfortable with the family-centered model's focus on them more than their infant.

EDUCATIONAL CONSIDERATIONS

Understanding and appropriately serving children who are hard of hearing has long been considered an unmet challenge in the education of children with hearing loss (Davis, 1990). Historically, these children have been an enigma to professionals who have tried to bridge the gap between what is known about their needs and the services that are actually provided to them. In 1996, the U.S. Department of Education reviewed the educational status of hard of hearing children in light of a 1976 task force on children's unmet service and educational needs (The Leadership Training Institute, 1976). After 20 years, no improvements were observed in the unacceptably low standard of service for hard of hearing children or in the preparation of professionals to adequately serve them.

Ironically, hard of hearing children's strengths are responsible in part for the failure of public education to adequately address their needs. Because many of them can learn to understand speech when wearing hearing aids, it is easy to assume that they will do "just fine." Families and professionals may even believe that once their child learns to talk, he or she will be okay. In fact, most of these children *do* develop intelligible speech as a result of focused listening and practice during their early years (Elfenbein, Hardin-Jones, & Davis, 1994; Yoshinaga-Itano & Sedey, 2000). The clarity of their speech leads the general public to assume that what children who are hard of hearing can hear is equally understandable. But often, it is not.

Partial hearing is dangerously deceptive. In a quiet setting with only one conversational partner, a young child who is hard of hearing may hear very well. But homes, preschools, and social settings tend to be noisy, often with competing conversations and multiple speakers, putting the young child with hearing loss at a considerable disadvantage. In a noisy group setting, even with the best amplification, much of the message may be inaudible for children who are hard of hearing, and often it is difficult for these children to determine who is talking. Young hard of hearing children eager to participate in family conversations at mealtime or informal discussions in preschool discover that, by the time they figure out who is talking by using speechreading for clarification, the conversation has switched to another speaker. They often do not know what was said and miss their opportunity to contribute. Conversations are important language learning situations for young children; the hard of hearing child may miss many of them.

STATUS OF HARD OF HEARING CHILDREN

In planning services for hard of hearing infants, toddlers, and preschoolers, there is an alarming tendency for professionals and family members to consider these losses identified at birth not serious enough to justify intensive programming from the moment of identification. In fact, some states require a documented language delay in addition to hearing loss in order to determine eligibility for services (K. White, personal communication, January, 2001). The performance of those hard of hearing children identified around or after age 2, the average age before UNHS, illustrates the consequences of this ill-founded practice.

Prior to the advent of UNHS, late identification of hearing loss was a particularly harmful barrier to normal linguistic, social-emotional, and cognitive development for hard of hearing children. People sometimes assume that with hearing aids (often bringing thresholds within the normal range), these children will soon catch up to their peers linguistically and do well in school. Research indicates, however, that this frequently does not happen (Bess, Dodd-Murphy, & Parker, 1998; Davis, 1990; Ross, 1990). The linguistic challenges of these children are compounded throughout their school years by often-compromised acoustic environments. If environmental accommodations and support services are not available, performance continues to lag, gaps in academic achievement widen, and children tend to continue to struggle academically, socially, and emotionally (Cappelli, Daniels, Durieux-Smith, McGrath, & Neuss, 1995).

Academic Performance

Nothing about hearing loss should prevent any hard of hearing child from achieving academically at or above the level of his or her hearing peers; thus, the academic outlook for hard of hearing children ought to be extremely positive. On average, however, hard of hearing children are at risk for underachievement in school. Research results indicate that large numbers of children who are hard of hearing without additional disabilities, even those with mild hearing loss, fall significantly below age norms academically. Multiple investigations of the academic performance of hard of hearing students reveal an average of 2- to 3-year delays beginning in the elementary grades (Bess et al., 1998; Davis, Elfenbein, Schum, & Bentler, 1986; English & Church, 1999; Ross, 1990; Yoshinaga-Itano & Downey, 1996).

In the absence of adequate programming, any degree of hearing loss can negatively affect school performance. In a study of 1,218 children with minimal sensorineural hearing loss (average pure tone thresholds between 20 and 40 dB [decibel] HL [hearing level], including children with high frequency loss, unilateral loss, and conductive loss), 37% of the children had failed at least one grade in school (Bess et al., 1998). English and Church (1999) found 24% of children with unilateral hearing loss achieving below grade level.

Language and Speech

The academic difficulties observed in many children who are hard of hearing are for the most part related to deficient language skills arising from limited auditory access to the linguistic message, which affects the children's development of vocabulary, syntax, pragmatics, and speech (Andrews, 1990). Early intervention programming strategies to prevent or mitigate these linguistic challenges are discussed later in the chapter.

Vocabulary   Hard of hearing children tend to have fewer words in their vocabulary than their hearing peers (Gilbertson & Kamhi, 1995; Ross, 1990), perhaps because their early word learning opportunities often are limited to quiet situations in which a speaker close to them directs conversation to them.

Syntax and Pragmatics   Because hard of hearing children often do not hear the complete linguistic message, phonological processing of the message, as well as subsequent phonological development, can be impaired. It is not surprising, then, that many children who are hard of hearing have more difficulty than their hearing peers with complex syntactic constructions that depend on minimal acoustic information (e.g., final /s/, final /t/ indicating past tense). Extensive listening experience is necessary in order to learn such elements. The most common pragmatic error (language within a communication context) made by children who are hard of hearing is in their responses to questions or dialogue, in which their ambiguity or failure to provide requested information demonstrates their difficulties either in comprehending the question or in assessing their conversational partner's knowledge base and gearing their response to it (Elfenbein et al., 1994).

Speech Production   Children who are hard of hearing can monitor their speech production fairly well using audition. Their most frequently observed errors are omission of final consonants, sound substitutions, and some distortions (Elfenbein et al., 1994; Ross, 1990). As hard of hearing children become more sophisticated listeners, they tend to self-correct and their speech improves. Yoshinaga-Itano and Sedey (2000) reported that children with mild to severe hearing losses were almost always understood by adults familiar to them by 5 years of age.

Social/Emotional Characteristics and Identity

Because ease of communication and interaction with others are important to developing a positive self-concept, the communication difficulties associated with partial hearing loss may interfere with social relationships and can readily be observed as early as preschool. The hard of hearing 3- or 4-year-old might withdraw from teacher-led discussions, have difficulty following directions, and feel left out of the fast-paced role negotiations and pretend play scenarios so common to the cooperative play of preschoolers. Reflections by adults on the childhood effects of their hearing loss suggest that many children who are hard of hearing struggle with the development of their identity as hearing, hard of hearing, or deaf individuals. Some remember going through school pretending they understood and working very hard to fit in, but much of the time they felt left out. Donald Grushkin (1996), a hard of hearing researcher who studied social and identity development in hard of hearing adolescents, reported being confused himself by an unclear sense of identity as he grew up. Described as functionally hard of hearing and interacting only with hearing individuals, his self-perception was as a hearing person who could not hear.

RESULTS OF AN EFFECTIVE EDUCATIONAL APPROACH

Although there are hard of hearing children who do well in inclusive early childhood placements with appropriate supports, and those attending oral programs for deaf and hard of hearing children who function very well (Moeller, 1997), it is interesting to consider children whose families have used *both* speech and signs. This approach is on the rise in the United States and abroad for both hearing and hard of hearing children. Proponents of the approach report an accelerated rate of language and speech acquisition over auditory-oral approaches alone (Carver, 1996; Daniels, 1993; Garcia, 1999; Graney, 1997; Preisler & Ahlstrom, 1997). Two regional educational programs for children with hearing loss in Oregon are following the development and academic performance of a number of hard of hearing children whose families, during the early childhood years, elected to communicate with them through speech and through speech with signs within comprehensive family-centered programs. Some families used Signed English and others used sign-supported speech (speech and American Sign Language signs) in their dual language program (Columbia Regional Program, 1998; Rushmer & Melum, 2002).

The most striking outcome for these children was an earlier and accelerated rate of language acquisition over that previously observed in hard of hearing children learning spoken language alone. The addition of signs appears to facilitate understanding of and memory for new language. Expressively, the children will often sign a new word first until they gain confidence in their spoken utterance. They then tend to drop the sign. By the age of 5 years, many of these hard of hearing children score at age level or above on standardized language tests for hearing children. By second grade, most enter their neighborhood schools where they successfully compete academically with hearing peers, still receiving support services or monitoring to be sure they remain on track. In fact, several of the older hard of hearing students studied, whose ages range between 9 and 16 years, scored from 1–4 years above grade level in reading (Columbia Regional Program, 1998).

There has long been a concern that the use of sign language with hard of hearing children would interfere with spoken language development (i.e., that attending early childhood programs with signing deaf children would not provide the level of access to hearing, talking peers that is critical to the hard of hearing child's speech development). Yoshinaga-Itano and Sedey (2000) reported that the use of sign language does not necessarily preclude the development of good speech. According to Marilyn Daniels (personal communication, February 21, 2000), there is absolutely no evidence that using sign language with deaf, hard of hearing, or hearing children delays their speech. There is much evidence to the contrary that shows it helps their speech as well as their ability to comprehend meaning and communicate.

Detractors of a dual language approach (ASL and spoken English and/or sign-supported speech) for children who are hard of hearing, and those supporters of bilingual learning who advocate always keeping the languages separate, voice strong objections, believing that exposure to a visually based language as well as an auditorily based language is too confusing for young children and will result in greater language delay. This fear may seem to be intuitively correct, but it is not supported by research or the achievements of the children. The work of Petitto and colleagues with hearing children (2001) indicates that the capacity to differentiate between two languages (signed and spoken) is well in place prior to first words. The children they studied did not confuse the two languages, and they achieved appropriate linguistic milestones in both languages at the same time.

THE NEEDS OF FAMILIES OF HARD OF HEARING CHILDREN

It is a misconception of professionals and some parents of *deaf* children that the discovery of a less severe hearing loss is easier to bear for families than the discovery of deafness, and that the families and children have fewer needs. Parents of hard of hearing children hear from parents of deaf children: "Oh, you are so lucky that she hears so much and talks so well" (Maxon & Brackett, 1992, p. 157). From the perspective of parents of young hard of hearing children, however, the effects of the loss are no less profound. Reporting on a survey of 218 families of hard of hearing children under the age of 7 years, Sass-Lehrer and colleagues (1999) noted the special concerns these families had for their children during the early childhood years: social development, speech and language development, use of hearing aids, cognitive development, placement and appropriate services, and changes in hearing abilities. Advice for professionals included a request for support groups, better communication with parents, a respect for parents' feelings, specification of options followed by appropriate referrals, and a need to be listened to. A parent of a hard of hearing daughter with epilepsy and cerebral palsy advised that professionals

Be willing to listen to parents and what their concerns are. And try to help the parent become better informed and more involved instead of just assuming that parents can't understand what the problem is . . . I've had some good experiences too, but . . . the specialists just see themselves as the authority and not just over the child and the condition, but over the parent. They need to spend more time helping the parent. A child who's just been diagnosed with something, try to inform the parent, giving them resources or asking them, "Would you like to learn more about this?" (Sass-Lehrer et al., 1999)

PROGRAM APPLICATION GUIDELINES FOR INFANTS, TODDLERS, AND PRESCHOOLERS WHO ARE HARD OF HEARING

The greatest impact of mild to severe hearing loss in young children is on developing communication and language. Recognizing that there can also be secondary effects on cognitive, academic, and social-emotional development, this section presents various guidelines to help parents and professionals improve the acquisition of auditory, vocal, visual-gestural, speech, and language skills in infants, toddlers, and preschoolers who are hard of hearing. These skills do not develop in isolation but in combination with other aspects of development; however, for purposes of this discussion, each area is dealt with separately. Strategies that parents and professionals can use to promote these skills are noted briefly, as are resources that describe them in detail.

It is important to note that even with identification and placement of amplification within the first weeks of life, hard of hearing infants do not hear normally. Families need regular and appropriate early support in order to help their children acquire communication and language skills commensurate with cognitive potential. Levels of support that families need and want may range from periodic consultation only to a more intensive regular service.

Guideline 1: A relationship-based approach to serving families supports the parent–child bond

Relationship-based intervention is a way of delivering services to young infants and their families that includes a focus on the importance of parent–child interaction and how the staff–family relationship influences family–child relationships (Heffron, 2000). Parents of infants newly identified as hard of hearing are often concerned that they do not know what to do for their infant. They may not know that they already have many intuitive skills for successfully helping their infant. When well-meaning professionals take over the interactions with the infant in order to model strategies for parents, they lose the opportunity to observe and reinforce the parents' intuitive skills. When they adopt an authoritative or expert role, this interferes with the parent–child interaction (Condon, 2000). These professionals who have traditionally been "in charge" of sessions with families need to relinquish control in order to sit back, observe, and support the nurturing and growing communication interaction between parent and child.

In a relationship-based approach, supportive comments from professional to parents that acknowledge the infant's and parents' responsiveness to one another and their success as communication partners serve to boost the parents' sense of competence and facilitate the bonding process between parent and child. The parents' growing relationship and dialogue with a supportive professional increases their confidence that they can understand, nurture, and communicate with their hard of hearing infant.

Guideline 2: Adults need to read and respond to the young child's messages

Infants and toddlers have much to "tell" the adults around them. By observing and understanding their infant's states of consciousness (sleep, alert, drowsy, crying), and by reading and interpreting prelinguistic cues and behaviors (sustained eye gaze, crying, frowning, eye widening, leg kicking, pushing away, facial brightening, quieting, smiling, lip grimace, gurgling, looking away), families can become skilled in *responding* to their children's messages, giving their infants a beginning sense of success as communicators as well as confidence in the caregivers who meet their needs. These early communication exchanges support the bond between parent and child and provide the foundation for the turn taking that is integral to subsequent communication and language growth.

Guideline 3: Acquisition of skills during early childhood tends to proceed in an orderly fashion

The most effective early childhood professionals utilize a developmental approach. This requires an in-depth knowledge of child development, assessment strategies for determining developmental levels, and the ability to promote subsequent skills. In working with young children who are hard of hearing, this approach implies that for any given activity the professional will tap into multiple developmental areas, using what is known about the child's motor, social-emotional, cognitive, and play skills, along with his or her auditory, vocal, and linguistic levels.

Guideline 4: Hearing aids, if recommended, should be worn consistently in order to facilitate auditory and speech development

It is important to make the case for immediate placement of hearing aids on newborns identified as having moderate to severe and severe hearing losses; clearly these infants will not hear or understand conversational speech without amplification. Convincing families and some professionals of the importance of aiding infants with mild hearing losses, however, may be a challenge. The professional's role is to help parents understand that infants with mild losses will hear and respond to speech; however, without amplification, they can miss the softer consonants that contain critical linguistic information. When families learn of their central role in their infant's acquisition of speech and language, an understanding that the child needs to hear as much as possible of the spoken message comes more easily. Some families have reported that listening to simulations of hearing losses on audio- or videotape was the key to understanding how much their child was missing.

Guideline 5: The child's acoustic environment must be monitored

Infants and young children who are hard of hearing and use amplification, those with unilateral hearing losses, and deaf children who have cochlear implants are especially affected by the presence of noise in the environment because background sound interferes with the speech signal, making it harder to decode the spoken message. Children can learn to ignore some background sounds in the environment if they can identify them and have opportunities to practice consciously tuning them out. Working to understand speech under a constant barrage of background sound, however, is exhausting. It is important to regulate household noise from stereos, televisions, and noisy appliances (Candlish, 1996), especially during family gatherings such as mealtimes. In child care and preschool settings that are expected to be language-learning environments, acoustic treatment of rooms is important in order to reduce reverberation. Effective sound-absorbing materials include carpets on floors, acoustic tile on ceilings, and corkboard on walls (Maxon & Brackett, 1992). Some families and their preschool-age children have found the use of FM systems beneficial during home conversations in the presence of background noise and in social situations such as preschool, shopping trips, or religious activities (Moeller, Donaghy, Beauchaine, Lewis, & Stelmachowicz, 1996). Digital programmable hearing aids also improve speech perception in noisy situations (see Chapter 13).

Guideline 6: When families know what the infant can hear, families can support the stages of auditory development

Hearing aids are only the first step for infants who are hard of hearing who, even with amplification, do not hear normally. These young children need the adults around them to systematically support their growing auditory and vocal awareness. In order to provide meaningful auditory experiences for an infant (e.g., those he or she is likely to hear and is interested in), families and professionals need to have sufficient information about the child's aided hearing. Knowledge of what the infant can hear is then related to the acoustic characteristics of the speech and common environmental sounds the infant will experience in order to determine what he or she actually hears. For example, are the tiny bells on the crib toy audible to the child with a sloping high frequency hearing loss? (There are ways to figure this out. For examples, see Schuyler & Rushmer, 1987; Schuyler & Sowers, 1998, p. 104.) With appropriate amplification and meaningful listening experiences, the hard of hearing infant can soon be on his or her way toward recognizing environmental sounds and speech.

Guideline 7: Home is an ideal place for the infant to learn to understand what he or she hears

Infancy is well suited to auditory development, and home is an ideal place for it to occur, as this is where parents spend much of their time with their infant. Adult caregivers are frequently very close to the infant when they talk and sing to him or her, increasing the likelihood of a clear auditory-verbal signal. Hard of hearing infants who have access to sufficient auditory information through this close, nurturing contact can become sophisticated listeners very early. Families also report that time spent in the car with their infants and toddlers can facilitate rich nonverbal and, later, verbal conversations.

Guideline 8: Speech development is based on hearing and is sequential

The development of vocalizations and speech are closely linked to development of auditory skills. For example, after a period of listening to the adults around them and to their own vocal sounds, hearing and hard of hearing infants begin to modify their own vocalizations in an attempt to match those of the adults. After 4 or 5 months of listening, consonants are added to the vowels in vocal play, babbling begins, and infants begin to show evidence of their developing auditory feedback mechanism. They listen to the sounds they produce, practice and refine them (i.e., they can monitor phoneme production), and compare their sounds with those of adult caregivers. Auditory feedback is at the core of speech development from this point on. Parents have intuitive skills that encourage their children's vocal behaviors through verbal turn-taking routines and vocal and verbal play interactions. Helpful guides for assisting families in continuing to promote the sequential acquisition of auditory, vocal, and speech skills in hard of hearing infants and young children are found in Cole (1992); Estabrooks (1994); Estabrooks and Marlowe (2000); Pollack, Goldberg, and Caleffe-Schenck (1997); Schuyler and Rushmer (1987); and Schuyler and Sowers (1998).

Guideline 9: The visual environment should be monitored

There is a common misconception that because hard of hearing infants and toddlers hear spoken language, they have the auditory perceptual skills to discriminate and comprehend the entire message (without the aid of visual cues). This often is not the case and can lead to difficulties throughout the child's development. Infants and young children who are hard of hearing utilize visual information from facial expressions, lip movements, and body language to attach meaning to the speech they hear. There will be times when the child receives clear linguistic information auditorily so that he or she need not look at the speaker, and times when he or she relies more on visual clues. Parents of hard of hearing toddlers and preschoolers know that their children rely on speechreading. Lighting on the speaker's face and the absence of bright light or distracting movement behind the speaker can enhance the child's ability to distinguish lip movements.

Guideline 10: Families promote communication and language growth both visually and auditorily

The process of language acquisition for hard of hearing children will sometimes resemble that of hearing children and at other times may resemble that of those deaf children who rely more on vision, depending on the degree and type of loss, age and appropriateness of amplification, and environmental conditions (e.g., distance from speaker, reverberation, background noise). Under noisy conditions, when there are multiple speakers or when at a distance, the child may not hear well enough to understand. It is this pattern of hearing and then not hearing that can interfere with language acquisition. It is important for families to know when their child needs to have the verbal message supported with visual information such as pointing, pantomime, good access to the face for speechreading cues, or sign language.

Guideline 11: Adults can use child-directed language that is both auditory-verbal and visual

Hearing and deaf parents intuitively use child-directed language or "motherese/parentese" (i.e., "baby talk") with their infants and toddlers. "Parentese" is an adult conversational style that promotes language acquisition. There are many parallels between the child-directed language used by hearing parents and those strategies that deaf parents use (see Table 8.1). Families who use both speech and signs with their hard of hearing infants and toddlers have access to both hearing and deaf parents' "parentese" strategies. The visual communication techniques deaf parents use (Mohay, 2000; Swisher, 2000) along with auditorily based strategies characteristic of hearing parents (Cole, 1992) can be very effective at sustaining the infant's interest and engagement with the adult.

Guideline 12: Joint attentional focus is established auditorily and visually

Extended periods of adult–child "joint attentional processes" scaffold children's early language development (Tomasello, 1988). By 6 months of age, infants will look toward the object of their parents' gaze, and by 9 months, infants alternate looks between the adult and the object of the adult's gaze. These periods of joint attention, coupled with the adult's verbal labels or descriptions, help the child figure out the relationship between the spoken or signed word and the referent (object, person, or event).

Auditory-oral approaches have long advised parents with children who are deaf and hard of hearing to talk both while the child is looking

Table 8.1. Characteristics of child-directed language: "Baby talk"

Hearing parents' baby talk	Deaf parents' baby talk
1. Higher pitch than adult conversation; exaggerated intonation with vowel prolongation.	1. Exaggerated size of signs; positive facial expression (70–80% of time).
2. Talking about the "here and now."	2. Same. Referent object is brought directly into conversational space.
3. Prolonged gazing.	3. Prolonged gazing; eye contact.
4. Nonverbal communication signals.	4. Interspersing nonverbal affective acts with language (e.g, tickling, tapping).
5. Short, simple, but grammatically correct sentences.	5. Majority of utterances consist of one word at a time, generally in citation form.
6. Much repetition of words and phrases.	6. Repetition of signs, as well as movement within signs. Orientation of signs may be changed to facilitate perception.
7. Numerous questions (up to 50% of adult's utterances).	7. Extensive use of point (up to 50% of signs in parents' utterances).
8. Longer than normal pauses between sentences and phrases.	8. Longer than normal pauses between periods of signing.
9. Special words ("baby talk").	9. Special words ("baby talk").
10. Imitation, expansions, and prods.	10. Imitation, expansions, and prods.
11. Changes in type and quality of language input depending on capabilities of child.	11. Grammatical ASL and fingerspelling not introduced until 2 to $2^1/2$ years. (Before then, noun-verb pairs are undifferentiated and verbs not modulated).

From Rushmer, N., & Hatfield, N. (1993). Promoting early communication II: The role of the family. In V. Schuyler (Ed.), *Early intervention series* (p. 19). Portland, OR: Portland Center for Hearing and Speech; reprinted by permission.

and when he or she is not looking. The intent is to build auditory comprehension in children who have usable residual hearing. Parents of hard of hearing infants and toddlers who use both auditory-oral and signed communication with their children utilize both auditory and visual strategies for establishing joint attention, just as they use both auditory and visual forms of child-directed language. At times, adults can talk while their infant is scanning the environment, and at other times they can wait until the child looks back to them before they provide both spoken and signed information. Or they may use speech alone while the infant is looking away and reinforce the concept with signs when the child looks back to them.

Guideline 13: Using signed and spoken language can accelerate the rate of language acquisition

Parents who utilize both speech and ASL or a signed system with their children who are hard of hearing report that the use of signs serves as a "bridge" to meaning and then to language and speech (interviews with Oregon parents, 2000). When children are toddlers, and they don't know the spoken word for something or their speech is still unintelligible, signs allow the toddlers to clearly express their needs and wants, thereby reducing frustration. Parents report that the ability to sign allows more natural communication with their hard of hearing child throughout the day. This is especially true in situations in which the hearing aid is malfunctioning or not worn, for example, in the bathtub, when swimming, in noisy environments (restaurants, Sunday school, at home when the radio or television is on), and at a distance (in the park, in a shopping center, during soccer games, on family outings).

As children who are hard of hearing get older and begin to understand most of their families' spoken language, their families tend to sign less and less, except in situations involving distance or background noise, when they want to explain complex or abstract concepts, or when the meaning is unclear to their child. Jamie, a hard of hearing preschooler whose language scores are *above* age level, cited this difficulty in her response to her audiologist when asked if she could hear better with her new digital hearing aids: "Yes, I can hear better, but I still need sign language to understand." Although Jamie could hear better in some situations, she still needed sign language to augment the verbal message in noise or with complex new concepts.

Guideline 14: Families and teachers can continue to improve preschoolers' language skills with language-rich activities

Hard of hearing preschoolers who received effective early intervention and have developed intelligible speech can still be at risk for linguistic problems and later academic impairments. It is easy to assume that they are doing better than they are when their grasp of colloquial language is good. The clear speech of hard of hearing children attending inclusive preschools and those in classes with deaf children may mask language gaps such as reduced vocabulary and difficulty with abstract concepts, complex sentences, and pragmatics.

Even when language is age appropriate or better and communication throughout the day goes fairly smoothly, the work of parents and teachers is not over. Children's language skills and world knowledge must be continually broadened in order to support later academic success. With more severe hearing losses, children need extensive and repeated exposure to linguistic forms and vocabulary in order to deduce increasingly complex language rules (Maxon & Brackett, 1992).

Achievement of specific linguistic targets during the preschool years is crucial to later academic success. These include broadening concepts, introducing multiple meanings of words, expanding vocabulary, modeling compound and complex sentences, and modeling question forms, including when, why, how, how far, how long, what kind, and which one. Preschoolers also need to master temporal terms (e.g., before, after, yesterday, next week, in a few days) and the language related to beliefs, knowledge, and feeling states of themselves and others. They should be able to maintain a topic over several turns in conversation, using revision, topic changing, and clarification (using awareness of what the listener knows to provide clarification). Four- and five-year-old preschoolers should also be able to make inferences and use figurative language, metaphorical language, and the language of hypothetical conversations.

These linguistic targets can effectively be addressed through home and school learning activities that have significant visual, hands-on, and experiential elements such as science experiences that promote the language of problem solving, predicting, making inferences and thinking abstractly; dramatic play that can promote role taking and more abstract conversation; and narratives (made up or retold stories or accounts of personal experiences). Experience with narratives through exposure to children's literature, listening to storytellers, and telling one's own stories is highly related to language acquisition and literacy. As adults read stories again and again, children are exposed to complex syntactical forms, world knowledge, nuances of meaning, figurative language, story grammar, and information about the internal mental states of characters. Gray and Hosie (1996) found that hard of hearing children have difficulty in understanding and retelling stories. There are, however, highly successful preschool programs for hard of hearing children that address this need by emphasizing narratives. These programs can produce graduates with age-appropriate language (Moeller, 1997).

Guideline 15: Hard of hearing children can be served effectively within a variety of educational models and approaches

Comprehensive early childhood programs for young children who are hard of hearing support all major developmental areas—auditory, language, speech, social-emotional, cognitive, and motor—and screen for and address other special needs. They may provide occupational and physical therapy, sensory integration therapy, vision services, and support for children with other disabilities, such as autism spectrum disorders, cerebral palsy, attention-deficit/hyperactivity disorder, Down syndrome, and developmental delay. Hard of hearing children can receive appropriate services within the same range of models and communication approaches as do deaf children. These include inclusion models such as the co-education model (Kreimeyer, Crooke, Drye, Egbert, & Klein, 2000), bilingual/bicultural models, and inclusion with support (see Chapter 9).

Guideline 16: Hard of hearing
preschoolers in inclusive settings need support

Preschoolers who are hard of hearing or deaf with cochlear implants who have age-appropriate language and communication skills need accommodations to allow them to thrive educationally in the regular classroom. Necessary supports include the environmental accommodations mentioned earlier (acoustic treatments such as carpeting and acoustic tile on the ceilings, good lighting, reduction of the effects of glare, seating close to instructors), peers with whom the child can communicate comfortably, and staff who are oriented to and proficient at making learning activities visual as well as auditory. Teachers and other adults in the classroom must be knowledgeable about strategies for making language accessible in a classroom environment, and be prepared to provide all the repetition and clarification that is needed. Ideally, itinerant teachers and speech-language specialists should provide support by consulting with the general education preschool staff on the special accommodations children who are hard of hearing need. All too often, due to funding or other programmatic constraints, these specialists are available only on a limited basis, if at all, and this task then falls on the family.

One mother of a hard of hearing child designed an orientation program for her daughter Leela's inclusive preschool staff that worked so well she used it throughout her schooling. Because of Leela's sloping high frequency hearing loss, her behavior was confusing to her educators, who believed that because Leela heard and understood some things, she must hear and understand everything. This mother adapted the "speech banana" lesson[1] she had received in her parent–infant program and reworked the phonetic aspects of typical phrases as her child was likely to hear them. She says: "It worked like a charm! Leela's teachers would say, 'Oh!' "

This mother's experience facilitating her daughter's passage through school is similar to that described in *Overcoming the Expectation Gap* by Daniel Simmons, parent of a hard of hearing daughter. In his chapter, Simmons spells out the strategies he used to foster understanding and ensure appropriate accommodations throughout his daughter's school years. He asserts, "mainstreaming a hard of hearing child without adequate support services is tantamount to child abuse" (Simmons, as cited in Davis, 1990, p. 61).

---

[1]The "speech banana" is a banana-shaped region of the audiogram where speech sounds fall based on their intensity and frequency. A child's aided audiogram can be plotted on a form with this acoustical information about speech included in order to illustrate which individual sounds that child is likely to hear.

Guideline 17: Families with
hard of hearing children have as great a need
for support and information as do parents of deaf children

The goal of infant-family services for hard of hearing infants and toddlers is to provide families with the support they need to be a family, provide the tools to facilitate their infant's learning and growth, and, later, to help them take an advocacy role when their child is school age. This assistance begins with clear information about the implications of hearing loss coupled with emotional support.

Adjusting to the realization of a future that is different from the one they had envisioned for their infant is a process that requires time for parents of hard of hearing and deaf children. The adjustment is eased by access to information as well as by opportunities to share feelings and concerns with accepting listeners, in particular, with other parents. Parent support groups in programs that serve *both* deaf and hard of hearing children have much to offer parents of hard of hearing children. Learning about the variety of experiences and life choices open to individuals with all degrees of hearing loss better prepares parents to make choices for their child and begin to build new hopes and dreams for their child's future. At the same time, families with children who are hard of hearing have reported that, although they benefit greatly from their association with deaf adults and parents of deaf children, they also appreciate time spent with other parents of hard of hearing children.

Guideline 18: Working across cultures
requires sensitivity and can involve interpreters

There is a strong likelihood that professionals will encounter families of hard of hearing children whose cultural backgrounds, beliefs, and values differ from their own. Lynch and Hanson (1998) offered guidelines for cross-cultural work, beginning with an understanding of the cultural basis of one's own behaviors, beliefs, and values, followed by the acquisition of other culture-specific information and experiences. In some cultures, for example, including some native cultures in Alaska, children learn to show respect for adults by making minimal eye contact. Given that eye contact is central to the social interactions and communication that accompany language acquisition for hard of hearing children, these issues need to be addressed with families and accommodations made that respect cultural practices.

The wishes of non–English-speaking families must be respected, in terms of whether one language is focused on first or the child is exposed to both English and his or her native language. Language difference between the early childhood program and home can be a significant challenge for children who are hard of hearing and is deserving of a major focus in the development of resources to assist educators who work with families. Specialists must be trained to work effectively with interpreters and to be sensitive to the issues each family faces in order to ensure that the family's goals are understood and respected and that the needs of the child are also met (Ohtake, Milagros-Santos, & Fowler, 2000).

Guideline 19: The needs of families whose children have multiple developmental issues must be addressed

Professionals serving children who have multiple developmental needs and their families must have transdisciplinary skills and be prepared to work collaboratively with specialists at other agencies. When parents must go to a variety of agencies to get the different kinds of help their children need, the stress can be overwhelming and the services fragmented. For example, one mother, whose infant, Leela, had cerebral palsy and possible cognitive delays in addition to hearing loss, was seeing four different specialists for a time because of Leela's multiple needs. Her mother reports

Each specialist gave me assignments every week and when they gave a new one, they didn't remove the old one. They never talked to each other. Our whole life revolved around doing all the therapies Leela needed. The day I realized I was feeling guilty for taking time out to gas up the car, I knew something had to change. (B. Davis, personal communication, July 2000)

This mother, in fact, rebelled! She decided herself what was most important for her daughter during each developmental stage, and that is what she focused on, a practice she continued for many years. Some might argue that Leela's mom might have been better served had she and Leela met periodically with all the therapists together, or worked with a coordinator to design plans that were possible to carry out. But, testimony to parents' abilities to know what their children need, once they are given access to information, is Leela's success as a recent high school graduate, active in music and 4-H, boasting a 3.77 grade point average and the recipient of several honors, including a college scholarship.

SUMMARY

It is no longer necessary that hard of hearing children be referred to as "not deaf enough" (Candlish, 1996) or "our forgotten children" (Davis,

1990). This chapter has shown that much is known about what they need and about how to mitigate those needs, given early identification and early appropriate family-centered programming. Effective education of parents, teachers, and school officials can help avoid the pitfalls of assuming that after the placement of good hearing aids and the development of clear speech hard of hearing children will be just fine on their own, or of assuming that because they hear well sometimes they must hear well all the time. When families and educators pay careful attention to the needs and the development of the hard of hearing child in the areas of communication, school achievement, and social-emotional well-being, the child has the potential to do well in school while feeling comfortable with who he or she is.

LOOKING TO THE FUTURE

Identification of hearing loss at birth through UNHS is an important first step in overcoming the challenges faced by children who are hard of hearing and their families; however, it is just the beginning. If hard of hearing children are to reach their potential to achieve academically and to function in society with self-confidence and a sense of competence, additional changes to programs that provide services for children who are hard of hearing and their families must be made. Service delivery to hard of hearing infants and young children must be modified, professionals must be better trained to meet the needs of these infants and their families, and further research is needed. The following is just the beginning of a list of issues that still need to be addressed.

All hard of hearing infants and toddlers need to receive services based on individual needs

Already there are indications that, even with identification at birth, some communities do not consider hard of hearing infants eligible for early services if a language delay cannot also be demonstrated. Early, comprehensive, family-centered services must be in place for these children in order to mitigate the linguistic and academic effects of mild to severe hearing loss described earlier in this chapter.

There will be increased numbers of hard of hearing children in early childhood programs needing services from providers with specialized skills

Hard of hearing children, previously identified after the age of 2 years, will increasingly be identified at birth. The professional specialties that have traditionally served young hard of hearing children (deaf education, speech-language pathology, audiology, early childhood special education) will need to significantly increase the numbers of professionals trained and modify training to address the unique needs of families with infants and toddlers who are hard of hearing. In addition, with continued improvements in the technology of hearing aids and cochlear implants, there will be significantly greater numbers of children who, with assistive devices, are functionally hard of hearing.

Further investigations are needed to explore the similarities and differences between hard of hearing children, deaf children with cochlear implants, and hearing children

Regardless of cautions by cochlear implant centers, families and the general public often have expectations that every deaf child with a cochlear implant will function with the device as if he or she were "normally hearing." There are obvious pitfalls and heartbreaks should this turn out not to be the case. Further investigations are needed to explore the degree to which deaf children who receive cochlear implants early in life are *alike* and *unlike* hearing, hard of hearing, or deaf individuals without cochlear implants in order to provide realistic counseling to parents and eventually to the children themselves.

Families of hard of hearing children need to join together with families of deaf children with cochlear implants to require school programs to provide the supports both of these groups of children need

Increasing numbers of families with deaf children are deciding to get cochlear implants for their children. Many of these children share traits and needs in common with hard of hearing children in inclusive settings in that they profit from such supports as itinerant teachers, preferential seating, FM systems, information presented visually, and captioning on films. This significant increase in numbers of children needing these supports holds promise for more adequately serving hard of hearing children in inclusive environments.

The linguistic backgrounds of highly literate hard of hearing children should be investigated

Some children with moderate and severe hearing losses excel academically, reading several years beyond the average levels of hearing peers.

Some of these children's families used both spoken and signed communication with them from the earliest years. Does this dual language exposure provide a linguistic advantage to some hard of hearing children?

Families must learn to support the social-emotional well-being of their hard of hearing children through adolescence to young adulthood

Mental health referrals for young adults who are hard of hearing are high (M. Minkin, personal communication, March 23, 2000). Families with hard of hearing infants and young children need information about the social-emotional effects of mild to severe hearing loss in order to prepare from the earliest years to mitigate those effects. Most hard of hearing children are eventually educated in their public neighborhood schools in which they may be the only hard of hearing student in the school. By adolescence, interactions with peers are primarily verbal and identity is formed through these interactions and relationships. Some hard of hearing adolescents report that although they work hard to "fit in," they still feel different and at times isolated because of the challenges of understanding when there are multiple speakers in noisy situations. Inclusion in groups is difficult for students who are hard of hearing (Cappelli et al., 1995). These students and their families need counseling and support that will facilitate their transition through this period.

REFERENCES

Andrews, J. (1990). Partial hearing. In M.E. Vernon & J. Andrews (Eds.), *The psychology of deafness: Understanding deaf and hard-of-hearing people* (pp. 250–266). New York: Longman Publishing.

Bess, F., Dodd-Murphy, J., & Parker, R. (1998). Children with minimal sensorineural hearing loss: Prevalence, educational performance and functional status. *Ear and Hearing, 19*(5), 339–354.

Candlish, P.A.M. (1996). *Not deaf enough: Raising a child who is hard of hearing.* Washington, DC: Alexander Graham Bell Association for the Deaf.

Cappelli, M., Daniels, T., Durieux-Smith, A., McGrath, P., & Neuss, D. (1995). Social development of children with hearing impairments who are integrated into general education classrooms. *The Volta Review, 97*, 197–208.

Carver, R. (1996, March/April). To be visual or not to be visual: The hard of hearing child. *Deaf Children's Society of British Columbia Newsletter.*

Christensen, K. (2000). *Deaf plus: A multicultural perspective.* San Diego: Dawn Sign Press.

Cole, E. (1992). *Listening and talking: A guide to promoting spoken language in young hearing impaired children.* Washington, DC: Alexander Graham Bell Association for the Deaf.

Columbia Regional Program. (1998). *Position paper on hard of hearing students in early childhood.* Unpublished manuscript.

Condon, M. (2000, September). *On the journey to relationship-focused intervention.* Paper presented at the Conference on Relationship-Based Early-Intervention: How it Looks, How it Feels, Seattle.

Daniels, M. (1993). ASL as a factor in acquiring English. *Sign Language Studies, 78,* 23–29.

Davis, J. (1990). *Our forgotten children: Hard of hearing pupils in the schools.* Washington, DC: Self-Help for Hard of Hearing People.

Davis, J., Elfenbein, J., Schum, R., & Bentler, R. (1986). Effects of mild and moderate hearing impairments on language, educational and psychosocial behavior of children. *Journal of Speech and Hearing Disorders, 51,* 53–62.

Directors of Speech and Hearing Programs in State Health and Welfare Agencies Data Forms (DSHPSHWA). (2000). *Early hearing detection and intervention.* Atlanta, GA: Centers for Disease Control and Prevention, National Center on Birth Defects and Developmental Disabilities.

Elfenbein, J., Hardin-Jones, M., & Davis, J. (1994). Oral communication skills of children who are hard of hearing. *Journal of Speech and Hearing Research, 37,* 216–226.

English, K., & Church, G. (1999). Unilateral hearing loss in children: An update for the 1990's. *Language, Speech and Hearing Services in Schools, 30,* 26–31.

Estabrooks, W. (Ed.). (1994). *Auditory-verbal therapy for parents and professionals.* Washington, DC: Alexander Graham Bell Association for the Deaf.

Estabrooks, W., & Marlowe, J. (2000). *The baby is listening.* Washington, DC: Alexander Graham Bell Association for the Deaf.

Gallaudet Research Institute. (2001, January). *Regional and national summary report of data from the 1999–2000 Annual Survey of Deaf and Hard of Hearing Children & Youth.* Washington, DC: Author.

Garcia, J. (1999). *Sign with your baby: How to communicate with infants before they speak.* Seattle, WA: Northlight Communications.

Gilbertson, M., & Kamhi, A. (1995). Novel word learning in children with hearing impairment. *Journal of Speech and Hearing Research, 38,* 630–642.

Graney, S. (1997). ASL and spoken English: A bilingual program. *Perspectives in Education and Deafness, 16*(2), 6–8, 23.

Gray, C., & Hosie, J. (1996). Deafness, story understanding and theory of mind. *Journal of Deaf Studies and Deaf Education, 1*(4), 217–233.

Grushkin, D. (1996). *Academic, linguistic, social and identity development in hard of hearing adolescents educated within an ASL/English bilingual/bicultural educational setting for deaf and hard of hearing students.* Doctoral dissertation. Ann Arbor, MI: UMI Company.

Heffron, M. (2000). Clarifying concepts of infant mental health—promotion, relationship-based preventive intervention, and treatment. *Young Children, 12*(4), 14–21.

Joint Committee of the American Speech-Language-Hearing Association and the Council on Education of the Deaf. (1998, Spring). Hearing loss: Terminology and classification. *Asha,* 22–23.

Kavanaugh, K. (1995). Ear, nose, and sinus conditions of children with Down syndrome. In D. Van Dyke, P. Mattheis, S. Eberly, & J. Williams (Eds.), *Medical & surgical care for children with Down syndrome: A guide for parents* (pp. 155–174). Bethesda, MD: Woodbine House.

Kosma, C. (1995). Medical concerns and treatments. In K. Stray-Gundersen (Ed.), *Babies with Down syndrome: A new parents' guide* (pp. 1–36). Bethesda, MD: Woodbine House.

Kreimeyer, K., Crooke, D., Drye, C., Egbert, V., & Klein, B. (2000). Academic and social benefits of a co-enrollment model of inclusive education for deaf and hard of hearing children. *Journal of Deaf Studies and Deaf Education,* 5(2), 175–185.

The Leadership Training Institute/Special Education and the Bureau of Education for the Handicapped (U.S. Office of Education). (1976, March). *Serving hard of hearing pupils: Alternative strategies for personnel preparation.* Summary conference, Atlanta, GA.

Lynch, E.W., & Hanson, M.J. (Eds.). (1998). *Developing cross-cultural competence: A guide for working with children and their families* (2nd ed.). Baltimore: Paul H. Brookes Publishing Co.

Mason, S. (2000). *One mother's perspective.* Unpublished manuscript.

Maxon, A., & Bracket, D. (1992). *The hearing impaired child: Infancy through high-school years.* Woburn, MA: Butterworth-Heinemann.

Meadow-Orlans, K., Mertens, D., & Sass-Lehrer, M. (2003). *Parents and their deaf children.* Washington, DC: Gallaudet University Press.

Moeller, M. (1997). *Analysis of story narratives in two groups of preschool children.* Unpublished manuscript.

Moeller, M., Donaghy, K., Beauchaine, K., Lewis, D., & Stelmachowicz, D. (1996). Longitudinal study of FM system use in nonacademic settings: Effects on language development. *Ear and Hearing, 17*(1), 28–41.

Mohay, H. (2000). Language in sight: Mothers' strategies for making language visually accessible to deaf children. In P. Spencer, C. Erting, & M. Marshark (Eds.), *The deaf child in the family and at school: Essays in honor of Kathryn P. Meadow-Orlans* (pp. 151–166). Mahwah, NJ: Lawrence Erlbaum Associates.

Northern, J.L., & Downs, M.P. (1991). *Hearing in children* (4th ed.). Philadelphia: Lippincott Williams & Wilkins.

Ohtake, Y., Milagros-Santos, R., & Fowler, S. (2000). It's a three way conversation: Families, service providers and interpreters working together. *Young Exceptional Children, 4*(1), 12–18.

Petitto, L., Katerelos, M., Levy, B., Gauna, K., Tetreault, K., & Ferraro, V. (2001). Bilingual signed and spoken language acquisition from birth: Implications for the mechanisms underlying early bilingual language acquisition. *Journal of Child Language, 28*(2), 453–496.

Pollack, D., Goldberg, D., & Caleffe-Schenck, N. (1997). *Educational audiology for the limited hearing infant and preschooler: An auditory-verbal program* (3rd ed.). Springfield, IL: Charles C Thomas.

Preisler, G., & Ahlstrom, M. (1997). Sign language for hard of hearing children: A hindrance or a benefit for their development? *European Journal of Psychology of Education, 12*(4) 465–477.

Robards, C. (1991). *A nationwide study of parents of deaf and hard of hearing children during initial diagnosis: Implications for audiologists, physicians and educators.* Unpublished master's thesis, Western Maryland College, Westminster, MD.

Ross, M. (1990). Definitions and descriptions. In J. Davis (Ed.), *Our forgotten children: Hard of hearing pupils in the schools* (pp. 3–17). Washington, DC: Self-Help for Hard of Hearing People.

Rushmer, N., & Hatfield, N. (1993). Promoting early communication II: The role of the family. In V. Schuyler (Ed.), *Early intervention series* (p. 19). Portland, OR: Portland Center for Hearing and Speech.

Rushmer, N., & Melum, A. (2003). Columbia Regional Program, Portland, Oregon: Dual language learning in the early childhood years (birth to age eight). In D. Nussbaum, R. LaPorta, & J. Hinger (Eds.), *Cochlear implants and sign language: Putting it all together (identifying practices in educational settings)* (pp. 31–37). Washington, DC: Laurent Clerc National Deaf Education Center.

Schuyler, V., & Rushmer, N. (1987). *Parent-infant habilitation.* Portland, OR: Infant Hearing Resource.

Schuyler, V., & Sowers, J. (1998). *Parent-infant communication* (4th ed.). Portland, OR: Hearing & Speech Institute.

Shriberg, L., Friel-Patti, S., Flipsen, P., & Brown, R. (2000). Otitis media, fluctuant hearing loss, and speech-language outcomes: A preliminary structural equation model. *Journal of Speech, Language & Hearing Research, 43*(1), 100–120.

Simmons, D. (1990). Overcoming the expectation gap. In J. Davis (Ed.), *Our forgotten children: Hard of hearing pupils in the schools* (pp. 57–68). Washington, DC: Self-Help for Hard of Hearing People.

Swisher, V. (2000). Learning to converse: How deaf mothers support the development of attentional and conversational skills in their young deaf children. In P. Spencer, C. Erting, & M. Marshark (Eds.), *The deaf child in the family and at school: Essays in honor of Kathryn P. Meadow-Orlans* (pp. 151–166). Mahwah, NJ: Lawrence Erlbaum Associates.

Tomasello, M. (1988). The role of joint attentional processes in early language development. *Language Sciences, 10,* 69–88.

Yoshinaga-Itano, C., & Downey, D. (1996). The psychoeducational characteristics of school-aged students in Colorado with educationally significant hearing losses [Monograph]. *The Volta Review, 98*(1), 65–96.

Yoshinaga-Itano, C., & Sedey, H. (2000). Early speech development in children who are deaf or hard of hearing: Interrelationship with language and hearing [Monograph]. *The Volta Review, 100*(5), 181–211.

Reflecting on My Son Jared's First 5 Years

Tracy Weakly

I remember the very moment the doctors placed Jared in my arms. While everyone admired his beautiful dark hair and long eyelashes, I looked for something more. There they were, small slit-like holes on each side of his neck and pit-like holes near the top of each ear. "I'll bet he has a hearing loss, too," I thought to myself. Not that I was completely surprised. My mother is hearing impaired. My twin sister and I both had the same marks at birth, and we both have hearing loss. With a bit of sadness mixed with understanding, I handed Jared to my husband, Dwight. I wondered what little Jared's future would be.

The doctors confirmed that Jared had branchio-oto-renal syndrome, a rare disorder that was discovered about 10 years after I was born. Medical testing proved that other impairments of the syndrome did not affect Jared. The only thing to be determined was the degree of hearing loss. Oddly enough, Jared passed the auditory brainstem response (ABR) test. I was told his hearing was fine, with maybe a mild loss in the left ear only. Inwardly I couldn't believe Jared's hearing was okay. I pressed the audiologist for more testing that he finally agreed to when Jared was 9 months old.

Jared's first 3 months were exhausting. He had to be moving and facing outward all the time, constantly watching everything around him. He rolled over, sat, and crawled early, walking by 9 months. He was a bundle of energy and made loud noises, but he didn't really babble. People told me that Jared was a boy—boys don't talk. I knew better. I began signing to him. Eventual retesting showed a severe sloping to moderate hearing loss. It seemed that his loss was more severe than mine, but I was so relieved to learn the true status of Jared's hearing that I didn't care.

By age 2, Jared was receiving hearing and language services and knew well over 100 signs. His teachers told me he might never talk or if he did, it might not be understandable. I was willing to accept this possibility but inwardly I believed Jared would talk. Then came the surgeries. A month before Jared's second birthday he had surgery to remove the cysts in his neck. It was a heart-rending experience, but Jared recovered quickly and soon afterward began to talk. And then just before his fourth birthday a computerized axial tomography (CAT) scan revealed that both cochleas were leaking fluid into the inner ear and a cholesteatoma was growing in Jared's right ear. These conditions required two surgeries; the second to remove the cholesteatoma lasted 3 hours. It gave me lots of time to think. Once again I was faced with the fact that Jared might become deaf in one or both ears. The cholesteatoma could grow back. I could accept my son as either deaf or hard of hearing, but the back and forth was getting to me.

When Jared turned 3, the school system declared that he would have to go to a preschool where the teacher had never had a deaf or hard of hearing child. It was the only option. He would receive an FM system for the regular class and pull-out services for speech. Jared hated school. He didn't want to go. He stopped signing at home. When I observed the classroom, I found that the teacher and paraprofessionals talked down to him. Then my husband received a job transfer to a different state.

Jared was immediately placed in an early intervention preschool with two teachers trained in the education of deaf and hard of hearing students. Of the eight children in the class, half were hard of hearing and half were hearing. Jared blossomed. He wore his hearing aids and started signing again. Teachers told me Jared was intelligent, full of energy, and loved to participate in group discussions. It was a dream come true.

By age 5, Jared's speech and language were age appropriate and I decided to home school for kindergarten this year. Jared is thriving. He is learning to read and do simple math, and he takes various sports classes from the local Parks and Recreation Department, where he excels in gymnastics. As I watch the classes, I am aware of how much he observes and how much he misses. Currently, I am his advocate and interpreter, a role most mothers of deaf and hard of hearing children must play. He still receives periodic hearing tests and CAT scans. Presently, all seems well. The future is yet to be determined. To me, Jared is a normal, healthy, happy, energetic, and compassionate boy. Whether he remains hard of hearing or whether he becomes deaf is irrelevant. My wish is that Jared will be happy in what he chooses and successful in what he does and that he will find his special place in this world and make it better.

CHAPTER NINE

Inclusion of Young Children Who Are Deaf and Hard of Hearing

CAROL JACKSON CROYLE

Eight 4-year-old children are sitting in a classroom at a round table enjoying a Popsicle as a special treat. Tommy and Joe, who are sitting next to each other, are engaged in conversation, each signing and not using their voices. They are deaf. A boy, Steve, who is hearing, and a boy, Larry, who is deaf, are watching their reflections in a mirror that is set up behind the table as they lick their Popsicles. They copy each other's silly faces and laugh. A girl who is deaf, Bernadette, appears to be daydreaming as she eats her Popsicle; she has just woken from a nap. Cindy, a girl who is hearing, turns to another hearing girl, Alicia, who is sitting next to her and says, using voice only, "I love you." Pam, another hearing girl who is sitting across the table looks at Cindy and says, "You're not supposed to say that!" Cindy says, "Yes, you are supposed to tell your friends that you love them because it makes them feel good. That's what friends are for." Alicia says, "That's what friends are for!" Then Pam chimes in, "That's what friends are for!" The three hearing girls continue to chant, without signing, "That's what friends are for! That's what friends are for! That's what friends are for!"

These young children are being educated together in an inclusive preschool classroom at a school for the deaf. Enrolled in this program are an equal number of children who are deaf and children who are hearing. This is one example of the many types of inclusive programs. Inclusive programs can have different ratios of children who are deaf versus those who are hearing. Early education inclusive programs can be found in schools for the deaf as well as in general settings such as public schools, child care programs, neighborhood play groups, hospitals, libraries, community centers, and child development centers.

This chapter outlines the benefits and special challenges of educating infants, toddlers, and preschoolers who are deaf and hard of hearing in inclusive settings. Relevant research is reviewed, and recommendations are provided for improving the potential for success. This chapter also describes two early education programs that enroll children who are deaf, children who are hard of hearing, and children who are hearing, but differ in educational philosophy and communication methodologies.

THE LARGER CONTEXT OF INCLUSION

Most children who are deaf and hard of hearing, especially those born to hearing parents, are included in a hearing society from birth. The majority of children who are deaf and hard of hearing live in a home with hearing members, attend community events with mostly hearing people, attend hearing churches, and attend playgroups with hearing children. Therefore, a majority of deaf children live in an inclusive world. When describing her son's placement in a preschool program for children who are deaf, one mother stated, "This is the only place where my child can communicate with everyone. His whole life is mainstreamed; at church, in the neighborhood, everywhere we go." Because of the communication needs of this child and the lack of ability to communicate in environments outside of his preschool program, this mother chose a noninclusive early educational setting.

If early education programs are supposed to focus on the special needs of the children they support, why do many parents seek inclusive programs for infants, toddlers, and preschoolers who are deaf and hard of hearing? What are the advantages of providing services to these children in an environment that includes hearing children? Can the special needs of children who are deaf and hard of hearing be met in an inclusive program? Antia and Levine emphasized that "inclusion of children who are deaf or hard of hearing is an unusually difficult task that requires careful planning, adequate resources, and professional expertise" (2001, p. 365). To ensure successful programs, there must be collaborative efforts among early interventionists, educators, child care staff, program administrators, parents, and community leaders. Even with the efforts and hard work of all involved, successful inclusion of deaf and hard of hearing children with hearing children can be especially challenging (Leutke-Stahlamn, 1994; Walsh, Rous, & Lutzer, 2000). Various challenges may involve academic inclusion, social inclusion, and educating a diverse student population (Stinson & Antia, 1999).

RATIONALE FOR INCLUSIVE PROGRAMS

Inclusive programs for young children who are deaf and hard of hearing exist for a number of reasons, including sociopolitical context, federal and state legislation, theoretical principles, philosophical principles, and family concerns.

Sociopolitical Context

One of the historical foundations for the inclusion of children who are deaf and hard of hearing into classrooms with hearing children was the Civil Rights movement. In response to the Civil Rights movement in the 1950s and 1960s, American legislators acknowledged and addressed a wide range of social, educational, and economic inequities. Although most often associated with the issue of racial inequality, the Civil Rights movement also served as a critical foundation for policy changes in special education. The broad scope of the enacted legislation provided a foundation for attempts to address the educational needs of children who are deaf and hard of hearing.

Legislation

As a result of the 1954 Supreme Court decision in *Brown v. Board of Education,* a legal rationale was provided for the racial integration of public schools. The Civil Rights movement and the *Brown* ruling had an impact on the expectations and perceptions of many minority groups, including parents of children with special needs.

One group that began to speak out against inequality was the parents of children with mental retardation. Many of these children were institutionalized without access to an educational program. As a result of the Supreme Court's ruling in *Pennsylvania Association for Retarded Children (PARC) v. Commonwealth of Pennsylvania* in 1971, it was determined that children with disabilities had the right to a public education. On the basis of court cases and advocacy from parents of children with disabilities, Congress passed the Education for All Handicapped Children Act of 1975 (PL 94-142). This act required that children with disabilities be provided a free and appropriate public education in the least restrictive environment (LRE). The LRE has often been interpreted as meaning the same programs provided to typically developing children.

As early as 1989, revision of the law (which became Part C of the Individuals with Disabilities Education Act [IDEA] of 1990, PL 101-476) required early intervention services to take place in settings with children without disabilities. However, it was the amendments to and reauthorization of IDEA in 1997 (PL 105-17) that "strengthened the requirement that early intervention services be provided to infants and toddlers (birth to age 3) with disabilities in 'natural environments,' to the extent appropriate to the child" (Walsh et al., 2000). Any services sought by families with infants and toddlers with disabilities must be offered in "settings that are natural or normal for the child's age peers who have no disabilities" (34 C.F.R. Part 303.18). Natural environments include the child's home as well as community settings such as child care centers, play groups, nursery schools, neighborhood school classrooms, and other programs that are accessible to typically developing hearing children (Council for Exceptional Children, Division for Early Childhood, 2000). Services provided outside of these inclusive natural environments require written justification.

Along with PL 105-17, the Americans with Disabilities Act (ADA) of 1990 (PL 101-336) helped to ensure that individuals with special needs, including infants, toddlers, and preschoolers who are deaf and hard of hearing, have equal access to the same facilities and opportunities as their typically developing peers. However, research suggests that simply placing children who are deaf and hard of hearing in close proximity with hearing peers does not ensure successful social inclusion or acceptance from hearing peers (Lee & Antia, 1992; Solit, Taylor, & Bednarczyk, 1992). Programs, then, must make reasonable modifications to accommodate children with a hearing loss.

Within the domain of deaf education, the implementation of IDEA 1997 has been controversial. Many educators and parents of children with hearing losses are opposed to certain interpretations of the law. The stipulation in IDEA that children with hearing loss have access to a "free appropriate public education," must be educated in the "least restrictive environment," and that programming for infants and toddlers with a hearing loss be offered in "naturalistic settings" is often interpreted to mean that children who are deaf and hard of hearing can be educated only in those programs designed for a hearing population. Some would argue, however, that programs consisting of a majority of hearing children would in fact be considered a more restrictive environment because there is a lack of a shared language. As stated by Mowl,

> The need for a sense of belonging and comfort is very real. No matter how hard society pushes inclusion, especially in educational opportunities, people's acceptance of each other without regard to race, sex, or disability is a formidable task and this society has been trying to address it for years and years. The name change from mainstreaming to inclusion is like "old wine in a new bottle." The underlying issues remain unresolved. Inclusion does not guarantee acceptance. (1996, p. 239)

Another controversial issue concerns the number or proportion of children who are deaf and hard of hearing in a classroom. Leaders in the Deaf community feel that educational programs should enroll a critical mass of children who are deaf and hard of hearing and share a common language to enhance communication and socialization between peers. (See the Considerations for Placement section later in this chapter). Perhaps with the reauthorization of IDEA 1997 that is in progress as of 2003, these controversial issues concerning children with hearing loss will be addressed. (See Chapter 3 for a more in-depth discussion on legislation.)

Theoretical Principles

In addition to legal mandates, theoretical principles have driven the development of inclusion of children with disabilities with typically developing children. One theory holds that children with disabilities will demonstrate improved performance from exposure to and interaction with peers without disabilities. The rationale for placement of deaf and hard of hearing children in programs with typically developing hearing children is that students without disabilities will model relatively advanced social and linguistic behaviors for students with disabilities (Spencer, Koester, & Meadow-Orlans, 1994). In fact, research on children with disabilities nonspecific to deafness has shown that children with disabilities and their families benefit from the children's interaction with peers without disabilities. However, there has been no empirical evaluative research on the efficacy of inclusive programs for young children who are deaf and hard of hearing and their families.

In theory, including children who are deaf and hard of hearing in programs for hearing children can help the hearing children develop more positive attitudes toward children with hearing loss and allows hearing children to benefit from interactions with their deaf and hard of hearing peers. Research involving older children with disabilities not specific to deafness has shown that children without disabilities more readily accept peers with disabilities when given opportunities to interact with them (Voeltz, 1982) and also benefit from these experiences as they develop friendships with their peers with disabilities (Staub, 1998). Research results specific to deafness indicated that school-age students who were deaf were "well received socially" by hearing classmates in an inclusive educational program (Cambra, 2002). Positive outcomes for all children in an inclusive setting may include "companionship, growth in social understanding, increased positive sense of self, development of personal principles, and a sense of belonging" (Staub, 1998, p. 97). Research is needed to determine the outcomes for very young children who are deaf and hard of hearing when placed in inclusive programs.

Philosophical Principles

In our vastly diverse society, it is imperative that children learn to accept and tolerate differences in others. "Learning tolerance for those who are different is becoming an increasingly important goal for our society and our schools as our population becomes more diverse" (Cavallaro & Haney, 1999, p. 23). However, as Afzali-Nomani warned, "forced integration does not always result in greater acceptance of diversity" (1995, p. 396). Fuchs and Fuchs contended that one of the primary jobs of educators is to "help change stereotypic thinking about disabilities among normally developing children" (2000, p. 71). Through inclusive programs, children as well as other family members can learn about diversity of abilities as well as diversity in culture, language, communication, and values.

"The conviction is that inclusion is a morally defensible ideal; the imperative, that everyone must champion the cause of full inclusion and accept the underlying premises as well as the practical implications for programming because it is simply the right thing to do" (Winzer, 2000, p. 9). Early education specialists must take the lead and learn about the various cultures of the children and families they support. Sharing and celebrating Deaf culture is a necessity if children who are deaf and hard of hearing are included in an early childhood program. Inviting older students and adults who are deaf and hard of hearing into the classroom to read stories and interact with all members of the group can facilitate a better understanding of diversity and deafness.

Family Concerns

In addition to societal, legal, and theoretical principles involving inclusive programming for children with disabilities, there are also family concerns to consider. With the majority of families in the United States having both parents in the workforce, child care is a critical issue for families. "According to the latest estimates from the U.S. Census Bureau, 60 percent of the nation's children age 5 or younger now live in two-parent homes where both parents work or in single-parent households where that parent is employed" (Doherty, 2002, pp. 1–2).

In addition to seeking quality child care and preschool programs, families with children who are deaf and hard of hearing also need to ensure that the program includes adults and peers who can effectively communicate with and serve as role models to their children. Finding a child care program, whether private or public, with staff that can meet the needs of children who are deaf and hard of hearing and their families is problematic. Staff availability, staff competency, and having an appropriate number of peers who share similar communication preferences are issues that become paramount to program selection.

Location of programs available to families with children who are deaf and hard of hearing is another concern. Most programs are located in urban areas, making them less accessible to families living in rural areas. In an interview with a parent of two children with hearing losses, the mother reported that she placed one of her children in a preschool program in her neighborhood, while the younger child attended a center-based parent–infant program located a distance from their home. Doing this resulted in the ease of scheduling for the entire family. In this situation, the older child was able to ride the bus to the neighborhood preschool program while the mother was able to transport her younger child to the center-based parent–infant program. Scheduling conflicts and transportation issues often influence parents' selection of the most appropriate educational setting.

Aside from program concerns, most parents of children with disabilities want their child to be a part of the community in which they live. "Parents of children with disabilities often believe that inclusion can offer their child greater exposure to the real world, positive social contacts, opportunities to learn from children without disabilities, a wider variety of activities, and greater community support" (Wall, 2000, p. 203). Providing young children who are deaf and hard of hearing access to community events, such as storytelling at the local library, benefits all families living in the neighborhood. The young child who is deaf or hard of hearing gains added experiences and opportunities for learning. At the same time, other families living in the area have an opportunity to learn from the child (and his or her family) who has a difference in hearing ability and possibly a difference in mode of communication. Community programs can only be successful, however, if the appropriate services (e.g., fluent signer, oral interpreter, preferential seating) are made available to the child who is deaf or hard of hearing.

Parents also generally hope that their children will develop friendships with hearing children in the neighborhood. Parents may have experienced the development of friendships between their hearing children and other hearing children living in the neighborhood. Because of location, convenience, and the probability that the hearing children attend the same school and community programs, these friendships between hearing children occur very naturally. However, because of the relatively low incidence of children born with hearing loss, the likelihood of finding children who 1) are similar in age, 2) have a hearing loss, 3) share the same mode of communication, and 4) live within the same neighborhood is small. The possibility of friendships developing between children with hearing losses and children who can hear is increased when organizations and programs within the community provide special services to ensure inclusion of the child who is deaf or hard of hearing.

In many ways, friendships between children who can hear and children who are deaf and hard of hearing more easily occur when the children are young (Mundy, 2002). In a 2002 article in the *The Washington Post Magazine,* a deaf mother of two deaf children related her early experiences of friendships with peers who were hearing. She said, "Those friendships were relatively easy when [I] was young, riding bikes and running around, but became much harder in adolescence, where so much of friendship is conducted verbally, in groups, which are impossible to lip-read" (as cited in Mundy, 2002, p. 27). By providing inclusive programs (with appropriate special services) in the community of families with children who are deaf and hard of hearing, meaningful friendships can develop between toddlers and preschoolers, regardless of hearing status.

LITERATURE REVIEW

Although there are good reasons for integrating deaf and hearing children, little research has been published that specifically determines the efficacy of early inclusion. No studies have assessed the social, emotional, or cognitive domains of children in inclusive programs versus those in noninclusive programs through empirical research. Researchers who have examined young children with a hearing loss included with children who can hear have primarily focused on social inclusion of these children. More specifically, researchers have concentrated on the direct interactions between the two groups to determine success of inclusive environments.

For example, Spencer et al. (1994) conducted a study with young children who are deaf and hard of hearing and their hearing peers in which the primary focus was on the number of interactions between the two groups in order to assess the acceptance of children who are deaf and hard of hearing by their hearing peers. Eight children were selected on the basis of their hearing status, their parents' hearing status, their gender, and their age. Two children were deaf and had hearing parents, two were deaf with Deaf parents, two were hearing with Deaf parents, and two were hearing with hearing parents. The group included five girls, ages 28–36 months, and three boys, ages 29–30 months. The researchers limited their focus to communicative interactions of children in the classroom setting only. In a quantitative analysis of communicative interactions of deaf and hearing children in a child care setting, the researchers found that although there were interactions between the two groups, there was a tendency for deaf children as well as hearing children to communicate with their same hearing status peers.

Although this study provided valuable information, readers are left with many questions about the nature, content, context, and success of the communicative interactions that did occur between the deaf and hearing children. What is the meaning and importance of frequency counts as a measure within this context? Can frequency of communication between young children alone adequately describe or predict a social relationship or friendship or acceptance of deaf children by their hearing peers? The quality of communication and the success or failure of communication attempts between the two groups of children in this study was not determined.

Minnett, Clark, and Wilson (1994) were also interested in the inclusion of deaf and hearing populations in the educational system. Like Spencer et al. (1994), they studied the number of communicative interactions between preschoolers who were deaf and hard of hearing and hearing. In addition to frequency of communicative interactions, they investigated the number and types of play behavior the two groups engaged in. Descriptive information about the children's interactions, however, was not provided. The number of children participating in this research was substantially larger than in the Spencer et al. (1994) study. A total of 60 participants were included; there were 30 hearing students and 30 students who were deaf or hard of hearing in six different classrooms. The children ranged in age from 3 to 5 years and included children of cultural and ethnic diversity (African American, Caucasian, and Hispanic children were present in each group studied).

Another feature of the Minnett et al. (1994) study is the inclusion of deaf and hard of hearing children and their hearing peers from both auditory/oral communication inclusive programs and total communication inclusive programs. By comparing children enrolled in two different communication methodology environments, the researchers were able to capture levels of communication and play behaviors used with peers with different communication modalities or methodologies. The researchers found that nonsocial play and communication with peers did not differ significantly between the two communication environments. However, although children in the auditory communication environment were more likely to engage in solitary play, the children in the total communication environment were more likely to engage in parallel play.

The results of this quantitative research correspond with the Spencer et al. (1994) study. Both deaf and hearing children preferred to communicate with their same hearing status peers. Although both groups exhibited similar amounts of social play, the researchers concluded that "without exception, children were more likely to engage a peer of similar-hearing status in all levels of social play and communication" (p. 424).

Like Minnett et al. (1994), Esposito and Koorland (1989) studied the types of play behavior of two deaf preschool-age children. The children were observed in a self-contained preschool classroom and in their separate inclusive child care programs. Both children engaged in more associative play with the hearing children in the inclusive child care program than in their noninclusive preschool program. In the preschool program, the children engaged primarily in parallel play. The researchers concluded that the presence of hearing children helped promote interactive play in these preschool children who were severely to profoundly deaf.

Antia and Ditillo (1998) investigated the play behavior of preschool-age children in inclusive playgroups. Although the researchers were unable to determine the hearing status of the play partners when analyzing their data, as this information was not recorded, they were able to conclude that the deaf and hard of hearing children engaged in similar levels of positive peer interactions as their hearing peers.

While these studies focus on the socio-emotional and play benefits of inclusion, needed are studies that focus on linguistic and academic benefits of inclusion for deaf and hard of hearing children.

TYPES OF INCLUSIVE PROGRAMS

There are a variety of program development strategies for integrating children with special needs, including infants, toddlers, and preschoolers who are deaf and hard of hearing, into classrooms with typically developing peers. This section discusses two program models: inclusion and reverse mainstreaming.

Evolution of Terminology

Although many people in the field of special education use the terms mainstreaming and inclusion interchangeably, they have different meanings (Stinson & Antia, 1999; Winzer, 2000). Mainstreaming was a practice that was used in the past to integrate preschoolers with special needs, such as those who were deaf and hard of hearing, into programs with typically developing peers, while at the same time incorporating delivery of special services by early interventionists outside of the general classroom (typically called "pull-out" services) to ensure success. This practice came about with the implementation of PL 94-142. At the time mainstreaming began, most states did not provide publicly funded educational programs for any preschoolers; therefore, preschoolers who were deaf and hard of hearing, for example, usually received early intervention services in their homes and/or in center-based programs developed for children with special needs. This continues to be true today (Wolery & Odom, 2000).

Inclusion

Because children with special needs are included in the general classroom only part of the day with mainstreaming, many parents and educators involved in general education feel that inclusion is a more appropriate approach when integrating children with and without special needs. Although there is still controversy and confusion about inclusion (Heward, 2000), it is generally agreed that the practice involves placement of children with special needs and those without special needs together. Inclusion is described as programming that "extends beyond formal educational settings to a wide variety of family, child care, and community activities" (Wall, 2000, p. 198). As with mainstreaming, deaf and hard of hearing children, for example, are placed in programs that are composed of a majority of hearing children. Inclusion, however, is different from mainstreaming in that the children who are "included" receive special services and support within the inclusive setting. Special services such as speech-language therapy, occupational therapy, physical therapy, and play therapy are provided within the placement setting to enable the deaf child to succeed in this environment. "Under the principles of inclusion . . . children do not push into the mainstream because inclusive programs expect that all children will be based in the schools or classrooms that they would attend if they did not have a disability" (Winzer, 2000, p. 6). The advantage of receiving services within the classroom is that the children with special needs are full-time members of the class and are not perceived by the other students and teachers as "visitors" to the classroom. Many parents and educators believe that inclusion is a better practice "because it indicates that children with disabilities are naturally members of the general education classroom and belong there on a full-time basis" (Cavallaro & Haney, 1999, p. 21).

Reverse Mainstreaming

Another inclusive program model is reverse mainstreaming. Reverse mainstreaming can be defined by the inclusion of typically developing children within early intervention programs developed specifically to educate children with special needs. For example, reverse mainstreaming would include hearing children in programs designed specifically for children who are deaf and hard of hearing. Ratios of children who are deaf and hard of hearing and hearing children vary from program to program, but typically the majority are children who are deaf and hard of hearing. The presence of hearing children serves a number of purposes, including providing role models to the children who are deaf.

However, children who are deaf and hard of hearing often have unique communication needs, the solutions for which all hearing students may not be able to fully provide. To ensure ease of communication, many of the hearing children selected for reverse mainstreaming programs are children of Deaf adults (CODA) and siblings of children who are deaf and hard of hearing. There are potential benefits of this arrangement for the child with a hearing loss as well as for the hearing child and his or her family. Antia and Levine reported that teachers of kindergarten and first-grade students in an inclusive program "mentioned that sign language created a beneficial visual environment for all children in the classroom" (2001, p. 370). Many children of Deaf adults enter the program with fluent signing skills that facilitate direct and effective communication between the children who are hearing and the children who are deaf. Likewise, hearing siblings attending an early intervention preschool can benefit from the increased exposure to sign language that then enables them to communicate more effectively at home with their older brother or sister who is deaf (G. Solit, personal communication, 2002). This may be especially beneficial in families in which the parents are struggling to learn to sign.

Early intervention center-based programs serving deaf and hard of hearing infants and toddlers usually include non–school-age hearing siblings in play groups set up specifically for the deaf child in the family. At the preschool level, there is an effort to enroll hearing peers in classrooms designed for children who are deaf and hard of hearing. Under these circumstances, language access is central to the needs of the deaf child.

A Team Teaching Approach

Regardless of which model is utilized, a highly recommended practice for inclusive programs involves team teaching. Along with the general education preschool or child care teacher, children who are deaf and hard of hearing and children who can hear are taught by an early education specialist trained in Deaf education. This is also referred to as the co-enrollment model (Kreimeyer, Crooke, Drye, Egbert, & Klein, 2000) or co-teaching model (Kluwin, 1999). Ideally, in a team teaching situation, the early education specialist would be present in the early childhood setting at all times as described in the co-enrollment and co-teaching models. In reality, however, many times the deaf education specialist serves as an itinerant teacher and is available on a limited basis, primarily as a resource to the classroom teacher. It is important that the special education and general classroom teacher understand their respective roles and responsibilities regardless of the model they are working in (Antia, 1999; Jimenez-Sanchez & Antia, 1999).

Influences on Program Development

Adequate provision of appropriate services is essential to ensure success in an inclusive setting (Afzali-Nomani, 1995; Stinson & Antia, 1999). Although various inclusive programs have been defined, it should be pointed out that no two programs are exactly alike within each category. Differences in communication methodology choices, curriculum choices, and various program philosophies of educating children who are deaf and hard of hearing may have a great influence on program development. For example, two programs may call themselves bilingual and utilize American Sign Language (ASL) and English but approach the use of each language very differently. One program may primarily utilize ASL in face-to-face communication, while promoting the acquisition of English through exposure to print. Another program may use ASL during specific times of the day and a sign system such as manually coded English to teach English at other times. Yet another choice might be for some people in the child's environment to sign ASL, while others sign using manually coded English (Watkins, Pittman, & Walden, 1998).

Curriculum choices also create differences in inclusive programs. The are numerous curricula available to early educators, and curriculum choice often reflects the educational philosophy of the program. For example, an early intervention program incorporating the Reggio Emilia approach would look very different than one using the more structured Montessori curriculum and materials.

Another factor affecting inclusion involves the ratios of children in the setting; the ratios of children with a hearing loss and without a hearing loss can vary from program to program and may change over time. Inclusive programs may include children with other special needs as well. Some programs include interpreters as part of the team, and professionals trained to serve children who are deaf and hard of hearing may or may not be present in inclusive programs. Deaf adults may or may not be included in the early intervention team, depending on program philosophy and availability of Deaf adults in the community. Programs also vary in the amount of time infants, toddlers, and preschoolers receive services.

Families can also have a large impact on program development. By their very nature, home-based, family-centered early intervention programs can be considered inclusive programs.

> Family-centered services by design must focus on the complete family, not just the child who is deaf or hard of hearing. Within this concept there is an understanding that the definition of family can extend far beyond the traditional sense, and can involve anyone who cares for, loves, and is involved with the child's life. (Pittman, 2001, p. 9)

These programs may involve siblings of the child who is deaf and hard of hearing as well as extended family members (e.g., cousins, aunts, uncles, grandparents), and family support people. For example babysitters, neighborhood friends (including children), and others who are felt by the family to provide support are often encouraged to join the early interventionist when conducting a home visit.

COMMUNICATION ISSUES SPECIFIC TO YOUNG CHILDREN WHO ARE DEAF AND HARD OF HEARING

One of the primary challenges of child care providers, early interventionists, and others providing services to infants, toddlers, and preschoolers who are deaf and hard of hearing is ensuring that these children have access to language and communication. "The major difficulty faced by children who have a hearing loss is access to oral communication and the oral language of the community" (Antia & Levine, 2001, p. 367). Most deaf children experience difficulty understanding spoken language, and few hearing children are fluent in sign language. The challenges for all involved focus on three main issues: language differences, modality differences, and language competence.

The primary language of many deaf children is ASL, although most hearing children in the United States communicate through spoken English. This lack of a shared language creates barriers to effective communication, socialization, and building of relationships.

Modality differences between children who are deaf and hard of hearing and children who can hear occur because many children, especially those with profound hearing losses, do not readily acquire language through the auditory channel. They must have access to language through a visual channel. For these children, sign language or a sign system or cued speech is required for access to information. Although it may be easier for children who are deaf and hard of hearing to learn a visual sign language, these children often lack exposure to a community of fluent signers (Antia & Levine, 2001). Because of the low incidence of deafness, many inclusive programs are unlikely to have fluent signing teachers or early interventionists. Few hearing peers in early childhood programs understand or use sign language or cued speech, and many children who are deaf and hard of hearing experience difficulty in speaking. Therefore, there are few opportunities for deaf and hearing children to effectively communicate using a mutual language modality.

Although children who are deaf and hard of hearing and born to Deaf parents acquire language (through sign) at the rate and level of hearing children of hearing parents, many deaf children born to hearing parents have difficulty acquiring levels of language proficiency equal to these peers. This difference in language competency level contributes to the difficulty in successful inclusion of children who are deaf and hard of hearing with children who can hear. In essence, the primary challenges for professionals developing programs that integrate deaf and hearing populations involve the deaf and hard of hearing child's access to language, the basis for socialization, interaction, and cooperative learning.

PURPOSE OF AN INCLUSIVE
PROGRAM FOR CHILDREN WITH HEARING LOSSES

One might ask, "What is the purpose of setting up inclusive programs for very young children who are deaf and hard of hearing?" "The goal of inclusive programs that is most directly and firmly rooted in the ideology of inclusion relates to the nature of the social relationships that occur between children with and without disabilities" (Guralnick, 2001, p. 23). In describing a federal outreach grant program, Project Access, Solit and Bednarczyk (1999) listed three main objectives of the inclusive child care program: to create a social environment that facilitates acceptance of children who are deaf and hard of hearing by children who can hear, to enable friendships between children with and without hearing losses to develop, and to provide opportunities for children using different languages and communication modes and from different cultures to learn from each other.

Facilitating Acceptance

One of the primary ways to promote acceptance of differences is through modeling positive behaviors and attitudes. Afzali-Nomani (1995) found that programs that offered strong support from general teachers for full inclusion positively affected the success of the deaf and hard of hearing children. It is very important that early educators be given a choice to include a child with a hearing loss into the program and be willing to do so. It is also imperative that the provider demonstrates positive attitudes toward the child who is deaf and hard of hearing.

Diamond and Innes (2001) pointed out that children's literature, especially books that emphasize competence of children with special needs, can be used to promote positive attitudes toward children with differing abilities. Hands-on activities and opportunities for exploration can also foster the development of positive attitudes. In the case of the child who wears a hearing aid and is in an inclusive program, it would be helpful for the interventionist to explain the function of a hearing aid and allow the children to manipulate the aid (one borrowed from the district audiologist or hearing aid dealer). All children in the inclusive setting should be allowed to put the hearing aid on and take it off, listen to sound through the aid, insert and remove the batteries (under adult supervision), and be given information about deafness in terms they can understand.

Hearing children in the inclusive program with children who are deaf and hard of hearing should be introduced to the concepts of deafness and, if children are present who sign, taught sign language. This strategy is advantageous for children who can hear as well as the children who are deaf and hard of hearing (Afzali-Nomani, 1995). It is important for the child care provider to present accurate information in a positive way by discussing the uniqueness of the deaf individual. A positive approach to introducing deafness involves identifying the ways in which people with hearing losses are just like other people and emphasizing the abilities and many achievements of deaf and hard of hearing individuals as well as ways they compensate for their hearing loss. This avoids stereotyping and stresses the uniqueness of individuals (National Information Center on Deafness [NICD], 1991, p.8).

Friendships

Fuchs and Fuchs reported that

> Full inclusionists believe that one of the primary jobs of educators is to help children with disabilities establish friendships with nondis-abled persons . . . and that within the context of friendship mak-ing . . . educators should help children with disabilities develop social skills. (2000, p. 71)

Afzali-Nomani (1995) also found that success of inclusive programs is favorable if children who are deaf and hard of hearing receive social encouragement from teachers.

If, in fact, one of the main goals of inclusion is to help children with disabilities establish friendships, adaptations can be made in the environment to encourage socialization. For example, many programs for very young children make available a variety of learning centers for the children. It is important that young children are allowed to move about freely when making choices, selecting materials, and choosing places to play. By providing choices, a variety of learning centers enable children with similar interests to socialize and be involved in cooperative play. Antia (1994) suggested strategies for socializing young children who are deaf and hard of hearing with their hearing peers. These include 1) reducing teacher–child interactions, 2) changing classroom activity structure to be more child centered rather than teacher directed, 3) providing social skills intervention, 4) providing peer-mediated interventions, 5) increasing familiarity through intensive contact, and 6) providing peer orientation. Other suggestions for fostering friendships can be found in Table 9.1 (Staub, 1998).

Leutke-Stahlman (1994, 1995) also outlined strategies for both child-centered and adult-centered activities to promote social interactions between young children who are deaf and hard of hearing and their hearing peers. Several strategies for maximizing success of social interactions are 1) providing continuous facilitation by adults throughout the day, 2) including the child who is deaf or hard of hearing with hearing children during a majority of instructional time, 3) structuring groups so that they include both hearing children and children who are deaf and hard of hearing, and 4) having play be the primary medium through which intervention occurs (Leutke-Stalman, 1994).

Table 9.1. Strategies for fostering friendships

Create classroom communities that promote belonging and acceptance for all children.

Do not make friendships a big deal.

Respect personal boundaries.

Model behavior.

Encourage reciprocity and contribution.

Merge respect and help.

Emphasize empathy and social justice.

Encourage families to spend time with other families who have a child in the inclusive program separate from the early childhood setting.

Source: Staub (1998).

Different Language and Communication Modes

Another goal of inclusive programming for children with hearing losses is for all children, both hearing and Deaf and hard of hearing, to interact with each other and with deaf and hearing adults in order to learn various language and communication modes. Children learn language by interacting with people. Communication is a turn-taking endeavor and very interactive. Therefore, direct communication between all children and between the children and early childhood teachers is essential (Solit & Bednarczyk, 1999; Winston, 1994).

Because very young children who are deaf and hard of hearing are learning the rules of language and communication, reliance on a sign language interpreter is inadvisable. Interpreters are also not recommended for very young children because "there is not much knowledge of how young children perceive their interpreters, whether they understand that the teacher talk is being interpreted, and how interpreters facilitate or inhibit children's classroom participation" (Antia & Levine, 2001, p. 373). Antia and Levine stated that "language is learned through interaction and exposure. The interpreter can only provide exposure. . . . The young child may not understand that the interpreter is actually functioning as the hands for the teacher" (2001, p. 371). When attempting to incorporate the use of a sign language interpreter in an educational setting, the direct, interactive communication between the interventionist and the child is lost. The use of interpreters can cause confusion to very young children who are deaf and hard of hearing and are just beginning to learn the rules of language and communication.

Although the hearing children may automatically acquire some signs from exposure, Solit et al. (1992) advised the intentional teaching of signs to hearing children in early childhood programs in order for them to truly understand sign language. These authors also suggested incorporating activities that help children use their facial expressions and body language while communicating. The adults in the program should also ensure that hearing children in the classroom are aware of the visual needs of their classmates who are deaf and hard of hearing.

Deaf Culture

Antia and Levine contended that

> Children who are deaf face greater challenges for language acquisition than do those who are hard of hearing. Although children who are hard of hearing may benefit greatly from amplification, preferential seating, and other accommodations, they need access to the Deaf

community and signing because, such as children who are deaf, they grow up to be part of this community. (2001, p. 392)

A resource on Deaf culture for early interventionists who work on a team with Deaf adults is the *Deaf Mentor Curriculum* (Pittman, 2001). In addition to topics in Deaf culture, the *Deaf Mentor Curriculum* provides information on Deaf history and famous Deaf people. The *Deaf Mentor Curriculum* was developed for Deaf adults who serve as mentors to hearing families of children who are deaf and hard of hearing. In addition to teaching families about famous Deaf people, Deaf culture, and Deaf history, mentors also teach families ASL.

STRATEGIES FOR SUCCESSFUL INCLUSIVE EARLY CHILDHOOD PROGRAMS

As with most successes in programming, support is needed from the top. For successful inclusion to occur, administrators should be not only supportive, but must be actively involved. Therefore, early education specialists and parents need to enlist the support of directors and administrators of child care and early childhood programs. Positive outcomes, such as shared funding, benefit programs that are willing to include children with disabilities. Also, with the presence of the early education specialist, there is an added member and resource for the team of individuals working with young children in the inclusive program.

Because of the importance of the administrator in the success of inclusive early childhood programs, the NICD (1991) developed a comprehensive list of administrative responsibilities; roles of the administrator include

1. Working closely with parents in a team approach

2. Being aware of and willing to give the extra time to find appropriate support

3. Providing services, arranging for special transportation needs, and dealing with the other considerations of a mainstream placement

4. Consulting with experts in the education of students who are deaf and hard of hearing for information and guidance on hearing loss and the needs of students who are deaf and hard of hearing

5. Determining the range of resources available locally or in the district or state system and the means by which to tap these resources

6. Providing in-service orientations on hearing loss and the special needs of students who are deaf and hard of hearing for faculty, staff, students, and parents

7. Consulting with teachers prior to placing a child, and ensuring that the teacher who receives a child who is deaf or hard of hearing is willing, understanding, and has a teaching style utilizing strategies that complement the child's needs

8. Demonstrating support by personally attending in-service programs, meetings, and so forth, to show that students who are deaf and hard of hearing are important

9. Interacting personally with students who are deaf and hard of hearing and supporting staff

Aside from administrative support, professional training and family support are also crucial to inclusive programs for infants, toddlers, and preschoolers (Wall, 2000).

Professional Training

"Although it is not expected that the early education/child care workers become experts on deafness, they should have a basic understanding of the need for a visual environment, Deaf Culture, audiological aspects of deafness, communication modes, and assistive devices" (Solit et al., 1992, p. 11). As described previously, administrators have an important role in meeting the needs of early childhood personnel and child care workers. One of their most important roles is training staff in the needs of children who are deaf and hard of hearing.

Training for staff should include an orientation to hearing loss and its impact on an individual. Other topics addressed should cover 1) the possibilities and limitations of hearing aids and cochlear implants, 2) the potential impact of hearing loss on speech and language, 3) the differences and similarities between people who can hear and those who cannot, and 4) information about the achievements of deaf people (NICD, 1991, p. 12).

Parent Support and Involvement

Including all parents in training sessions is important because the more knowledge parents have, the better able they will be to help their children benefit from the inclusive experience. Marschark alluded to the communication abilities between parent and child as a primary factor in determining potential success of a child who is deaf and hard of hearing in an inclusive setting (1993). Afzali-Nomani (1995) reported that parental support has a favorable impact on the self-confidence/esteem of children who are deaf and hard of hearing in an inclusion program.

CONSIDERATIONS FOR PLACEMENT

Nowell and Innes stated, "The most important issues, when contemplating inclusion for a deaf individual, are related to language and communication" (1997, p. 4). Parents and professionals are encouraged by Nowell and Innes to consider the child's 1) specific communication needs; 2) preferred mode of communication; 3) linguistic needs; 4) severity of the hearing loss and ability to use residual hearing; 5) social, emotional, and cultural needs; and 6) opportunities for peer interaction and communication when choosing an inclusive program. Antia and Levine (2001) discussed concerns about inclusion from some members of the Deaf community, professionals who work with children who are deaf and hard of hearing, and parents with deaf and hard of hearing children. They stated

> With the movement toward full inclusion in schools and preschools, many believe that placement of young children who are deaf or hard of hearing in inclusive environments may be inappropriate for the development of communication and social skills. Professionals are concerned about placing these young children in inclusive programs without the support of teachers and peers who can enhance communication during the course of the entire school day. . . . Parents are often under great stress in trying to negotiate the service delivery system, the overwhelming developmental challenges presented by the presence of hearing loss in their child, and the confusion of having to make choices about communication and education. (p. 382)

Although the inclusion of children with hearing losses in programs developed for hearing children is controversial, the National Association of the Deaf (NAD) outlines very specific guidelines to consider when contemplating program placement for children who are deaf and hard of hearing. The NAD Position Statement on Inclusion (2001) stated that an appropriate placement is one that

1. Enhances the child's intellectual, social, and emotional development
2. Is based on the language of the child
3. Offers direct communication access and opportunities for direct instruction
4. Has a sufficient number of age-appropriate and level-appropriate deaf and hard of hearing children
5. Takes into consideration the child's hearing level and abilities
6. Is staffed by certified and qualified personnel trained to work with deaf and hard of hearing children
7. Provides full access to all curricular and extra-curricular offerings customarily found in educational settings
8. Has an adequate number of deaf and hard of hearing role models
9. Provides full access to support services
10. Has the support of informed parents
11. Is equipped with appropriate communication and learning technologies

The Division for Early Childhood (DEC) revised its Position on Inclusion statement in the year 2000. It stated, "Ultimately the implementation of inclusive practice must lead to optimal developmental benefit for each individual child and family." Many leaders in the Deaf community, professionals who work with children who are deaf and hard of hearing, and parents with children who are deaf and hard of hearing feel that the NAD guidelines for "appropriate programming" ensure "optimal developmental benefits."

ACTIVITIES PRIOR TO PLACEMENT

Before considering placement of a child who is deaf or hard of hearing in an early childhood program with hearing children, detailed information about the child must be obtained. Crucial to this process is input from the parents, those who generally know the child best. The parent can share essential background information, such as how and when the child became deaf or hard of hearing, the hearing status of other members of the family, and the communication preference of the child and family. Fundamentally, the parents are considered equal partners of the individualized family service plan (IFSP) team. As such, parents are able to state their goals for the child and family.

Once those who will be providing services to the child and family have an understanding of the communication needs of the child who is deaf or hard of hearing, strategies should be implemented that reflect the specific needs of the child in an inclusive setting. Services should be provided on the basis of the IFSP, rather than developing an IFSP on the basis of the availability of services and personnel. Afzali-Nomani (1995) found that placement made on the basis of children's needs, rather than on budgets, positively affected the academic achievement and social adjustment of children who are deaf and hard of hearing in inclusive programs. Likewise, Afzali-Nomani (1995) found that children who were permitted to use sign language showed better social adjustment and self-confidence/esteem. If a child uses sign language to communicate, it is essential that a fluent signer (a person with whom the child can communicate directly) be present in the inclusive setting at all times (Solit et al., 1992). Also, inclusion of Deaf teachers, aides, or volunteers is strongly recommended to serve as language and role models to children who are deaf and hard of hearing. This is especially critical in bilingual inclusive programs (Miller & Moores, 2000).

It is very beneficial for children who are deaf and hard of hearing to visit the program prior to their starting date (Solit et al., 1992). Oftentimes, parents are encouraged to stay with their child for the first several days so that their child can become familiar with the people and environment while in the presence of a familiar adult.

CLASSROOM ENVIRONMENT

The classroom environment is of utmost importance for any child who is deaf or hard of hearing, regardless of the communication modality being used. The classroom environment must be adapted to ensure access to communication taking place in the early childhood program. These adaptations involve visual considerations, auditory modifications, and attention-getting instructional strategies.

Visual Considerations

Because young children are small, it is important that the environment be furnished with low-standing furniture. Children, especially those relying on vision for communication, can communicate directly with other children and adults in the environment when there are no visual barriers. In addition, incidental learning can occur by observing other conversations from a distance. It is important to place any adult-sized furniture such as bookcases, storage bins, and desks along the walls of the room.

Aside from furniture, educators should consider the students' seating arrangements. During structured time, the seating arrangement should be circular. This allows all of the children to more readily see signs and/or lipread the person who is communicating with them at any given time. It is also helpful during these times for preschoolers to learn to raise their hands before communicating so that all children have equal access to communication.

The early interventionist should set up the environment so there are as many visual cues as possible. Photographs of children involved in various activities denoting the classroom schedule are important, as well as drawings or photographs of what happens in each area of the classroom. Labeling play areas as well as labeling shelves enables children greater independence (Solit et al., 1992) and is beneficial for all children.

Another important consideration is lighting. The learning environment should be well lit, with glare from windows minimized (NICD, 2001). Children who are deaf and hard of hearing should be given preferential seating when it comes to light distractions (Antia & Levine, 2001). In an early education setting, this usually means that children who are deaf and hard of hearing be placed in a position facing away from light coming through the window, which can interfere with lipreading and/or perceiving other's signs.

Visual distractions need to be considered as well and should be minimized as much as possible (Antia & Levine, 2001). Visual distractions that obstruct the children's vision include objects placed on tabletops and items such as mobiles or artwork that are hung from the ceiling. An object being held in the signer's hand while attempting to sign is another source of distraction for young children. The early education specialist who signs should also be cognizant of the distractibility of excessive or elaborate jewelry. Movement of people in the hallway can attract the attention of children when the door is left open. The number of visitors entering and exiting the classroom should also be minimized, as their movement is often distracting to young children. However this limitation should not interfere with the movement of the children, which is essential for active discovery and learning.

Last, it is important that the early education specialist attract the attention of all the children in the classroom during times of transition, for turn taking, before announcements are made, during movement activities, and when storytelling. Reliance on hearing (e.g., bells, buzzers, music), however, to alert children to transitions is not appropriate. Instead, visual techniques and strategies by the adults in the classroom should occur before giving instruction (Sass-Lehrer, 1998; Solit & Bednarczyk, 1999). "Appropriate attention getting techniques include touching a deaf person lightly on the shoulder, tapping the table, or waving one's hand" (Solit et al., 1992, p. 134). A strategy suggested by Solit et al. (1992) is role playing appropriate communication strategies with the children in the program. It is important to face the child while communicating so that there is an opportunity for lipreading. These visual strategies also benefit the hearing children in the classroom.

Auditory Modifications

In addition to visual adaptations, it is important to adapt the environment acoustically so that the child who is deaf or hard of hearing can more readily access others' communications. Caregivers, teachers, parent–infant specialists, speech pathologists, occupational therapists, and other service providers should have knowledge of how to set up the environment as well as how to most effectively communicate with children with hearing loss using spoken language. "Two issues are paramount in the discussion of access to spoken language: 1) the acoustic environment of the classroom and 2) the use and monitoring of appropriate amplification" (Antia & Levine, 2001, p. 373).

The learning environment should be made to be as sound absorbent as possible. Carpeting on the floors (in the hallways as well as in the classroom), curtains on the windows, and acoustic wall tiles on the ceiling all serve to reduce reverberation and background noise. Removal of rattling blinds is also advisable (NICD, 1991). The presence of corkboards and bulletin boards on the walls also decreases noise levels. Heaters, fish tanks, fans, and other appliances that make noise should be monitored.

If the child is wearing an FM system, the teacher should repeat comments made by the other children or pass the FM transmitter to the speaker (NICD, 1991).

Instructional Strategies

It is recommended that programs for young children follow the guidelines for appropriate practices of early education. The National Association for the Education of Young Children (NAEYC, n.d.) outlined programming that is appropriate for any young child. These guidelines, for example, are appropriate for children who are deaf and hard of hearing as well as hearing children. To ensure the quality of early childhood programs, particularly child care centers, it is important that the program adhere to the standards of and be accredited by NAEYC. To become an accredited program, standards must be met within the following domains:

- Interactions among teachers and children

- Curriculum

- Relationships among teachers and families

- Staff qualifications and professional development

- Administration

- Staffing

- Physical environment

- Health and safety

- Nutrition and food service

- Evaluation

Please visit the NAEYC web site at http://www.naeyc.org/accreditation/naeyc_accred/info_general-components.asp for specific guidelines within each category. Solit and Bednarczyk (1999) emphasized "developmentally and individually appropriate curriculum choices, the use of child-initiated and child-directed practices, hands-on and experienced-based activities, and assessments of the children who are deaf and hard of hearing that are sensitive to their individual abilities" (Solit & Bednarczyk, 1999, p. 87).

Exposure to age-appropriate curriculum is a primary benefit for children with hearing losses in inclusive programs. Curriculum should be available to the child with an emphasis on allowing the child many hands-on experiences (NICD, 1991). The NICD suggested that the curriculum include a sign language component. Following the example of teachers in Antia's case study (1999), this could be accomplished by setting up a learning center that incorporates age-appropriate activities and emphasizes sign language acquisition.

Reading to children is an integral part of any early childhood program. The Shared Reading Project, at the Laurent Clerc National Deaf Education Center at Gallaudet University, recommends 12 tips for parents when reading to their deaf child (see the Shared Book Reading Project section in Chapter 2). By reading and telling stories to young children who are deaf and hard of hearing, interventionists and educators introduce children to literacy. Deaf and hard of hearing children in bilingual programs are given opportunities to observe, through stories, how English and ASL are connected, which in turn promotes the development of English language skills (Erting & Pfau, 1997). Regardless of communication modality used, children can gain an understanding of how verbal or sign communication is related to print if adults in the program utilize adaptations and special techniques to accommodate the special needs of the deaf and hard of hearing children included in the program.

Early education specialists can learn a great deal from Deaf adults about techniques or strategies that have been found to be beneficial when reading or telling stories to children who are deaf and hard of hearing. The Shared Reading Project distributes a videotape and manual titled "Reading to Deaf Children: Learning from Deaf Adults." Although these principles in the videotape and manual were developed for hearing parents of children who are deaf and hard of hearing, they are also applicable to early childhood interventionists. Not all of the principles are applicable to early childhood teachers working in oral programs, but most of the principles are relevant to any person working with young children, regardless of the communication methodology being used. See Table 9.2 for an overview of these principles.

ORAL/AURAL AND BILINGUAL/BICULTURAL PROGRAMS

This section describes two programs that follow NAEYC guidelines and attempt to satisfy social and legislative biddings to educate children who are deaf and hard of hearing with hearing children. Both programs are designed for preschool-age children and are housed at a school for the deaf. Both face the challenges of educating children who are deaf and hard of hearing with hearing peers, while at the same time ensuring that the children who are deaf receive the structure and individual attention they need. Even though both programs have similar environmental setups with children's art and pictures on the walls, many children's books displayed around the room, dramatic play areas, art centers, science centers, and so forth, the program philosophy of educating children who

Table 9.2.   15 principles for reading to deaf and hard of hearing children

1. **Translate stories using American Sign Language (ASL):** Allow children to intake and process information in their first language so they may fully comprehend and enjoy it. Remember that all English words and phrases do not have signs that translate directly to ASL. When this is the case, do not "make up" a sign. Instead, fingerspell the word, and explain to insure that your child understands its meaning.

2. **Keep both ASL and English visible:** While you are signing in ASL, keep English print visible to children so they have an opportunity to identify relationships between signed and written language.

3. **Elaborate on the text as needed:** Since all English words and phrases do not translate directly to ASL, it is vital to children's comprehension to explain and describe those that don't. For example, consider a story about a horse named "Whinny." The story may reference the horse being or not being true to her name. It would be helpful, in this case, to explain that horses make noises when they are discontented that are referred to as "whinnying." This would help to increase a child's understanding of the story.

4. **Re-read stories on a story "telling" to story "reading" continuum:** The first several times reading a story to a child, add signs as needed to enhance comprehension. As the child becomes more familiar with the story, sign it closer and closer to the written text, still using ASL.

5. **Follow the child's lead:** Children let you know whether or not they are interested or "getting it." If today is not a good time, try tomorrow. If one story is boring him, try another. If your daughter loves stories about cowboys, take her to the library, seek them out, and check them out.

6. **Make what is implied explicit:** Young readers may not yet be familiar with English idioms. When you come across a phrase like "joined at the hip," be sure your child understands this means being good friends, feeling connected, and spending a lot of time together.

7. **Adjust sign placement to fit the story:** In order to maintain interest and variety, be creative with your signs. For example, move a classifier representing a hungry bear toward your child to make the story come alive.

8. **Adjust signing style to fit the character:** Be an actor! When you are speaking for a loud, ferocious giant in a story, be sure to sign in a bold and menacing way. When you are playing a part of a child who is frightened by the giant, your signs should communicate fear and apprehension.

9. **Connect concepts in the story to the real world:** Has the prince in the story been wronged by a friend? Has the dinosaur found his mother after being lost? Help your child relate these experiences to her own life. Talk about her responses and what she thinks and feels.

10. **Use attention maintenance strategies:** Anyone who has spent time with children knows they do not respond well to monotony. Use methods that work for your children to keep their attention, whether taking turns reading, assigning different readers to be different characters, varying your pace and tone to keep the story alive, reading for relatively short periods of time, or whatever else works for you.

11. **Use eye gaze to elicit participation:** When reading to children, looking them intently in the eyes has a "drawing in" effect. Few children can resist such one-to-one attention.

12. **Engage in role play to extend concepts:** Assign or let the child choose a role. This will help him become more involved in both the reading process and the story, and elevate the reading experience to another level.

(continued)

Table 9.2. *(continued)*

13. **Use ASL variations to sign repetitive English phrases:** Sayings such "Run, run, as fast as you can, you won't catch me, I'm the gingerbread man!" become tedious when signed and fingerspelled word for word in exact English. Instead, bring the story alive by alternating between the signs for "run," "escape," "took off," and "running" (with your arms moving). Translating phrases to ASL in a variety of ways makes stories catchy and fun.

14. **Provide a positive and reinforcing environment:** Encourage your child to share his ideas about the story. Ask what you think will happen next in the story, and validate your child's idea by saying things such as, "That's a good idea. . . . Let's keep reading and see what happens . . . "

15. **Expect the child to become literate:** Believe in your deaf child's abilities to read and write. Don't worry about reading to teach English or to instruct reading; just read to share a love of books, and the rest will follow.

are deaf and hard of hearing differs for these two programs; one program adheres to a bilingual philosophy and the other a monolingual philosophy. The bilingual program advocates a visual/spatial language (i.e., ASL) as the most effective way to communicate with children who are deaf and hard of hearing. Conversely, the oral/aural program advocates the use of residual hearing to help the child who is deaf or hard of hearing learn to acquire language and to control the features of his or her own speech.

Oral/Aural Preschool Program

Four children arrive at school and go into the preschool program, all between the ages of 3 and 4 years. All children have a hearing loss, and three of the children are wearing personal ear-level hearing aids. One child has a cochlear implant. A teacher and an assistant teacher, both specialists in early childhood education, greet the children. An audiologist is also present and will remain in the classroom for 30–45 minutes. Upon arrival in the classroom, the children hang up their coats, put on their harnesses and pouches, and proceed to the "auditory table," where they take off their hearing aids and put on their FM system, which are provided by the school. (FM systems are checked with and without transmitter before the children come to school.) The students' personal hearing aids are left with the audiologist in a bag labeled with their name. The child with a cochlear implant has his or her magnets and processors checked daily.

One hour after the children who are deaf and hard of hearing arrive, six additional children, all hearing, enter the classroom. At this time, all of the children engage in self-directed activities that they choose from a variety of learning centers (cognitive area, math area, art area, constructionistic play area, science area, food preparation area, sensorimotor area). As the children play, the adults move from group to group to facilitate cooperative play and social interaction.

The remaining 30 minutes are spent in large group activities or gross motor activities that are usually held outdoors. The children who are deaf and hard of hearing remove their FM systems prior to outdoor play, as it is the last activity of the morning and the FM systems remain at school. Once their outdoor activities are over, all of the children are dismissed from the playground to the bus. Field trips are also an integral part of the program.

In an oral/aural approach to inclusive programming, much emphasis is placed on proper maintenance of hearing devices so that the children receive optimal benefits. On-site audiological services are a fundamental component of the program. This permits daily observation of auditory behavior; daily sharing of information between parents, teachers, and the audiologist; and immediate response to equipment failure, suspected changes in hearing, and middle ear function.

Bilingual/Bicultural Preschool Program

The children arrive at school and enter the classroom. Members of the classroom include six children who are deaf and hard of hearing and three hearing children between the ages of 4 and 5 years. A hearing teacher, who has been trained as a teacher for children who are deaf, a Deaf teacher trained in early childhood education, and a Deaf assistant compose the teaching team in the classroom. The adults greet the children with big smiles and sign, "good morning" without using their voices. One hearing child runs up to the hearing teacher and, using spoken English only, says that her dad drove her to school. The teacher responds in ASL, "Do you like when your dad drives you to school?" The girl responds in spoken English and signs, "yes," and proceeds to hang up her coat.

After the children settle in by putting away their backpacks and coats, the teacher begins the day with a group discussion. Sitting on mats in a semi-circle with the teacher in the front, the teacher asks the children what is inside their heads. One hearing child responds, "ice cream." The teacher asks why the child thinks ice cream is inside her head. The child responds in sign and spoken English, "because when I eat ice cream, it gets cold right here," and points to her forehead. Another child responds with "food." A third child who is deaf signs, "bones," and a fourth child who is hearing pipes in using only his voice: "a brain."

Throughout the morning, the adults in the classroom communicate among themselves and with all of the children using ASL. The hearing children use a mixture of ASL and spoken English. One hearing boy signs without voice when he communicates with both Deaf and hearing adults and peers. One hearing girl signs and speaks English simultaneously, regardless of the recipient's hearing status. Another hearing girl speaks mostly in English to the hearing teacher and her hearing peers; however, she signs when directly communicating to Deaf adults and peers. One hard of hearing child primarily signs to all the adults in the classroom and deaf peers but occasionally uses spoken English only when communicating with hearing peers. The other deaf children primarily sign in ASL and occasionally vocalize when communicating.

In this program, two languages are being used in the classroom. However, for the purposes of providing access to language for all of the children and adults in the classroom, ASL is the primary mode of communication desired in face-to-face communication. Even though all of the hearing children, as well as the child who is hard of hearing, use spoken English to communicate with each other, access to this spoken communication is not apparent for the children with profound hearing losses when not accompanied by sign. Therefore, a primary goal of this program is to encourage the hearing children to sign as much as possible, even when not directly communicating with a peer or adult who is deaf or hard of hearing.

If one of the primary purposes of educating young children is to eventually have the child read and write English, then how will the child who is exposed only to ASL acquire this ability? The bilingual/bicultural program teaches English literacy through exposure to and interaction with English print (i.e., reading books to children and having children take part in early writing projects). The contention is that preschool children who are deaf learn to be bilingual as they not only become literate in English but at the same time become literate in ASL (Erting & Pfau, 1997). Photos of the children and drawings by them, along with written descriptive sentences (captions), cover almost every surface. Children are asked to tell about their experiences and artwork. The stories are translated from ASL to English so that the children can see print reflecting their communications. It is not uncommon for children, during transitions, to go to the various displays and read the captions.

Children's books are an integral part of the preschool classroom. Stories are first told to the class in ASL. Later, the stories are told incorporating more and more English words and the teacher points out English words printed on the page. Fingerspelling is an integral part of storytime. The teacher fingerspells a word by placing a hand configuration on each letter of the printed word being spelled. Then the teacher provides the sign for the word.

Home-Based Bilingual/Bicultural Program

The Deaf Mentor Project resulted from a U.S. Department of Education grant received by the SKI-HI Institute in 1993. This project allows families with young children who are deaf and hard of hearing to receive the services of a Deaf Mentor, in addition to a Parent Advisor, in their homes. Although the parent advisor is typically hearing, Deaf mentors are selected from the Deaf community in the state of Utah.

In this early intervention bilingual/bicultural approach, the parent advisor visits the home and is responsible for providing families with information regarding their child's hearing loss, early communication and language development, hearing aids, auditory skill development, and speech development. The parent advisor teaches family members a sign system, manually coded English, in which individual signs are presented in English word order. Meanwhile, the Deaf mentor provides the family with information regarding effective early visual communication, ASL, the Deaf community, and Deaf culture. Not only do the Deaf mentors communicate directly with family members using ASL, they also provide direct instruction of the language. Through the Deaf mentor's presence, the family is exposed to Deaf culture. For example, the Deaf mentor shares his or her personal experiences and demonstrates assistive devises (e.g., flashing lights for the doorbell and telephone, use of the TTY, vibrating alarm clocks, pagers) that they use in daily living. The Deaf mentor also teaches the family about famous Deaf adults and about Deaf History.

Many professionals working with children who are deaf and hard of hearing "agree that Deaf children of all ages should be exposed to Deaf adults and to cultural aspects of the Deaf community" (Miller & Moores, 2000, p. 227). This is an especially critical component of a bilingual/ bicultural program. In addition to providing fluent language to the child and his or her family and serving as role models for the children who are deaf and hard of hearing, Deaf adults also have a tremendous impact on hearing parents. In a videotaped interview that serves as a training tool for SKI-HI Institute, a hearing mother of a 4-year-old girl who is profoundly deaf and participated in the Deaf Mentor Program stated,

We didn't have any idea what Deafness was. We didn't have any idea what that meant to an individual. We had never heard of Deaf Culture. I don't think we knew there was a Deaf Center here in our city. I don't know if we ever met a deaf person. We didn't have any frame of reference at all. And now, we realize that there is a whole community of support for us. That especially being the parents of a deaf daughter, the Deaf people we meet welcome us. I think they sense some of our struggle. We realize the potential inside of her and inside of all people that are Deaf to fulfill whatever dreams they have—of having a home or a family or college—that these are accessible to them. I think we went from thinking, 'Can she speak?,' which was our first concern, to 'She can go to college!' We've been involved with this; well we've known for 3 years that she was deaf—about 3 years. And we've gone from 'Can we even teach her language?' to having been very confident that

our daughter could go to college and graduate and choose a career and be
whatever she wanted to be; by watching the lives of other Deaf people.

—*Renee Evans, 1999*

CONCLUSION

In 1991, the NICD stated, "Finding the least restrictive environment for children with hearing losses will probably always be a complex task, requiring the sorting out of multiple factors—including social, academic, linguistic, and cultural factors—on a case-by-case basis" (p. 22). This prediction still holds. There are many factors to consider when deciding placement of children in inclusion programs. However, the primary consideration should focus on communication issues specific to each child who is deaf or hard of hearing. Not all children who are deaf and hard of hearing have identical needs, making it imperative that a full range of placement options be available to children who are deaf and hard of hearing (Afzali-Nomani, 1995; Siegel, 2000; Wilson, 1997), including inclusive programs (Fuchs & Fuchs, 2000).

In considering the individual child who is deaf or hard of hearing, it is worth contemplating Siegel's viewpoint:

> There is not one way to communicate or one placement for all deaf and hard of hearing children. This is particularly true with technological advances and increased respect for the vibrancy of spoken and signed language. What is common for all these children is the importance of communication—an effective, communication-driven system will meet the needs of all deaf and hard of hearing children. It is time inclusion and communication become educational siblings, diverse but equally vibrant, valuable and supported. (2000, pp. 3, 5)

IDEA has made a difference for many children with disabilities, including children who are deaf and hard of hearing. A hearing mother of two young deaf children pointed out that difference by saying,

I think acceptance is the key. I think that in this day and age, people are
definitely more accepting, more understanding of differences. And we see
it more in our community. So I'm just so glad that they were born actually
in this day and age than when we were children.

—*Nancy Dexter, 1999, SKI-HI training videotape*

FUTURE PERSPECTIVES

With universal newborn hearing screening, more children are being identified as having a hearing loss at an earlier age. At the same time, more children who are deaf are receiving cochlear implants at an earlier age. It is important that these children and their families are provided a wide spectrum of program choices, from programs developed specifically to meet the needs of infants, toddlers, and preschoolers who are deaf and hard of hearing to total inclusion. There is a lack of understanding about the nature of relationships between young children who are deaf and hard of hearing and hearing children at a critical age when the child is becoming more independent and utilizes friendships to enhance social and emotional growth. If the placement of children who are deaf and hard of hearing in programs with hearing children continues, research is needed to identify successful communication interactions and classroom culture that promote friendships between these populations. There is a need for empirical research, which looks at the efficacy of specific strategies utilized to facilitate socialization of young children who are deaf and hard of hearing and hearing children. There is also a need for empirical research that focuses on the efficacy of inclusive programs in terms of language, cognitive, emotional, and "academic" growth of infants, toddlers, and preschoolers who are deaf and hard of hearing when they are included in programs with children who can hear.

Researchers should examine the quality and effectiveness of language interactions not only between classroom teachers and children who are deaf and hard of hearing, but also between children with differing hearing abilities within inclusion programs.

REFERENCES

Afzali-Nomani, E. (1995). Educational conditions related to successful full inclusion programs involving deaf/hard of hearing children. *American Annals of the Deaf, 140,* 396–401.

Americans with Disabilities Act (ADA) of 1990, PL 101–336, 42 U.S.C. §§ 12101 *et seq.*

Antia, S. (1994). Strategies to develop peer interaction in young hearing-impaired children. *The Volta Review, 96,* 277–290.

Antia, S. (1999). The roles of special educators and classroom teachers in an inclusive school. *Journal of Deaf Studies and Deaf Education, 4,* 203–214.

Antia, S., & Ditillo, D. (1998). A comparison of the peer social behavior of children who are deaf/hard of hearing and hearing. *Journal of Children's Communication Development, 19,* 1–10.

Antia, S.D., & Levine, L.M. (2001). Educating deaf and hearing children together: Confronting the challenges of inclusion. In M.J. Guralnick (Ed.), *Early childhood inclusion: Focus on change* (pp. 365–398). Baltimore: Paul H. Brookes Publishing Co.

Brown v. Board of Educ., 347 U.S. 483 (1954).

Cambra, C. (2002). Acceptance of deaf students by hearing students in regular classrooms. *American Annals of the Deaf, 147,* 1.

Cavallaro, C.C., & Haney, M. (1999). *Preschool inclusion.* Baltimore: Paul H. Brookes Publishing Co.

Council for Exceptional Children, Division of Early Childhood. (2000). *Position on inclusion.* Denver, CO: Author.

Diamond, K.E., & Innes, F.K. (2001). The origins of young children's attitudes toward peers with disabilities. In M.J. Guralnick (Ed.), *Early childhood inclusion: Focus on change* (pp. 159–177). Baltimore: Paul H. Brookes Publishing Co.

Doherty, K.M. (2002). Children attend variety of settings. *Education Week on the Web, 21*(17), 21. Retrieved from http://www.edweek.org

Education for All Handicapped Children Act of 1975, PL 94-142, 20 U.S.C. §§ 1400 et seq.

Esposito, B., & Koorland, M. (1989). Play behavior of hearing-impaired children: Integrated and separated settings. *Exceptional Children, 55,* 412–419.

Erting, L., & Pfau, J. (1997). *Becoming bilingual: Facilitating English literacy development using ASL in preschool.* Washington, DC: Pre-College National Mission Programs, Gallaudet University Press.

Fuchs, D., & Fuchs, L. (2000). Inclusion verses full inclusion. In W.L. Heward, *Exceptional children* (pp. 72–74). Columbus, OH: Merrill.

Guralnick, M.J. (2001). A framework for change in early childhood inclusion. In M.J. Guralnick (Ed.), *Early childhood inclusion: Focus on change* (pp. 3–35). Baltimore: Paul H. Brookes Publishing Co.

Heward, W.L. (2000). *Exceptional children.* Columbus, OH: Merrill.

Individuals with Disabilities Education Act Amendments of 1997, PL 105-17, 20 U.S.C. §§ 1400 et seq.

Jimenez-Sanchez, C., & Antia, S. (1999). Team-teaching in an integrated classroom: Perceptions of deaf and hearing teachers. *Journal of Deaf Studies and Deaf Education, 4,* 215–224.

Kluwin, T. (1999). Coteaching deaf and hearing students: Research on social integration. *American Annals of the Deaf, 144,* 339–344.

Kreimeyer, K., Crooke, P., Drye, C., Egbert, V., & Klein, B. (2000). Academic and social benefits of a co-enrollment model of inclusive education for deaf and hard-of-hearing children. *Journal of Deaf Studies and Deaf Education, 5,* 174–185.

Lee, C., & Antia, S. (1992). A sociological approach to the social integration of hearing-impaired and normally hearing students. *The Volta Review, 95,* 425–434.

Leutke-Stahlman, B. (1994). Procedures for socially integrating preschoolers who are hearing, deaf and hard of hearing. *Topics in Early Childhood Special Education, 14,* 472–487.

Leutke-Stahlman, B. (1995). Classrooms, communication, and social competence. *Perspectives in Education and Deafness, 13,* 12–16.

Marschark, M. (1993). *Psychological development of deaf children.* New York: Oxford University Press.

Miller, M., & Moores, D. (2000). Bilingual/bicultural education for deaf students. In M. Winzer & K. Mazurek (Eds.), *Special education in the 21st century* (pp. 221–237). Washington, DC: Gallaudet University Press.

Minnett, A., Clark, K., & Wilson, G. (1994). Play behavior and communication between deaf and hard of hearing children and their hearing peers in an integrated preschool. *American Annals of the Deaf, 139,* 420–429.

Mowl, G. (1996). Raising deaf children in hearing society: Struggles and challenges for deaf native ASL signers. In I. Parasnis (Ed.), *Cultural and language diversity and the deaf experience* (pp. 232–245). New York: Cambridge University Press.

Mundy, L. (2002, March 31). Deaf like me. *The Washington Post Magazine,* pp. 22–29, 38–43.

National Association of the Deaf (NAD). (2001). *NAD position statement on Inclusion.* Silver Spring, MD: Author.

National Association for the Education of Young Children (NAEYC). (n.d.). NAEYC accreditation: About accreditation. 10 components. Adapted from the *Accreditation criteria & procedures of the National Association for the Education of Young Children.* Retrieved February, 5, 2003, from http://www.naeyc.org/accreditation/naeyc_accred/info_general-components.asp

National Information Center on Deafness (NICD). (1991). *Mainstreaming deaf and hard of hearing students.* Washington, DC: Gallaudet University Press.

Nowell, R., & Innes, J. (1997). Educating children who are deaf or hard of hearing: Inclusion. *ERIC Digest, #E557,* 1–4.

Pennsylvania Association for Retarded Children (PARC) v. Commonwealth of Pennsylvania, 334 F. Supp. 1257 (1971).

Pittman, P. (Ed.). (2001). *Deaf mentor curriculum.* North Logan, UT: HOPE.

Sass-Lehrer, M. (1998, December). *Components of appropriate and inappropriate practices for inclusion of deaf and hard of hearing youngsters.* Material distributed at the International DEC Conference, Chicago.

Siegel, L. (2000). *The educational & communication needs of deaf and hard of hearing children: A statement of principle regarding fundamental systemic educational changes.* Washington, DC: Gallaudet University, National Deaf Education Project.

Solit, G., & Bednarczyk, A. (1999). *Issues in access.* Washington, DC: Pre-College National Mission Programs, Gallaudet University Press.

Solit, G., Taylor, M., & Bednarczyk, A. (1992). *Access for all.* Washington, DC: Pre-College National Mission Programs, Gallaudet University Press.

Spencer, P., Koester, L., & Meadow-Orlans, K. (1994). Communicative interactions of deaf and hearing children in a day care center. *American Annals of the Deaf, 139,* 512–518.

Staub, D. (1998). *Delicate threads.* Bethesda, MD: Woodbine House.

Stinson, M., & Antia, S. (1999). Considerations in educating deaf and hard-of-hearing students in inclusive settings. *Journal of Deaf Studies and Deaf Education, 4,* 163–175.

Voeltz, L. (1982). Effects of structured interactions with severely handicapped peers on children's attitudes. *American Journal of Mental Deficiency, 86,* 380–390.

Wall, S. (2000). Inclusion of infants, toddlers, and preschoolers with disabilities. In M. Winzer & K. Mazurek (Eds.), *Special Education in the 21st Century* (pp. 198–220). Washington, DC: Gallaudet University Press.

Walsh, S., Rous, B., & Lutzer, C. (2000). The federal IDEA natural environments provision: Making it work. In S. Sandall & M. Ostrosky (Eds.), *Young exceptional children monograph series: No. 2. Natural environments and inclusion* (pp. 3–16). Longmont, CO: Sopris West.

Watkins, S., Pittman, P., & Walden, B. (1998). The deaf mentor experimental project for young children who are deaf and their families. *American Annals of the Deaf, 143,* 29–34.

Wilson, C. (1997). Mainstream or "deaf school?" Both! say deaf students. *Perspectives in Education and Deafness, 16,* 10–13.

Winston, E. (1994). An interpreted education: Inclusion or exclusion? In R.C. Johnson & O.P. Cohen (Eds.), *Implications and complications for deaf students of the full inclusion movement* (pp. 55–62, Gallaudet Research Institute Occasional Paper 94-2). Washington, DC: Gallaudet University Press.

Winzer, M. (2000). The inclusion movement: Review and reflections on reform in special education. In M. Winzer & K. Mazurek (Eds.), *Special education in the 21st century* (pp. 5–26). Washington, DC: Gallaudet University Press.

Wolery, R., & Odom, S. (2000). *An administrator's guide to preschool inclusion.* Chapel Hill: University of North Carolina, Frank Porter Graham Child Development Center, Early Childhood Research Institute on Inclusion.

Early Childhood Programs

Gail Solit, Coordinator,
Early Childhood Programs,
Laurent Clerc National
Deaf Education Center

In the Laurent Clerc National Deaf Education Center Early Childhood Programs, we integrate deaf, hard of hearing, and hearing children in various classrooms. There are two early childhood programs at the Clerc Center:

1. The Child Development Center (CDC) addresses the needs of young children and their working parents and is the campus child care center on Gallaudet University's campus. This program serves children 19 months through kindergarten, as well as children through age 9 after school and in the summer.

2. The Early Childhood Education Team (ECET), a team at the Kendall Demonstration Elementary School (KDES), serves children in the Parent–Infant Program (birth through 2¹/2 years old), Nursery Classes (2¹/2–4 years old), Prekindergarten (4 years old), and the Kindergarten program (5 years old).

Both programs provide children who are deaf and hard of hearing opportunities to play, learn, and grow together. Teachers and staff also create opportunities that maximize child development in social, emotional, motor, cognitive, and language domains.

The CDC has been integrating deaf and hard of hearing toddlers through second grade since 1986. The amount of hours that deaf and hard of hearing children are at CDC has changed as the programmatic needs of KDES have changed over the years. Deaf and hard of hearing children may attend CDC for the full week or as little as 2 hours after school every afternoon. For example, the youngest children may be at CDC, every day, all day, except for two mornings a week when they and their parents attend the center-based program of the Parent–Infant Program, whereas the deaf children in kindergarten may only be in CDC after school or when KDES is not in session. Other deaf and hard of hearing school-age children from KDES attend CDC after school and/or in the summer.

In the CDC integrated classrooms, the majority of children are hearing. About half of the hearing children have deaf parents or other deaf family members. The other half are children of families who reside in the Washington, D.C., area who live in close proximity to the school or they have heard of the program and choose it on the basis of its educational success or because they would like to expose their children to a bilingual/bicultural approach to learning. There are deaf and hearing teaching teams in each class. American Sign Language (ASL) and English are used throughout the day. Sometimes languages are used simultaneously, and sometimes teachers do not use their voices to encourage everyone to use sign language. Other times, if a deaf teacher is leading an activity, he or she may be only using ASL, and the children use or are encouraged to use ASL in response. Other times, if a small group is all hearing, only English may be used. The goal is to ensure that all children have access to each language at all times.

Aside from providing access to two different languages, these classrooms also bring hearing, hard of hearing, and deaf children together for social reasons. Deaf and hearing children learn about each other, about each other's culture, and language. Some deaf, hearing, and hard of hearing children develop friendships with each other, others are learning to accept each other, while others are simply being exposed to different people other than themselves and their families.

The teachers create activities that encourage interactions between deaf and hearing children. They create games and projects so that partnerships between children are encouraged. Hearing children need to learn signs to communicate with the deaf children. All need to learn to be patient and take the time to truly listen to each other. The environment and all the learning activities are made visual, so that everyone will understand what is occurring throughout the day.

Children, teachers, and parents are learning about each other's cultures in a natural way in a setting that respects and teaches about each other's cultures. A child learns to tap on another child's shoulder to get his or her attention. When there is a fire drill, strobe lights and alarms go off. Old or broken teletypewriters (TTYs) are found in each dramatic area, as are telephones, so that all children can pretend to call their parents and friends in the manner in which they are accustomed at home. The CDC believes that when deaf and hard of hearing children need early education and care, the job of the child care staff is to create an environment that meets the children's needs and teaches children how to successfully interact with hearing peers.

The ECET at Kendall started to integrate hearing children from the CDC into the deaf and hard of hearing prekindergarten and kindergarten classes in 1999. The classes are composed of approximately 12 children, with more deaf than hearing children. The teaching teams are deaf and hearing adults. For the most part, the main languages of instruction are ASL and written English. At a specific time during the day, the hearing children in the prekindergarten and kindergarten classes are taken out of the classroom and work on literacy skills that depend on listening (phonics, rhyming, sound games). The emphasis for these classrooms is different than at CDC. The reason for the establishment of these classes at ECET is more for academic success for deaf and hard of hearing children. Our thinking is that deaf and hard of hearing 4- and 5-year-olds will benefit from being integrated with hearing children who are involved in literacy activities at an age-appropriate level. Our hope is that if the deaf and hard of hearing children are exposed to hearing peers who are doing prewriting and writing activities, they too will engage in such activities. All of the hearing children in these classrooms have deaf parents or siblings. Therefore, for all of the hearing children, especially those who have deaf parents, they have been using sign language since birth. Many of the deaf children have hearing parents, and therefore sign language is new to everyone in the family. For hearing children with deaf siblings, we want their signing to improve so they can bring more signs into the home for the benefit of their deaf siblings and their parents. There are also social and emotional benefits in the ECET classrooms, as all the children discuss the importance of access to language, respect for various cultures, and appreciating similarities and differences between themselves.

Though there has not yet been any formal research about the success of these classrooms, the anecdotal information and feedback from all the parents has generated great praise. The parents of the hearing children are seeing much better signing from their hearing children. The parents of the deaf children are very pleased that their children are interacting with hearing peers in a very positive setting.

Another aspect of our Early Childhood Programs is the coordination between the two programs. The majority of deaf, hard of hearing, and hearing children who are in integrated classrooms participate in both programs: the CDC and the ECET. We have created many methods for the teaching staff in both programs to communicate with each other and with the parents so that everyone knows the educational goals for all the deaf and hard of hearing children, we all know about how the children interact and behave in various settings, and we can all share curriculum ideas.

Questions and challenges that the teaching staff continually address in both settings include the following:

- How do we ensure that all the deaf children have access to language at all times in either setting? Which languages should be used? When? How much time with which language for what period of time during the day is appropriate?
- How do we ensure that the hearing children, within a deaf school, get their needs met?
- Should there be specific criteria for either group of children in the various settings?

- What is the appropriate training and orientation the teachers and staff need to work with the children?
- What kind of curricular activities need to occur to facilitate friendships and respect between children?
- How much time do the hearing children in the deaf school need with just spoken language activities?

Though it is a challenging endeavor to integrate hearing children and children who are deaf and hard of hearing, the Early Childhood Program teachers and staff believe that integrated classrooms, when done appropriately, are very beneficial for children who are deaf and hard of hearing. The critical components for a successful classroom are having 1) more children who are deaf and hard of hearing than hearing children; 2) all teachers sign fluently; 3) deaf and hearing teaching teams; 4) collaborative relationships among parents, teachers, specialists, and administrators of all programs involved; 5) appropriate educational programming for children who are deaf and hard of hearing; and 6) equal access to all languages used by children.

CHAPTER TEN

Educating Young
Deaf Children with
Multiple Disabilities

THOMAS W. JONES AND JULIE K. JONES

Anna was born prematurely, which resulted in her having a bilateral sensorineural hearing loss, cerebral palsy, and developmental delays. At 4 years of age, she neither hears, speaks, nor walks. She and her parents began receiving Part C special education services when she was an infant. Speech, occupational, and physical therapists, plus an infant special educator with background in deafness provided in-home therapies and instructions to her parents during weekly visits. For example, they helped her parents learn proper positioning and handling to manage Anna's cerebral palsy. They also helped her parents begin to learn and use signs with Anna. When Anna turned 2, her parents had the option of sending her to a noncategorical preschool program or a program for children who are deaf and hard of hearing. Her parents opted to continue with in-home services. When she turned 3, they decided she was ready to go to school. Their options remained the same, a noncategorical special education preschool in an elementary school or a preschool program for deaf and hard of hearing children in another elementary school. The noncategorical preschool program could address Anna's need for an augmentative communication system as well as address her physical disabilities and developmental delays in a fully inclusive environment. Unfortunately the personnel in the program had a limited knowledge of signing. They communicated with the other children and each other orally. The preschool program for deaf and hard of hearing children could address her needs stemming from the deafness. The interventionists and aides, as well as the bus drivers and bus aides serving the program, were all fluent signers. The deaf children signed, as did many of the hearing interventionists and children in the school. They, however, had no knowledge of or experience with augmentative communication systems. Neither were they experienced with managing the physical needs of young children with cerebral palsy, nor did they have training in teaching children with developmental delays. Linguistic input with no output system or a viable output system without an input system from which to develop language—these are the options available to Anna and many children like her.

Service delivery to young children who are deaf with multiple disabilities presents a conundrum to families and service providers. Problems occur regardless of the type of disability accompanying deafness (physical disabilities, cognitive delay, vision impairment, autism, or other disabilities). As a result, early educators face numerous challenges when working with young children who are deaf and hard of hearing with multiple disabilities and their families. These challenges range from characteristics of the children themselves and their impact on their families, to shortcomings in early intervention programs, to the lack of a professional venue for exchanging information concerning this small, diverse, and complex subpopulation. In spite of the many challenges, however, agencies and programs focused solely on hearing loss appear to be in a better position to effectively serve children with multiple disabilities and their families than are programs focused on other disabilities.

Although the proportion of children with multiple disabilities is large among the deaf and hard of hearing population (Holden-Pitt & Diaz, 1998), research and publications concerning this subgroup are extremely scarce. In addition, little has been done to assemble the resources needed to serve children who are deaf and hard of hearing with multiple disabilities effectively.[1] A major difficulty appears to be that, due to the widely varying characteristics and needs of young children who are deaf or hard of hearing with multiple disabilities, paradigms of education and special education service delivery underlying early intervention services create barriers to effective service delivery to a population consisting of individuals with extremely diverse and unique needs. Specific challenges include the following:

---

[1]An exception is children with deafblindness, a very small subgroup for whose educational services significant amounts of federal and private monies have been provided since 1969.

- The American education system has traditionally been structured around homogeneity, the idea that children with similar needs and abilities should be educated together, following the same curriculum and benefiting simultaneously from the same teaching methods. This concept, however, left out children with unique combinations of needs and characteristics, such as those with multiple disabilities. Unfortunately, with regard to these children, this situation persists today.

- Perhaps one of the most important elements of the American special education system is the connection of disability to primary service providers or placement. Special education agencies, early interventionists, schools, and classes are all organized to provide services related to specific disabilities, rather than any combination of disabilities.[2] When a disability is diagnosed, the child and family are referred to a particular agency or placement with expertise related to the disability. Because of the scarcity of expertise related to multiple disabilities, however, subjective personal characteristics of an individual primary service provider—open-mindedness, creativity, and problem-solving skills, for example—may provide a better basis for a referral than the disability focus of the agency or school. In addition, single-disability focal points create boundaries and barriers separating agencies and service delivery systems, making it difficult for agencies to collaborate in serving children with multiple disabilities and address their families' needs.

- Federal laws incorporated into the special education guidelines of most states define disabilities (including multiple disabilities) in ways that create barriers to identification, diagnosis, and appropriate service delivery for children with multiple disabilities (discussed later).

- In 1975, Wolfensberger described mainstream American culture as tending to reject, marginalize, and devalue (or even dehumanize) individuals with disabilities. With this emphasis on exclusivity (Emerton, 1998) and preoccupation with boundaries (Padden, 1998), this may be even more true for the American Deaf culture today, especially when the disabilities are visible, severe, or multiple. Similarly, interventionists working with students who are deaf may have negative attitudes toward the inclusion of students with disabilities (Lampropoulou & Padeliadu, 1997).

- Although children with multiple disabilities are considered separately (or as "footnotes") from children with single disabilities in many

---

[2]Even the recently "de-hyphenated" term *deafblindness*—seen with increasing frequency in the professional literature—appears to have been put forth to promote the idea of a single disability, rather than a combination of disabilities.

contexts, and in spite of the fact that children with multiple disabilities present unique needs, intervention services that separate children with multiple disabilities from other children have limited effectiveness for them (Jones & Ross, 1998).

- Because of these issues and the fact that children who are deaf and hard of hearing with multiple disabilities are a heterogeneous and poorly defined subgroup, research on this group is scarce, and many existing publications are of questionable validity. In addition, the professional literature has not addressed major questions concerning definition, diagnosis, identification, assessment, and intervention for children who are deaf and hard of hearing with multiple disabilities.

MARIBEL'S INTERVENTIONIST

As a graduate of a program specializing in deaf students with multiple disabilities, I was hired to start a deafblind program at a residential school for the deaf. Money for supplies and refurbishing a classroom suite was readily available. I was PSYCHED! I thought that this was a job too good to be true. When I arrived, I soon learned the secret, NO ONE wants to interact with deaf students (or their interventionists) with multiple disabilities. My classroom was placed in an abandoned dorm. My young charge, Maribel, was scheduled to live in the classroom/dorm by herself, with the exception of a round-the-clock houseparent. Lest you think this was 1960, it was not! This was an eye-opening experience for me. Not only did I refuse to allow Maribel to live by herself, I made sure that she was included with other deaf students at least 75% of the time. It took the two of us all of that first year to force our way into each and every class that we struggled to enter. The cafeteria used to deliver a tray of food to my classroom to "help" Maribel "save time" by not having to walk all the way to the cafeteria. By the time the tray arrived, the food was always cold. So I decided that Maribel and I would start taking the tray back to the cafeteria to ask for hot food. (We used this return trip as an opportunity for mobility training by balancing the full plate and tray.) The other interventionists complained constantly to the principal that their students should not have to be in Art, P.E., or even recess with Maribel. I tricked them all! I started inviting other young children to spend the day in my cool classroom. Of course the other interventionists liked that. By the end of the first year Maribel had a core group of eight other young friends that she regularly interacted with. Although I cannot say that I enjoyed the isolation and rejection from the other interventionists that lasted most of the first year, I refused to back down and leave this little girl in isolation.

In spite of these challenges, children with multiple disabilities continue to be identified at birth (even before birth, in some cases) and throughout their early years in growing numbers (U.S. Department of Education, 1995, 2000). Their disabilities are diagnosed, their strengths and weaknesses are assessed, and they receive early intervention services that may or may not be able to meet their needs. In order for these services to benefit young children with multiple disabilities optimally, issues in a number of areas need to be considered: definition, diagnosis, locating services, and service delivery—as well as issues related to multiple disabilities themselves. Considering challenges in these areas could result in recommendations for improved early intervention services for children who are deaf and hard of hearing with multiple disabilities and their families, among others.

DEFINITION CHALLENGES

At first glance, disability category definitions are not relevant to early intervention programs because eligibility for early intervention under the Individuals with Disabilities Education Act (IDEA) Amendments of 1997 (PL 105-17) does not require a defined disability (§ 303.16). Disability categories and their definitions, however, become important for preschoolers who are deaf and hard of hearing with multiple disabilities because, while their hearing loss has already qualified them for early intervention services, their other disabilities set them apart. Even though the federal definitions of multiple disabilities and learning disabilities have problematic aspects for deaf educators, both are particularly relevant, especially given the interest in identifying learning disabilities or mild learning problems in young children who are deaf and hard of hearing (Mauk & Mauk, 1992, 1993).

Federal definitions of disabilities are important not only because they are found in federal law and regulations overarching special education service delivery systems in the United States, but also because most states have incorporated the federal definitions into their state special education guidelines. (This facilitates demonstrating each state's eligibility for federal special education monies.) These disability definitions are extremely important because they provide a basis for identification, diagnosis, and intervention that is intended to benefit children and their families.

The meaning of the term *multiple disabilities* appears to be self-evident: the presence of more than one disability in an individual. In reality, however, a number of issues obscure both the meaning of the term and a conceptualization of the children being defined. The federal definition of *multiple disabilities* is

> Concomitant impairments (such as mental retardation-blindness, mental retardation, orthopedic impairment, and so forth), the combination of which causes such severe educational needs that they cannot be accommodated in special education programs solely for one of the impairments. The term does not include deafblindness. (IDEA 1997, § 300[c][7])

Aside from the seemingly paradoxical exclusion of deafblindness (to prevent counting children for two separate sources of funds), the federal definition of multiple disabilities contains several problematic elements. Specifically, this definition

- Describes no characteristics of the children the definition is intended to define (other than that "they cannot be accommodated"; in effect, the definition fails to define)
- Presupposes failure, or the expectation of failure, in single-disability programs as an eligibility criterion, rather than endogenous child characteristics like other disability definitions presuppose
- Opens the way for programs organized around single disabilities—as almost all special education services are—to determine that they cannot "accommodate" children with multiple disabilities (a provision that is in conflict with the spirit and intent of IDEA 1997)
- Appears to weigh a program's inability to "accommodate" at least as heavily as the severity of the child's disability in determining eligibility for services (also in conflict with IDEA 1997)
- Implies the availability of programs and services tailored for children with multiple disabilities, although such services are extremely rare

Because of these shortcomings, the federal definition creates barriers to identifying and serving children with multiple disabilities, rather than providing the basis for identification and service delivery that most disability definitions provide.

Even more directly than the federal definition of multiple disabilities, the federal definition of specific learning disabilities restricts access to educational services for children with multiple disabilities. The definition includes a phrase called the "exclusion clause," specifying that children are to be excluded from the learning disabilities category when their "learning problems" are primarily the result of visual, *hearing*, or motor disabilities; mental retardation; emotional disturbance; or environmental, cultural, or economic disadvantage" (IDEA 1997, § 300[c][7]; emphasis added). Although it is likely that causes of hearing loss as well as the effects of it can result in learning disabilities (Sabatino, 1983), the exclusion clause has been incorporated into many states' special education guidelines and has been interpreted to mean that children who are deaf and hard of hearing cannot simultaneously have a learning disability (Jones, 1998; Mauk & Mauk, 1992, 1993).

While eligibility for early intervention under IDEA 1997 does not require a defined disability, it does require that the child have a developmental delay, established risk, diagnosed condition from which developmental delay is highly probable, or biological or environmental risk that may significantly compromise the child's health or development without early intervention (§ 303.16). Even in early intervention programs, however, less formal definitions, policies, and eligibility criteria may work against identifying and serving children who are deaf and hard of hearing with *multiple* disabilities. Many schools and agencies focused on serving children who are deaf and hard of hearing, for example, proclaim publicly or privately that their mission is to serve children whose "primary" disability is deafness or hearing loss. The implication is that if another disability is "primary" (and, by implication, that the child's hearing loss is "secondary") then the child should be excluded and served elsewhere. In the context of disabilities, however, *primary* and *secondary* typically refer to a relationship in which one disability results from another, not where one is predominant. One might say, for example, that a child's language disorder is secondary to cognitive delay, or self-esteem issues are secondary to learning disabilities, implying a cause-and-effect relationship with no implication that one condition is more serious than the other or has a greater effect on the child (Hanson & Lynch, 1995). In proclaiming deafness as a "primary" disability, school and agency personnel, however, imply the weighing or comparing of the severity of educational needs related to hearing loss with the severity of educational needs resulting from another disability. Although such a comparison appears superficially to be logical—especially from the perspective of schools and agencies focused on a single disability—the comparison or weighing of disabilities rarely is possible. No tools or protocols exist to compare the severity of any disability and its resulting educational implications with the severity of a hearing loss and its sequelae. Such comparisons only allow programs focused on serving children who are deaf and hard of hearing (and other single-disability service providers) to exclude children with multiple disabilities, especially when the effects of disabilities other than deafness are severe (Flathouse, 1979).

DEMOGRAPHIC CHALLENGES

Given that federal and state definitions of multiple disabilities do not adequately define the condition and create barriers to identification, it is difficult to describe numbers of children with multiple disabilities with great confidence.

In *To Assure the Free Appropriate Public Education of All Children with Disabilities: Twenty-Second Annual Report to Congress on the Implementation of the Individuals with Disabilities Education Act,* the U.S. Department of Education (2000) reported that 107,591 school-age children with multiple disabilities were served during the 1998–1999 school year (compared with 70,813 deaf and hard of hearing students)—ratios that can be extrapolated to preschool children. (Also reported in 1998–1999 were 1,602 children with deafblindness, not included in the multiple disabilities category.) The number of children with multiple disabilities at the time of this report was double what it was in 1979 (U.S. Department of Education, 1982).

Numbers that the U.S. Department of Education (USDOE) reports annually to Congress are generated by state education departments to determine their allocation of Title VI-B funds through IDEA 1997. As a result, these numbers are believed to be comprehensive. The resulting report, however, does not provide incidence data on preschool children in different disability categories. It also does not differentiate among hearing, deaf, and hard of hearing school-age children in the multiple disabilities category. Similarly, it does not distinguish between multiple disabilities and severe disabilities, a special education category used by many states but not in USDOE statistical tables. Nevertheless, the USDOE report to Congress provides clear evidence that the number of children with multiple disabilities continues to grow significantly, a phenomenon that would seem to apply to children who are deaf and hard of hearing as well as to hearing children, and to preschool children as well as to school-age students.

The annual survey data reported by the Center on Assessment and Demographic Studies (CADS) is based on voluntary participation by programs serving children who are deaf and hard of hearing throughout the United States (Holden-Pitt & Diaz, 1998). Although the results may not be quite as comprehensive as the USDOE data, they provide considerably more detail (see Tables 10.1 and 10.2).

Table 10.1. Prevalence rates of selected additional disabilities

Disability	Percentage of deaf and hard of hearing children
Vision impairment	4%
Mental retardation	8%
Emotional/behavioral problem	4%
Learning disability	9%
Unspecified	9%
Total	**34%**

Source: Holden-Pitt & Diaz (1998).

Table 10.2. Leading causes of deafness

Cause	Percentage among deaf and hard of hearing children
Heredity	13%
Meningitis	7%
Prematurity	5%
Otitis Media	4%
Cytomegalovirus	2%
All remaining causes	69%

Source: Holden-Pitt & Diaz (1998).

The CADS data indicate not only a high incidence of additional disabilities among children who are deaf and hard of hearing, but also demonstrate that children with two disabilities are more likely than children with one disability to have any additional disabilities (Wolff & Harkins, 1986). In addition to statistics on multiple disabilities, the CADS annual survey data provide information on the causes of hearing loss in children (see Table 10.2) (Holden-Pitt & Diaz, 1998).

Similarly, Howell (1992) reported substantial gains in the number of preschool children who were deaf or hard of hearing in the 1970s and 1980s with etiologies of prematurity, birth trauma, cytomegalovirus, and parental drug abuse. With the possible exception of otitis media, all of these causes of deafness are also known to cause disabilities in hearing children. Very often, those disabilities are severe and include vision impairment, cognitive delay, and cerebral palsy. In addition, it appears that increasing numbers of children who are deaf or hard of hearing are born with other disabilities—perhaps most notably autism—for which the cause at present is unknown (Happé, 1998).

Although the CADS data are detailed, several questions make their accuracy uncertain. For example, how are differences among the disability category definitions provided by CADS and the varying definitions in state special education regulations handled by the interventionists and administrators who fill out the CADS survey? Anecdotal accounts indicate that some interventionists report disabilities—especially learning disabilities—based on clinical impression rather than official eligibility criteria or the category definition that CADS provides. Regardless of such questions, the CADS data have been stable over many years, indicating that about one third of all children who are deaf and hard of hearing have disabilities other than hearing loss.

Perspectives differ on whether the reported numbers of children who are deaf and hard of hearing with multiple disabilities are undercounted or overcounted. Those believing that the numbers are low point to definition problems, the lack of reliable and valid diagnostic and assessment instruments and procedures for this population, and the broadly pervasive potential of the damaging causes of hearing loss (Mauk & Mauk, 1992, 1993; Sabatino, 1983). In fact, Karchmer and Allen (1999), using the construct of "functional limitations" rather than disability definitions and eligibility criteria, estimated that one half to two thirds of all children who are deaf and hard of hearing have a functional disability. Similarly, interventionists report the incidence of learning disabilities among children who are deaf and hard of hearing at a level triple that reported by their school administrators (Elliott, Powers, & Funderburg, 1988).

Those who say that the numbers are inflated believe that many children who are deaf and hard of hearing counted as having developmental delays are reported falsely because the delays they exhibit are due to exogenous factors outside the child rather than endogenous or organic factors within the child. These exogenous factors include late diagnosis and intervention and experiential shortcomings or deprivations—especially including inadequate opportunities to receive language visually. This point of view notwithstanding, a fairly well-resolved issue in special education—particularly in early intervention programs—is that environmental risk factors are a legitimate reason for a disability label and special education intervention.

CHALLENGES IN DIAGNOSING DEVELOPMENTAL AND OTHER DISABILITIES IN CHILDREN WHO ARE DEAF AND HARD OF HEARING

Although professionals and laypeople alike view disability diagnoses as negative, such diagnoses are intended to serve a positive purpose in the special education field. Specifically, disability diagnoses serve as "tickets" to specialized services and professionals reserved for children with documented disabilities. For example, diagnosing a motor delay or disability should lead to the services of a physical or occupational therapist. If the diagnosis is delayed, the therapy also may be delayed. In addition, if the diagnosis of a disability is made early, the resulting intervention should be more effective than it would have been with a later diagnosis (Bronfenbrenner, 1975; Yoshinaga-Itano & Apuzzo, 1998). As a result, early diagnosis of additional disabilities in children who are deaf and hard of hearing should be sought, so that the family can seek specialized services to ameliorate or compensate for the disability and optimize the benefits of those services.

Physical and vision disabilities are diagnosed relatively directly by medical and physical examinations. Aside from some relatively minor communication difficulties, diagnosing physical and vision disabilities in children who are deaf and hard of hearing is not substantially different from doing so in hearing children. As a result, the diagnostic process for vision and physical disabilities does not require special expertise in hearing loss or in multiple disabilities.

Diagnosing cognitive, linguistic, social, emotional, and behavior delays—such as mental retardation or autism—is complicated in young *hearing* children, although increasingly reliable instruments, criteria, and protocols have been developed for doing so. Diagnosing such disabilities in young children who are deaf and hard of hearing, however, encounters serious complications and often yields results that spark more questions than they answer, as described below. Diagnosing children who are deaf and hard of hearing with other disabilities may lead to temporary or permanent deferral of appropriate intervention programs with deleterious effects on the children involved. For example, Jure, Rapin, and Tuchman (1991) reported that autism was diagnosed an average of 4 years later than the diagnosis of hearing loss for young children with both conditions.

Deafness May Mask Other Disabilities

In spite of having educational programs in the United States since the early 1800s, a remarkable number of children who are deaf and hard of hearing continue to demonstrate delays that may persist through adulthood. These delays particularly relate to the mastery of written English. The incidence of developmental delays frequently (some would say "typically") exhibited by children with a hearing loss may "mask" the diagnosis of a disability in a child who is deaf or hard of hearing (Jure et al., 1991; Moeller, 1985). Specifically, faced with a child who is deaf or hard of hearing with an obvious developmental delay in the areas of language and communication, the interdisciplinary teams responsible for diagnosing disabilities may be reluctant or unable to diagnose a disability other than hearing loss. Especially given the lack of reliable and valid assessment instruments for this purpose, they may be unable to differentiate between delays that are attributable to hearing loss versus other disabilities.

Moeller (1985) used the term "synergistic consequences" to describe how other disabilities interact with hearing loss and confound the diagnostic process. The difficulty or reluctance to diagnose a developmental disability may be especially pronounced soon after a hearing loss is diagnosed, because even obvious delays present at that time could have resulted from the failure to recognize the child's hearing loss earlier.

Other Disabilities May Mask Deafness

Developmental disabilities such as mental retardation, autism, and other forms of pervasive developmental disorders typically include significant delays in communication and language. As a result, diagnosis of hearing loss in such children may be delayed or even overlooked entirely as a possibility. In addition, if other disabilities are diagnosed first, children may be placed for early intervention services in programs in which professionals do not have the experience or training to recognize hearing loss. Ironically, even the genetic syndrome associated with the largest numbers of children with hearing loss—Down syndrome—is widely described as a mental retardation syndrome (a conceptualization in itself that is not fully accurate) and almost never as a syndrome associated with hearing loss (Pruess, Vadasy, & Fewell, 1987). Other disabilities may complicate the diagnosis of a hearing loss directly, as well. Passive diagnostic tests for hearing loss, such as auditory brainstem response (ABR), have poor or unknown reliability in children with documented brain injury (Abdala, 1999). In addition, disabilities such as motor impairments, cognitive delays, or autism may interfere with a child's responses in hearing screenings or examinations requiring active responses on the part of the child.

The Nature of Early Intervention Services
May Impede Diagnosis of Multiple Disabilities

Early intervention services are provided noncategorically to those young children who qualify under their states' and federal eligibility guidelines for such services. Noncategorical early intervention programs rest on the assumptions that avoiding categorical disability labels will prevent stigma and a negative self-fulfilling prophecy. In addition, many developmental disabilities—such as mental retardation, learning disabilities, emotional disorders, autism, Asperger syndrome, and fragile X syndrome—are difficult to diagnose in young children and their developmental consequences are ambiguous in the early years. Nevertheless, the noncategorical nature of early childhood special education may prevent diagnosing specific disabilities in young children who are deaf and hard of hearing, delay appropriate intervention, and exacerbate the difficulties the child encounters.

A Second Disability May Be Harder to Accept

Families of most children who are deaf and hard of hearing typically experience a grieving process, including denial, after their child is diagnosed with a hearing loss. The denial may delay intervention temporarily, but, with professional support, parents usually learn to accept their child's integrity and to support early intervention services wholeheartedly. Although this area has not received much attention in professional literature, it appears that some parents facing a diagnosis of a second disability find the second disability even harder to accept than the first, so that denial may be prolonged and intervention for the second disability delayed much longer than it should (Meadow-Orlans, Smith-Gray, & Dyssegaard, 1995; Schuyler & Rushmer, 1987).

Professionals also are vulnerable to denial of disabilities in children, especially second disabilities. For example, Meadow-Orlans, Mertens, Sass-Lehrer, and Scott-Olson (1997) found that program personnel reported a 24% incidence of "at-risk" conditions, compared with parental reports of 32%. Too frequently professionals will tell parents concerned about a child's obvious delay that the child "will grow out of it," or the professional will assume that a marked delay, indicative of perhaps cognitive delay or autism, is due to hearing loss, instead of initiating a referral or diagnostic process for another disability.

Professionals in deaf education especially may resist the idea of additional disabilities in children who are deaf and hard of hearing. The history of deaf people and deaf education reflects a long, intense, and emotional struggle to demonstrate that individuals who are deaf and hard of hearing are as capable as hearing people (i.e., that they do not have a disability). The historical resistance to a disabled identity appears to be another factor leading some professionals in deaf education to refuse to consider the diagnosis of a disability in a child who is deaf or hard of hearing. Professionals may fear the stigmatizing effects of assigning a child who is deaf or hard hearing a disability label.

In any case, either parental and professional reluctance or denial—or both—may be important factors in delaying appropriate diagnosis and intervention for children with multiple disabilities much longer than the delay for children with single disabilities (Lampropoulou & Padeliadu, 1997).

Assessment Tools Are Inadequate

Diagnosing any but the most severe or visibly apparent developmental delay in very young *hearing* children is difficult. Although standardized intelligence tests normed on young hearing children do exist, their reliability generally is weak. As a result, diagnoses of mild cognitive delay and learning disabilities in hearing preschool children are tentative at best. Standardized test scores are assumed to reflect the effects of a disability, and children's scores are supposed to be comparable to norms (Gordon, Stump, & Glaser, 1996), but these assumptions have not been studied for young children who are deaf and hard of hearing with multiple disabilities. As a result, interpretations of the meaning of their performance on standardized tests are open to question.

In contrast to standardized intelligence tests, developmental assessment tools and protocols used to identify developmental disorders in young children show increased validity with hearing children. The reliability and validity of those same assessment tools, however, are unstudied and unknown when the children being assessed are deaf and hard of hearing.

Although unnecessary early intervention has never been shown to harm a child, parents and professionals are reluctant to pursue intervention until they are confident of the diagnosis. Delays in intervention when it is needed, however, may make the intervention much less effective than earlier intervention (Bronfenbrenner, 1975). Complications in diagnosing multiple disabilities in young children—especially when they are deaf and hard of hearing—create significant problems and delays for families and early interventionists. Because of the lack of reliable and valid diagnostic tools, uncertain diagnoses of disabilities are more likely in children who are deaf and hard of hearing than they are in hearing children. The uncertainty in diagnosis frequently experienced by families of children with multiple disabilities also delays parental acceptance of the disability (Harris, 1983; Meadow-Orlans et al., 1995). As a result, children with multiple disabilities and their families may experience delays or denials of appropriate referrals and the initiation of beneficial services.

CHALLENGES IN FINDING SERVICES FOR CHILDREN WITH MULTIPLE DISABILITIES

Even when a child's multiple disabilities diagnoses are unquestioned, parents and professionals may have difficulty in locating beneficial early intervention services, especially to address developmental, communication, and cognitive needs, rather than treatment of medical issues related to disabilities. Programs, of course, usually can be found that address one disability, but they are not likely to have personnel with expertise related to the other disabilities a child with multiple disabilities may have. Known as "falling between the cracks," this is a source of great frustration for caregivers and advocates for young children with multiple disabilities for several reasons:

- Very few professional preparation programs for early interventionists and other professionals in the deaf education field include information on disabilities other than hearing loss. As a result, the number of deaf education professionals prepared to work with children with multiple disabilities is extremely small (D'Zamko & Hampton, 1985; Luckner & Carter, 2001). Conversely, programs preparing early childhood special educators rarely include more than a lecture or a chapter on hearing loss.

- As a result of their preparation to work with a single disability, most professionals in the deaf education field are unprepared to serve children and their families with developmental issues resulting from disabilities other than hearing loss. Because they know they lack expertise related to multiple disabilities, programs focused on providing services to children who are deaf and hard of hearing may exclude children with multiple disabilities or refer them for service by agencies with no expertise in hearing loss.

- Tendencies of American Deaf culture to exclude various categories of people (Emerton, 1998; Padden, 1998) make it likely that children with multiple disabilities are excluded from programs with a Deaf culture emphasis. As a result, children who are deaf and hard of hearing with multiple disabilities may be exposed to fewer deaf role models and competent signed language users. They may be denied esteem-building opportunities through a Deaf cultural identity and may have fewer opportunities and options for linguistic and social skill development than children who are deaf and hard of hearing with no other disabilities (Calderon & Greenberg, 1999; Watkins, Pittman, & Walden, 1998).

CHALLENGES IN IMPLEMENTING INTERVENTION FOR YOUNG CHILDREN WITH MULTIPLE DISABILITIES

Even when they are willing to serve young children who are deaf and hard of hearing with multiple disabilities, programs focused on providing services to children with hearing loss find that working with these children and their families is extremely challenging. Aside from the shortage of specialized professional expertise related to disabilities other than hearing loss, programs encounter unique challenges in serving deaf and hard of hearing children with multiple disabilities.

Modality Issues

Most programs serving young children who are deaf and hard of hearing and their families utilize the child's vision to facilitate intervention, especially in the critical areas of language and communication. Instruction for caregivers may focus on getting and maintaining the child's visual attention and using vision to compensate for hearing loss. Children with multiple disabilities, however, may have impaired vision, autism, cognitive impairments, or brain injury—conditions that can interfere with children's ability to receive or process information visually. Early educators and caregivers of young children who are deafblind may need to learn to use the tactile modality for play—this modality may be unfamiliar to educators of children who are deaf and hard of hearing—and to foster communication and language (Appell, 1988). The paradox resulting from these examples is that deaf educators—trained to use the child's vision as the primary pathway for intervention—may not recognize the need to utilize alternative modes for developing and maintaining the attention of the child with multiple disabilities, interacting with the child, and facilitating development.

Deaf educators who rely on strategies to compensate for hearing loss visually rather than to develop residual hearing also may not realize that residual hearing is more important to children with multiple disabilities than it is to children whose senses other than hearing are intact. Alternatively, deaf educators may not realize that children with some disabilities, such as autism, reject amplification systems because of hypersensitivity to sound (Rosenthal, Nordin, Sandstrom, & Gillberg, 1999).

Conversely, the preparation of professionals for early intervention with children having disabilities other than hearing loss—such as vision impairment, cognitive delay, learning disabilities, and autism—includes the use of sound and hearing to compensate partially or fully for the disabilities the children may have and to facilitate their development. Special education interventionists, for example, may be prepared to facilitate prereading skills via auditory means. As a result, when special educators not prepared in the area of hearing loss are responsible for a child who has disabilities and is deaf, they may lack the understanding of how to facilitate the child's development through visual means (i.e., through a means for which they were not prepared). Some of these problems can be avoided by early childhood special educators and early childhood deaf educators problem-solving together, each contributing a perspective based on their professional preparation and clinical experience. In many cases, systematically experimenting with different modalities and multimodal approaches should identify the approach that is most effective for each individual child with multiple disabilities.

Interactive and Instructional Pacing Challenges

Conversational and educational contexts for children (and adults) who are deaf and hard of hearing often require a time lag or "wait time." Because the children may be relying on vision to receive manual signs or to speech read, they must first scan the environment—unlike hearing children—in order to identify the person communicating to them. Most early educators working with children who are deaf and hard of hearing are accustomed to this factor and, in fact, train parents and caregivers to incorporate this understanding into their family interactions.

Deaf educators may be unaware that a similar time-lag factor exists with other disabilities, however. Cognitive delays and disabilities such as autism, for example, interfere with communication to a significant degree (Batshaw, 2002). For children with such disabilities, increased time—beyond that typically required by children who are deaf and hard of hearing—may be needed to attract and maintain the child's attention for each communicative interaction. In addition, the time needed for interactions with children who have some cognitive and learning disabilities may need to be increased even further beyond that needed for children who are deaf and hard of hearing, in order to allow them to "process" the information they are receiving and to formulate a response. Similarly, infants and young children who are deafblind and dependent on the tactile modality may need an even longer "wait time" (Downing & Siegel-Causey, 1988).

Issues of pacing become even more complicated when interacting with children who are deaf and hard of hearing and who also have attention deficits. Although it seems intuitive that they too would benefit from a slower instructional or interactive pace, in many cases it appears that rapid interactions are more effective in maintaining their interest and engaging them in participation (Carmine, 1976; Munk & Repp, 1994).

Like many issues in working with children with multiple disabilities, instructional pacing is best approached without preconceived notions about how to interact with the child. In the seemingly atypical instances that actually may be characteristic of children with multiple disabilities, interventionists and caregivers are well advised to use systematic trial and error to discover the pace of interaction that is effective for each child.

Instructional Availability Challenges

Particularly during infancy and the early childhood years, many children with multiple disabilities have health and therapy needs that require multiple appointments with a variety of professionals. The number of appointments appears to be directly proportional to the number of disabilities the child has. Not only does transporting the child to multiple professionals in different sites significantly reduce the time available for educational intervention activities, but it also drains the energy of the caregiver for interacting with the child. In some cases, when the parents' time has been so thoroughly consumed in meeting the health needs of a child with multiple disabilities, they leave to care for personal needs when an early childhood educator makes a home visit, rather than remaining for an instructional session (Fletcher & Browne, 1986). Such issues require understanding by early childhood educators working with families of children with multiple disabilities. In some cases, the problems can be reduced by serving the child and family with a transdisciplinary team that reduces the number of therapies and appointments.

Behavioral Challenges

Sometimes at even a very young age, children with multiple disabilities exhibit recurrent severe problem behaviors including biting, hitting, scratching, screaming, and destruction of materials. In addition, about 35% of children who are deaf and hard of hearing with multiple disabilities exhibit repetitive stereotypical behaviors (e.g., rocking, head banging, hand biting) (Murdoch, 1996). In a few cases, such severe problem behaviors are a natural consequence of a very rare genetic syndrome such as Rett syndrome or Lesch-Nyan syndrome (Batshaw, 2002). Much more typically, however, the behaviors recur because they serve a communicative purpose for the child. Children who are deaf and hard of hearing with multiple disabilities are especially vulnerable to such problems when their disabilities interfere with their ability to communicate their needs and desires and prevent them from being able to make choices. In such cases, an assessment process called "functional analysis" can determine the communicative intent underlying the behavior and result in a plan to facilitate replacement behaviors that help the children communicate their needs in ways that are socially acceptable (Durand, 1990; O'Neill, Horner, Albin, Storey, & Sprague, 1990; Webber & Scheurmann, 1991).

In contrast to aggressive or acting out behaviors, some children with multiple disabilities exhibit behaviors that may be described as passive or withdrawn (e.g., needing to be told to eat before each bite of food). In some cases, the passivity appears to be the result of overcompensation for the children's disabilities. The resulting condition, called "learned helplessness" (Seligman, 1983), can unwittingly be fostered by early intervention specialists (Schuyler & Rushmer, 1987).

Family Systems Challenges

Increasing numbers of children with disabilities come from families with multiple risk factors, including serious economic, medical, mental health, and social problems (Children's Defense Fund, 2000; Greenspan, 1982). Many of these children do not have intact family systems to support child rearing and responsiveness to early intervention programs. Families with a child who is deaf with multiple disabilities show either high levels of stress (Hintermair, 2000) or very low stress scores that could reflect repressed stress (Meadow-Orlans et al., 1995). Similarly, the frequency of divorce, separation, and desertion appears to be higher among families of children with disabilities than it is in the general population (Mori, 1983). All of these factors may make involvement in early intervention programs very difficult for parents and caregivers and may be exacerbated when the children have multiple disabilities. In fact, Meadow-Orlans et al. (1995) found that mothers of infants with multiple disabilities are younger, have less education, and have a lower socioeconomic status than parents of other deaf and hard of hearing infants. Early childhood educators working with families of children with multiple disabilities need to be sensitive to the likelihood of these factors and to recognize that they may need to provide support to the family and referrals to appropriate specialists before early intervention can directly benefit the child (Meadow-Orlans et al., 1995).

Instructional Planning and Curriculum Challenges

A developmental approach following predictable developmental sequences often provides the basis for instructional planning and curriculum sequencing in early childhood programs for children both with and without disabilities (Schuyler & Rushmer, 1987). In this context, preliteracy and literacy are familiar goals. For many children with multiple disabilities, however, a major goal may be the less familiar functional outcomes of independence, semi-independence, or interdependence. As a result, early childhood special education programs increasingly are utilizing a criterion-referenced approach called ecological assessment, in which the curriculum is based on the skills typically utilized in the particular environments that the child experiences and in which the skills the child acquires have immediate meaning and application (Thurman & Widerstrom, 1990).

An ecological approach may not be familiar to early intervention personnel in programs for children who are deaf and hard of hearing, but this approach is well suited for children with multiple disabilities (Jones & Ross, 1998). An ecological approach facilitates identifying the

skills necessary for children with multiple disabilities to function independently in their immediate environments. It also avoids several problems
that may be encountered when a strictly developmental approach is used
to plan intervention for children with multiple disabilities. These problems
may include the following:

- "Developmentally appropriate" skills can be so low level that they
  might not be functional for children with significant developmental
  delays.
- The development of some children with multiple disabilities may be
  so atypical that typical developmental sequences are difficult to apply.
- Long-range planning is difficult because the multiplicity of the children's disabilities prevents predicting their developmental outcomes
  with confidence.

The difficulty that some early intervention programs experience in
goal-setting for children with multiple disabilities is complicated by the
fact that parental goals for these children may initially be more ambiguous
than they are for children who are deaf and hard of hearing whose
development follows typical patterns and sequences. As a result, early
intervention personnel should utilize "person-centered planning" to facilitate parental goal setting as part of the instructional planning process
for children with multiple disabilities.

Person-centered planning is the general term applied to a group of
approaches for identifying, organizing, and guiding truly individualized
education programs (O'Brien & Lovett, 1992). Examples are Personal
Futures Planning (Mount, 1991), MAPS (Forest & Pearpoint, 1992; Forest & Snow, 1987; Vandercook et al., 1993), and PATH (Pearpoint,
O'Brien, & Forest, 1994). Each approach has some unique features, but
all focus on bringing together those who are important in the life of the
child at the center of the planning (e.g., parents, siblings, grandparents,
friends, interventionists or teachers, therapists, administrators). These
individuals come together in a series of meetings to discuss and learn as
much as possible about the child, identify the immediate and long-range
goals they have for the child, determine what is needed to make these
goals a reality, make a plan for doing so, and commit to implementing
the plan. Person-centered planning, done correctly, requires that those
involved remain committed to overcoming barriers to the desired outcomes (O'Brien & Lovett, 1992). Such an approach can involve the entire
school community in planning an inclusive goal-oriented program for the
child with multiple disabilities.

Affective Challenges

Professionals in early childhood programs for children who are deaf
and hard of hearing, without special preparation in the area of multiple

disabilities, may have a layperson's reaction to cognitive, physical, behavioral, or other disabilities. These affective reactions can include fear for their own illness or injury, pity for the child or family, overprotection, and infantilization (Wolfensberger, 1975). Unprepared early childhood personnel also can be preoccupied with fears of their own inadequacy. As a result of such reactions, early interventionists may be much less effective than they should be in advising, counseling, and partnering with parents of children with multiple disabilities. Collaborating with professionals accustomed to disabilities that may be multiple or severe may help the interventionist recognize and avoid averse reactions to the child's disabilities so that neither the family- nor child-centered aspect of their intervention will suffer (Campbell, 1987).

Child-Related Challenges

Beyond the systemic challenges addressed previously, a number of characteristics of some children with multiple disabilities present special challenges to their families and the personnel working with them. Some children may be medically fragile with multiple health problems including degenerative disorders and terminal illness. Many children receive multiple prescription medications every day to manage seizures, attention, or behavior. Some children with multiple disabilities require medical procedures throughout the day, such as naso-gastric, jejeunal, or gastric feeding; suctioning tracheostomies; bladder catheterization; and seizure management (Mulligan-Ault, Guess, Struth, & Thompson, 1988). As a result of such needs, one early intervention program for children who are deaf and hard of hearing reported having to provide personnel training in the areas of cardiopulmonary resuscitation and coping with viruses such as hepatitis, cytomegalovirus, and HIV (Howell, 1992).

Even as preschoolers, some children with multiple disabilities engage in dangerous self-abusive behaviors (e.g., eye poking, hand biting). Others may be so aggressive that they pose a threat to children and adults at home and in early intervention programs. Others may have such severe disabilities that interventions may be required with which the specialist in deaf education may be unfamiliar. These may include fairly esoteric instructional techniques such as partial participation (Ferguson & Baumgart, 1991), applied behavior analysis (Jones, 1993), or positive behavior supports (Boulvaare, Schwartz, & McBride, 1999; Koegel, Koegel, & Dunlap, 1996).

Still other children may have cognitive or physical disabilities that limit their expressive communication. Compensation for such limitations often can be achieved with augmentative communication systems (Beukelman & Mirenda, 1998), which also may be unknown to deaf educators.

Although all of the above conditions are unusual in programs focused on children who are deaf and hard of hearing, they are familiar in early childhood special education programs, especially those for children with severe disabilities. They also are increasingly familiar in the "mainstream" as more young children with severe and multiple disabilities are placed in community programs rather than in special education early intervention programs. As a result, several options are available for early childhood educators working with deaf and hard of hearing children to acquire specialized skills needed by their cases with multiple disabilities. These opportunities include

- Preservice special education courses at universities with special education programs or in a distance education format
- In-service training
- Collaboration with special educators, therapists, and medical personnel who have the necessary knowledge and skills

The challenges in providing early intervention services to children who are deaf and hard of hearing and their families tempt many programs focused on hearing loss to refuse service to children with multiple disabilities and their families, even though the children may have significant hearing losses. As programs begin to recognize and overcome the challenges and to serve all deaf and hard of hearing children regardless of the multiplicity or severity of their disabilities, they find that children with multiple disabilities achieve far beyond anyone's expectations for them (Jones & Ross, 1998). This is especially true when the children with multiple disabilities are fully included with their deaf and hard of hearing peers, rather than segregated from them, and when the interventionists implement child-centered cooperative learning strategies rather than traditional interventionist-directed instruction (Jones & Ross, 1998).

MARCO'S INTERVENTIONIST

The classroom in which I worked had a young deaf child named Marco, who had significant developmental delays. Marco's parents were very proactive about his education. They were very, very involved in the IEP process and daily classroom instruction. The school located and hired an interventionist who was a proficient signer with a degree in deaf education and who had almost completed her degree in mental retardation. What better combination could you ask for?

This young child had the "perfect" program placement with the "perfect" interventionist. Money was of no consequence at school or at home.

Marco's parents were well educated, very proactive, and proficient signers themselves. Yet, Marco did not thrive in this particular environment. He was physically separated from his same-age peers—both hearing and deaf. His language did not progress. He needed friends his own age. A lonely little boy, Marco had little to motivate his language development.

Children who are deaf or hard of hearing should not be segregated to a special placement due to their mental impairment. Granted, certain accommodations may have to be made in both the physical setting (e.g., bathroom) and in the academic instruction. A skilled interventionist with the help of an aide or a multiple disabilities specialist can accommodate these in a less restrictive setting.

Practical strategies for integrating students with multiple disabilities with other children are found in a variety of sources (Brown et al., 1991; Downing, 2002; Ferguson, Meyer, Jeanchild, Juniper, & Zingo, 1992; Jones & Carlier, 1995; Jones & Ross, 1998; Luiselli, Evans, Luiselli, DeCaluwe, & Jacobs, 1995; Rogers, 1994). The highly positive results of such inclusion probably are attributable to the fact that children who need communication and social skills can learn those skills much better in environments in which there are socially competent peer models using a language fluently that they can perceive, than in environments in which they are grouped with other children with severe deficiencies in social and communication skills.

PROFESSIONAL CHALLENGES

Professionals working in the field of multiple disabilities and deafness face the challenge of finding materials that address the unique needs of this diverse group of learners. What little there is available either does not address young children, focuses on only a subgroup of this population, or is quite dated. For example, even at the beginning of the 21st century, no professional association or periodical publication exists in the area of multiple disabilities. The short life of the privately published *Journal of the Multihandicapped Person* indicates the difficulties of organizing a professional forum focusing on a relatively small and highly diverse sub-disability group (or sub-sub-disability, if one considers only deaf and hard of hearing children with multiple disabilities). Perhaps the most relevant association for early educators working with children with multiple disabilities is TASH (formerly The Association for Persons with Severe

Handicaps). Its conference and journal, *Research and Practice for Persons with Severe Disabilities* (formerly *JASH, Journal of The Association for Persons with Severe Handicaps*), however, address issues related to moderate to severe multiple disabilities but not mild to moderate disabilities, the largest part of the deaf and hard of hearing children population (Wolff & Harkins, 1986). The Conference of American Instructors of the Deaf (CAID) has a special interest group for multiple disabilities, but it is currently inactive. Just a few books have been published addressing the education of deaf and hard of hearing children with multiple disabilities (Cherow, 1985; Prickett & Duncan, 1988; Tweedie & Shroyer, 1982). Although also not of recent vintage, curriculum guides have been prepared for deaf students with multiple disabilities (Foster, Levy, & Cullison, 1972; Hyde & Engle, 1980; Mahoney, 1981), including one focused on young children (Clark & Morgan, 1984).

Perhaps the greatest degree of professional structure related to multiple disabilities has been in the very small and specialized sub-field of deafblindness. Title VI-C federal funds that have supported programs and services for deafblind children since 1969, including D-B Link, a clearinghouse on deafblindness, and the Conrad N. Hilton Foundation, which has endowed the Hilton/Perkins Program of training and periodic conferences for professionals in the deafblindness field, have facilitated this structure. A coalition of parents and professionals formed an organization that focuses on the CHARGE association, a condition that includes hearing loss along with vision, mental, and physical disabilities (Jones & Dunne, 1988). The extent of professional structures in the field of deafblindness has resulted in several texts that address early intervention with children who have vision impairments and other disabilities (Chen, 1999; Goetz, Guess, & Stremel-Campbell, 1987; McInnes & Treffry, 1993) as well as instructional materials designed especially for this population (Ferrell, 1996).

PROGRAM APPLICATIONS

Although early educators face numerous challenges in working with young children who are deaf and hard of hearing with multiple disabilities and their families, agencies and programs with expertise related to the single disability of hearing loss appear to be in a better position to serve these children and their families effectively than are programs focused on other disabilities. It appears to be much easier to incorporate special education practices into a program for children who are deaf and hard of hearing than it is to meet the communication and language needs of children who are deaf and hard of hearing with multiple disabilities in a special education program. The special education practices that appear to have the greatest potential for enabling early intervention programs for children who are deaf and hard of hearing to effectively serve children with multiple disabilities and their families include the following:

1. Schuyler and Rushmer (1987) suggested approaching children who are deaf and hard of hearing with multiple disabilities as positively as possible, a recommendation that cannot be overstated. In order to achieve this goal, early intervention programs for children who are deaf and hard of hearing with multiple disabilities should address attitudes and misconceptions about a range of disabilities. An understanding and resolution of affective issues related to disability probably will need to include the professionals involved and should extend in ever-widening circles to the families, peers, neighbors, and associates of the children involved.

2. Early intervention for children with multiple disabilities can be fragmented, leading to both ineffective services and unnecessary family stresses. To avoid such problems, Meadow-Orlans et al. (1995) suggested that case managers are more important for families whose child has multiple disabilities than for other families. They also recommended that the intervention involve a holistic approach, instead of addressing the child's disabilities separately. Orelove and Sobsey (1996) similarly advocated for a transdisciplinary model for serving children with multiple disabilities, in which one professional is the primary facilitator of all services and other team members act as consultants.

3. Rather than disability categories and labels, individual characteristics and educational needs of each child separately should provide the basis for decisions concerning placement, curriculum, instructional methods, and other facets of early intervention (Jones, 1984).

4. Early childhood educators should collaborate across the disability emphases of their schools and agencies to problem-solve, plan, and deliver early intervention services to children who are deaf and hard of hearing with multiple disabilities and their families (Campbell, 1987; Rainforth & York-Barr, 1997).

5. Groups of children should be conceptualized, served, and educated as a collection of unique individuals, rather than a group with more similarities than differences. In effect, the diversity of the group or "class" should be viewed as spread along a continuum rather than clustered around an average. Not only is such a conceptualization more likely to be accurate when young children who are deaf and

hard of hearing are involved, but hopefully it will facilitate accepting, including, and better meeting the needs of children with more extraordinary characteristics (Jones, 1984).

6. Intervention should be both family centered and child centered and never interventionist directed. Early interventionists who are most concerned about "covering" information will find themselves unable to meet the needs of diverse learners. Interventionists who are responsive to the unique characteristics and interests of each child and family, however, will find themselves effectively meeting the needs of a broad range of children and families, including those with multiple and complex needs.

7. Preparation to work with children with multiple disabilities and their families should be a part of every professional preparation program in deaf education. The knowledge and skills competencies suggested by Luckner and Carter (2001) should provide a strong basis for such programs. Such programs should include a significant amount of content, experience, and skill development related to multiple disabilities. This has been accomplished in the field of vision impairments for many years but is equally important in the preparation of professional personnel for children who are deaf and hard of hearing.

8. Early intervention services for children who are deaf and hard of hearing with multiple disabilities need to be prepared to provide the much greater logistical and emotional support that many of these children's families need.

9. Early intervention programs for deaf and hard of hearing children with multiple disabilities should base children's developmental and educational goals at least as much on ecological assessment as on developmental assessment.

10. A long-term goal of early intervention for children who are deaf and hard of hearing with multiple disabilities should be the development of healthy lifelong support systems in the communities and cultures to which the children have a natural affinity (Carpenter, 1995) rather than artificial disability-focused environments such as sheltered workshops and mental retardation institutions.

Demographics indicate that a large proportion of children who are deaf and hard of hearing have multiple disabilities. Unfortunately, adequately diagnosing their needs and finding appropriate placements remain elusive. Diagnosing developmental and other disabilities in young children is difficult. Doing so in young children who are deaf and hard of hearing is even more so. Often, their developmental delays are attributed to deafness. When developmental disabilities have already been diagnosed, they may mask the existence of a hearing loss. Screening and assessment instruments do not address this population of young children. Finding programs that can address all of their educational needs, whether deafness related or other disability related, is difficult. Ethical and educational, if not legal, imperatives indicate that programs for children who are deaf and hard of hearing are often in the best position to provide effective services for these children and families with many complex needs. Many challenges exist that make this effort difficult, however. Few personnel preparation programs in the field of deafness, for example, provide information and training on working with disabilities other than deafness. At the same time, few personnel preparation programs in other disability fields include preparation to teach children whose disabilities include deafness. In spite of these challenges, the remedies are clear. When they are undertaken, the potential is great for programs and agencies organized around hearing loss to facilitate optimal development in children with multiple disabilities.

REFERENCES

Abdala, C. (1999). Pediatric audiology: Evaluating infants. In D. Chen (Ed.), *Essential elements in early intervention: Visual impairment and multiple disabilities* (pp. 246–284). New York: AFB Press.

Appell, M. (1988). Mother–child interaction and the development of preverbal communication. In M. Bullis & G. Fielding (Eds.), *Communication development in young children with deafblindness: Literature review* (pp. 129–142). Monmouth, OR: Teaching Research Division.

Batshaw, M.L. (Ed.). (2002). *Children with disabilities* (5th ed.). Baltimore: Paul H. Brookes Publishing Co.

Beukelman, D.R., & Mirenda, P. (1998). *Augmentative and alternative communication: Management of severe communication disorders in children and adults* (2nd ed.). Baltimore: Paul H. Brookes Publishing Co.

Boulvaare, G., Schwartz, I., & McBride, B. (1999). Addressing challenging behaviors at home: Working with families to find solutions. In S. Sandall & M. Ostrosky (Eds.), *Young exceptional children monograph series: Practical ideas for addressing challenging behaviors* (pp. 29–40). Denver, CO: Division for Early Childhood.

Bronfenbrenner, U. (1975). Is early intervention effective? In B.Z. Friedlander, G.M. Sterritt, & G.E. Kirk (Eds.), *Exceptional infant: Assessment and intervention* (pp. 449–475). New York: Brunner/Mazel.

Brown, L., Schwartz, P., Udvari-Solner, A., Kampschroer, E.F., Johnson, F., Jorgensen, J., et al. (1991). How much time should students with severe intellectual disabilities spend in regular education classrooms and elsewhere? *Journal of The Association for Persons with Severe Handicaps, 16,* 39–47.

Calderon, R., & Greenberg, M.T. (1999). Stress and coping in hearing mothers of children with hearing loss: Factors affecting mother and child adjustment. *American Annals of the Deaf, 144,* 7–18.

Campbell, P.H. (1987). The integrated programming team: An approach for coordinating professionals of various disciplines in programs for students with severe and multiple handicaps. *Journal of The Association for Persons with Severe Handicaps, 12,* 107–116.

Carmine, D.W. (1976). Effects of two interventionist presentation rates on off-task behavior, answering correctly, and participation. *Journal of Applied Behavior Analysis, 9,* 199–206.

Carpenter, B. (1995). Across the lifespan: Educational opportunities for children with profound and multiple learning difficulties. *Early Child Development and Care, 109,* 75–82.

Chen, D. (1999). *Essential elements in early intervention: Visual impairment and multiple disabilities.* New York: AFB Press.

Cherow, E. (Ed.). (1985). *Hearing-impaired children and youth with developmental disabilities: An interdisciplinary foundation for service.* Washington, DC: Gallaudet University Press.

Children's Defense Fund. (2000). *The state of America's children: Yearbook 2000.* Washington, DC: Author.

Clark, T.C., & Morgan, E.C. (1984). *The INSITE model: A parent-centered, in-home, sensory intervention, training and educational program.* Logan, UT: Project INSITE.

Downing, J.E. (2002). *Including students with severe and multiple disabilities in typical classrooms: Practical strategies for teachers* (2nd ed.). Baltimore: Paul H. Brookes Publishing Co.

Downing, J.E., & Siegel-Causey, E. (1988). Enhancing the nonsymbolic communicative behavior of children with multiple impairments. *Language, Speech, and Hearing Services in Schools, 19*(4), 338–348.

Durand, V.M. (1990). *Severe problem behaviors: A functional communication training approach.* New York: Guilford.

D'Zamko, M., & Hampton, I. (1985). Personnel preparation for multihandicapped hearing impaired students: A review of the literature. *American Annals of the Deaf, 130,* 9–14.

Elliott, R., Powers, A., & Funderburg, R. (1988). Learning disabled hearing-impaired students: Interventionist survey. *The Volta Review, 90,* 227–228.

Emerton, R.G. (1998). Marginality, biculturism and social identity of deaf people. In I. Parasnis (Ed.), *Cultural and language diversity and the deaf experience* (pp. 136–145). New York: Cambridge University Press.

Ferguson, D.L., & Baumgart, D. (1991). Partial participation revisited. *Journal of The Association for Persons with Severe Handicaps, 16,* 218–227.

Ferguson, D.L., Meyer, L., Jeanchild, L., Juniper, L., & Zingo, J. (1992). Figuring out what to do with the grownups: How interventionists make inclusion "work" for students with disabilities. *Journal of The Association for Persons with Severe Handicaps, 17,* 218–226.

Ferrell, K.A. (1996). *Reach out and teach: Meeting the training needs of parents of visually and multiply handicapped young children.* New York: AFB Press.

Flathouse, V.E. (1979). Multiply handicapped deaf children and Public Law 94-142. *Exceptional Children, 45,* 560–565.

Fletcher, M.A., & Browne, C.W. (1986). *The neonatal experience.* Washington, DC: The George Washington University Infant Educator Programs.

Forest, M., & Pearpoint, J. (1992). Commonsense tools: MAPS and circles. In J. Pearpoint, M. Forest, & J. Snow (Eds.), *The inclusion papers: Strategies to make inclusion work* (pp. 52–57). Toronto: Inclusion Press.

Forest, M., & Snow, J. (1987). *The MAPS Process.* Toronto: Frontier College.

Foster, E., Levy, J., & Cullison, S. (1972). *Let the sunshine in!: Learning activities for multiply handicapped deaf children.* Indianapolis: Indiana School for the Deaf.

Goetz, L., Guess, D., & Stremel-Campbell, K. (1987). *Innovative program design for individuals with dual sensory impairments.* Baltimore: Paul H. Brookes Publishing Co.

Gordon, R.P., Stump, K., & Glaser, B.A. (1996). Assessment of individuals with hearing impairments: Equity in testing procedures and accommodations. *Measurement and Evaluation in Counseling and Development, 29,* 111–118.

Greenspan, S.I. (1982). Developmental morbidity in infants in multi-risk-factor families: Clinical perspectives. *Public Health Reports, 97*(1), 16–23.

Hanson, M.J., & Lynch, E.W. (1995). *Early intervention: Implementing child and family services for infants and toddlers who are at risk or disabled.* Austin, TX: PRO-ED.

Happé, F. (1998). *Autism: An introduction to psychological theory.* Cambridge, MA: Harvard University Press.

Harris, G. (1983). *Broken ears, wounded hearts: An intimate journey into the lives of a multihandicapped girl and her family.* Washington, DC: Gallaudet University Press.

Hintermair, M. (2000). Children who are hearing impaired with additional disabilities and related aspects of parental stress. *Exceptional Children, 66*(3), 327–332.

Holden-Pitt, L., & Diaz, J.A. (1998). Thirty years of the Annual Survey of Deaf and Hard-of-Hearing Children & Youth: A glance over the decades. *American Annals of the Deaf, 143,* 72–76.

Howell, R.F. (1992). A profile of family education/early intervention services at the Maryland School for the Deaf. *American Annals of the Deaf, 137,* 79–84.

Hyde, S., & Engle, D. (1980). *The Potomac program: A curriculum for the severely handicapped deaf, hearing impaired, non-verbal.* Beaverton, OR: Dormac.

Individuals with Disabilities Education Act Amendments of 1997, PL 105-17, 20 U.S.C. §§ 1400 *et seq.*

Jones, M.M., & Carlier, L.L. (1995). Creating inclusionary opportunities for learners with multiple disabilities: A team-teaching approach. *Journal of Special Education Technology, 13,* 16–35.

Jones, T.W. (1984). A framework for identification, classification and placement of multihandicapped hearing impaired students. *The Volta Review, 86,* 142–151.

Jones, T.W. (1993). Best practices in classroom management of deaf students with multiple disabilities. In R.H. Eliott & A.R. Powers (Eds.), *Deaf and hard-of-hearing students with mild additional disabilities* (pp. 1–24). Tuscaloosa: The University of Alabama.

Jones, T.W. (1998). Can a deaf student have a learning disability?: The exclusion clause and state special education guidelines. In H. Markowicz & C. Berdichevsky (Eds.), *Bridging the gap between research and practice in the fields of learning disabilities and deafness* (pp. 113–118). Washington, DC: Gallaudet University Press.

Jones, T.W., & Dunne, M.T. (1998). The c.h.a.r.g.e. association: Implications for interventionists. *American Annals of the Deaf, 133,* 36–39.

Jones, T.W., & Ross, P.A. (1998). Inclusion strategies for deaf students with special needs. *The Endeavor, 37,* 2–22.

Jure, R., Rapin, I., & Tuchman, R.F. (1991). Hearing impaired autistic children. *Developmental Medicine and Child Neurology, 33,* 1062–1072.

Karchmer, M.A., & Allen, T.A. (1999). The functional assessment of deaf and hard of hearing students. *American Annals of the Deaf, 144,* 68–77.

Koegel, L.K., Koegel, R.L., & Dunlap, G. (Eds.). (1996). *Positive behavioral support: Including people with difficult behavior in the community.* Baltimore: Paul H. Brookes Publishing Co.

Lampropoulou, V., & Padeliadu, S. (1997). Interventionists of the deaf as compared with other groups of interventionists: Attitudes towards people with
disabilities and inclusion. *American Annals of the Deaf, 142,* 26–33.
Luckner, J.L., & Carter, K. (2001). Essential competencies for teaching students
with hearing loss and additional disabilities. *American Annals of the Deaf,
146,* 7–15.
Luiselli, T., Evans, J., Luiselli, J.K., DeCaluwe, S.M., & Jacobs, L.A. (1995).
Inclusive education of young children with deaf-blindness: Technical assistance
model. *Journal of Visual Impairments and Blindness, 89,* 249–256.
Mahoney, D. (1981). *Survival skills for the deaf.* Washington, DC: Precollege
Programs.
Mauk, G.W., & Mauk, P.P. (1992). Somewhere out there: Preschool children
with hearing impairment and learning disabilities. *Topics in Early Childhood
Special Education, 12,* 12–18.
Mauk, G.W., & Mauk, P.P. (1993). Compounding the challenge: Young deaf chil-
dren and learning disabilities. *Perspectives, 12,* 12–17.
McInnes, J.M., & Treffry, J. (1993). *Deaf-blind infants and children: A develop-
mental guide.* Toronto, Ontario: University of Toronto Press.
Meadow-Orlans, K.P., Mertens, D.M., Sass-Lehrer, M.A., & Scott-Olson, K. (1997).
Support services for parents and their children who are deaf or hard of hearing:
A national survey. *American Annals of the Deaf, 142,* 278–288.
Meadow-Orlans, K.P., Smith-Gray, S., & Dyssegaard, B. (1995). Sources of stress
for mothers and fathers of deaf and hard of hearing infants. *American Annals
of the Deaf, 140,* 352–357.
Moeller, M.P. (1985). Developmental approaches to communication assessment
and enhancement. In E. Cherow (Ed.), *Hearing-impaired children and
youth with developmental disabilities: An interdisciplinary foundation
for service* (pp. 171–198). Washington, DC: Gallaudet University Press.
Mori, A.A. (1983). *Families of children with special needs: Early intervention
techniques for the practitioner.* Rockville, MD: Aspen.
Mount, B. (1991). *Making futures happen: A facilitator's guide to Personal
Futures Planning.* Manchester, CT: Communitas.
Mulligan-Ault, M., Guess, D., Struth, L., & Thompson, B. (1988). The implementa-
tion of health-related procedures in classrooms for students with severe multi-
ple impairments. *Journal of The Association for Persons with Severe Handi-
caps, 13,* 100–109.
Munk, D.D., & Repp, A.C. (1994). The relationship between instructional variables
and problem behavior: A review. *Exceptional Children, 60,* 390–401.
Murdoch, H. (1996). Stereotyped behaviors in deaf and hard of hearing children.
American Annals of the Deaf, 141, 379–386.
O'Brien, J., & Lovett, H. (1992). *Finding a way toward everyday lives: The
contribution of person centered planning.* Harrisburg: Pennsylvania Office
of Mental Retardation.
O'Neill, R.E., Horner, R.H., Albin, R.W., Storey, K., & Sprague, J.R. (1990). *Functional analysis of problem behavior: A practical assessment guide.* Sycamore, IL: Sycamore Publishing Company.
Orelove, F.P., & Sobsey, D. (1996). *Educating children with multiple disabilities: A transdisciplinary approach* (3rd ed.). Baltimore: Paul H. Brookes
Publishing Co.
Padden, C. (1998). From the cultural to the bicultural: The modern deaf community. In I. Parasnis (Ed.), *Cultural and language diversity and the Deaf
experience.* New York: Cambridge University Press.
Pearpoint, J., O'Brien, J., & Forest, M. (1994). *PATH: A workbook for planning
positive possible futures.* Toronto: Inclusion Press.

Prickett, H.T., & Duncan, E. (Eds.). (1988). *Coping with the multi-handicapped hearing impaired: A practical approach.* Springfield, IL: Charles C Thomas.

Pruess, J.B., Vadasy, P.F., & Fewell, R.R. (1987). Language development in children with Down syndrome: An overview of recent research. *Education and Training in Mental Retardation, 22*(1), 44–55.

Rainforth, B., & York-Barr, J. (1997). *Collaborative teams for students with severe disabilities: Integrating therapy and educational services* (2nd ed.). Baltimore: Paul H. Brookes Publishing Co.

Rogers, J. (Ed.). (1994). *Inclusion: Moving beyond our fears.* Bloomington, IN: Phi Delta Kappa.

Rosenthal, U., Nordin, V., Sandstrom, G.A., & Gillberg, C. (1999). Autism and hearing loss. *Journal of Autism and Developmental Disorders, 29,* 349–357.

Sabatino, D. (1983). The house that Jack built. *Journal of Learning Disabilities, 16,* 6–27.

Schuyler, V., & Rushmer, N. (1987). *Parent-infant habilitation: A comprehensive approach to working with hearing-impaired infants and toddlers and their families.* Portland, OR: IHR Publications.

Seligman, M. (1983). *The family with a handicapped child: Understanding and treatment.* New York: Grune & Stratton.

Thurman, S.K., & Widerstrom, A.H. (1990). *Infants and young children with special needs: A development and ecological approach* (2nd ed.). Baltimore: Paul H. Brookes Publishing Co.

Tweedie, D., & Shroyer, E.H. (Eds.). (1982). *The multihandicapped hearing impaired: Identification and instruction.* Washington, DC: Gallaudet University Press.

U.S. Department of Education. (1982). *To assure the free appropriate public education of all children with disabilities: Fourth annual report to Congress on the implementation of the Individuals with Disabilities Education Act.* Washington, DC: Author.

U.S. Department of Education. (1995). *To assure the free appropriate public education of all children with disabilities: Seventeenth annual report to Congress on the implementation of the Individuals with Disabilities Education Act.* Washington, DC: Author.

U.S. Department of Education. (2000). *To assure the free appropriate public education of all children with disabilities: Twenty-second annual report to Congress on the implementation of the Individuals with Disabilities Education Act.* Washington, DC: Author.

Vandercook, T., Tetlei, R.R., Montie, J., Downing, J., Levin, J., & Glanvill, M. (1993). The McGill Action Planning System (M.A.P.S.): A strategy for building the vision. *Journal of the Association for Persons with Severe Handicaps, 14,* 205–215.

Watkins, S., Pittman, P., & Walden, B. (1998). The deaf mentor experimental project for young children who are deaf and their families. *American Annals of the Deaf, 143,* 29–34.

Webber, J., & Scheurmann, B. (1991). Accentuate the positive—Eliminate the negative! *TEACHING Exceptional Children, 24,* 13–19.

Wolfensberger, W. (1975). *The origin and nature of our institutional models.* Syracuse, NY: Human Policy Press.

Wolff, A.B., & Harkins, J.E. (1986). Multihandicapped students. In A.N. Schildroth & M.A. Karchmer (Eds.), *Deaf children in America* (pp. 55–81). San Diego: College-Hill Press.

Yoshinaga-Itano, C., & Apuzzo, M.L. (1998). Identification of hearing loss after 18 months is not early enough. *American Annals of the Deaf, 143,* 380–387.

A Parent's Perspective

Ashley's Father

Deciding on placement for a child with multiple disabilities truly becomes a matter of choosing the least inappropriate setting. Short of finding a residential school with a large enough population of deaf students to support a program in multiple disabilities, the options are few and far between. The trend toward identifying the dominant disability and letting that guide placement is a farce. Our daughter is deaf and has mental retardation. With her, whatever disability is underserved becomes her dominant disability. Serve the deafness with an HI [hearing impairment] placement, and her developmental needs rise up and cry out for help. Likewise, place her in a developmentally based environment without adequately addressing her communications needs as a deaf person, and she cannot even access the opportunities.

Parents must fight for services for the whole child. Placing children who are deaf or hard of hearing with multiple disabilities in a developmental program at first is dangerous because you may never know what effect the lack of communication will have on their cognitive abilities. We just toured a developmental center that has six children who are deaf or hard of hearing who have never been provided sign language! Who knows how much of their condition is caused by mental retardation and how much by a lack of access to communication.

Businessmen say there is price, quality, and service, and that you can only get two out of the three at any given time. If you get quality and price, the service lacks. If you get the service and price, the quality is lacking. In seeking a program that will address the unique needs of children who are deaf or hard of hearing with multiple disabilities, one cannot afford to get two out of three. The disabilities are like engines that run side by side. They must both be fed together. You cannot have two wheels moving and two wheels standing still. They also feed off each other.

I tend to look at the world as a hearing world. Schools are by and large designed for hearing people. Hearing people with disabilities have so many choices: classes for learning disabilities, autism, severe disabilities, emotional disabilities, and so forth. Deaf people only have one class. The assumption is that the only thing wrong with you is that your ears don't work. All the other special education classes are foreign to a deaf child because of the language issues. The only classes available to children who are deaf or hard of hearing as they approach school age focus on academics. If deciding that such a placement is not appropriate due to the lack of emphases on developmental issues, do not throw the baby out with the bath water. People readily accept the communication needs of children who are deaf or hard of hearing who have no other problems. Add other problems and people think the child can hear! People act as if all the problems a deaf child would have in the hearing world no longer are important when the child has other disabilities. I can accept what happened to my daughter as an act of nature. I could not accept what might happen to her as a result of others' indifference, ignorance, prejudice, or my own lack of involvement. Fight for your whole child, not just the part that fits in the box.

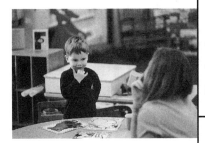

Language and Communication

CHAPTER ELEVEN

Parent–Child Interaction

*Implications for
Intervention and Development*

PATRICIA E. SPENCER

J ason (4 months old) sits in an infant chair that has been placed on a
table. He looks around the room at lights and objects hanging from
the ceiling. His mother sits facing Jason and watches him intently.
When Jason looks at her, his mother gives a bright smile and, tilting her
head from side to side, takes Jason's feet in her hands and moves them up
and down alternately. Jason matches his mother's bright smile. His mother
releases the baby's feet and signs, "Hello, hello. What are you looking for?
What are you looking for?"

My introduction to the issues discussed in this chapter occurred when I worked in the
Center for Studies in Education and Human Development of the Gallaudet Research Insti-
tute, Gallaudet University. My research on these issues was supported by grants from 1)
U.S. Public Health Service, Office of Maternal and Child Health, Grant Number MCJ-110563,
Kathryn P. Meadow-Orlans, Principal Investigator, and 2) U.S. Department of Education,
Office of Special Education and Rehabilitation Services, Grant Number HO23C10077, Donald
F. Moores, Principal Investigator. I want to thank Kathryn P. Meadow-Orlans for her guidance
and for many years of discussions about the topics and information presented in the chapter.
I also want to thank Amy Lederberg for helping me think about these issues and for providing
helpful comments on an earlier version of this chapter.

Parent–child interactions can occur at many times, including during routine caregiving activities, during special moments of face-to-face communication and play, and during conversations in which language is used. The activities, and even the feelings, of one participant in an interaction affect and are affected by those of the other. Of course, infants cannot express their needs and feelings explicitly because they do not have the language skills to do so. This means that parents and other adults who interact with an infant must interpret the meaning behind the infant's activities by attending to body tone and movements, direction of eye gaze, facial expressions, and vocalizations. Although this may sound like an almost impossible task, parents have been observed often to "intuitively" or spontaneously use behaviors and strategies with young infants in ways that seem designed to match their physical, social, and attentional needs (Papousek & Papousek, 1987). For example, hearing parents tend to position themselves so that their young infants can see them easily, touch their infants gently and often, and raise the pitch of their voice when speaking to infants. Parents talk to their infant as though they are having a conversation in which the infant is also taking turns. All of these apparently spontaneous modifications, or changes from adults' typical communication behaviors, have been shown to increase hearing infants' attention and participation during interactions early in life.

Participation in interactions with caregivers provides an important basis for infants' later development. Through such interactions, infants begin to learn whether their world is secure and whether people can be trusted to comfort them and meet their needs. They also begin to acquire cognitive skills such as understandings of cause and effect and sequencing. In addition, interactions throughout infancy and the toddler years provide input and practice for developing communication and language skills.

What happens, however, when an infant is born with a significant hearing loss and is not able to receive or process the caregiver's vocal communications during interactions? Can infants and toddlers who are deaf and hard of hearing learn from interactions with adults in the same way that hearing children do? What special kinds of modifications can parents make in their typical communication behaviors to best meet the needs of young children with a hearing loss? This chapter reviews information gathered from research with parents, hearing and deaf, and their deaf and hard of hearing children during the earliest years of life. This chapter also provides suggestions for intervention to help parents and interventionists "fine-tune" interactions with infants and toddlers who have hearing loss.

CHARACTERISTICS OF INTERACTIONS
BETWEEN INFANTS AND TODDLERS WHO ARE DEAF
OR HARD OF HEARING AND THEIR PARENTS OR CAREGIVERS

Interactions promote, and are subsequently affected by, children's developing communication behaviors as well as social-emotional bonding, or attachment, between children and caregivers. Many of the aspects of early interactions between caregivers and young children who are deaf or hard of hearing are similar to those of caregivers and young hearing children. However, some additional interactive characteristics, especially caregiver sensitivity to visual communication needs, are important for optimal support of development of deaf children.

Caregiver Sensitivity and Children's Participation

The phenomenon of caregiver sensitivity, or general responsiveness, during interactions with infants and young children has been extensively investigated and has been found to directly affect children's development. For example, researchers who have studied young hearing children and their mothers report that high levels of maternal sensitivity are associated with quicker development of play and language skills (Baumwell, Tamis-LeMonda, & Bornstein, 1997; Dunham & Dunham, 1992; Slade, 1987a; Smith, Adamson, & Bakeman, 1988). Similar associations have been found for deaf and hard of hearing children, including relations between maternal sensitivity and children's development of symbolic play, language, and visual attention skills (Meadow-Orlans & Spencer, 1996; Pressman, Pipp-Siegel, Yoshinaga-Itano, & Deas, 1999; Spencer & Meadow-Orlans, 1996; Wilson & Spencer, 1997).

In the vignette at the beginning of this chapter, the mother demonstrated sensitivity to her infant by attending carefully to his actions and direction of gaze, by responding to the infant with a positive emotional display when he looked at her, and by producing language related to what she perceived the infant to be doing. Researchers across studies have defined the general construct of sensitivity in a variety of ways. For example, Meadow-Orlans (1997) characterized maternal sensitivity as a combination of the following: 1) willingness to respond to and continue child's activity or interest; 2) flexibility, or willingness to accept child's indications of interest or disinterest in an activity; 3) consistency of interactive characteristics; 4) overall affect; and 5) level of involvement in the interaction. In contrast, Pressman et al. (1999) characterized maternal sensitivity by using a scale that measured the "emotional availability" of mothers during interaction. Others have focused on just one aspect of maternal sensitivity—"topic responsiveness," or the tendency to follow a child's lead and join in play or communication topics in which the child has expressed interest through eye gaze, action, and prelinguistic or linguistic communication (Spencer, Bodner-Johnson, & Gutfreund, 1992; Wilson & Spencer, 1997).

Whether the more general construct of sensitivity or the more specific one of topic responsiveness has been used, consistent differences have been found in studies when mothers and their children shared the same hearing status compared with those in which mothers and their children had a different hearing status (Jamieson, 1994a, 1994b; Lederberg & Prezbindowski, 2000; Meadow-Orlans, 1997; Meadow-Orlans & Spencer, 1996; Schlesinger & Meadow, 1972; Spencer et al., 1992; Spencer & Gutfreund, 1990; Waxman, Spencer, & Poisson, 1996). That is, greater maternal sensitivity and responsiveness have been reported, on average, in studies in which both mother and child are hearing or both are deaf than when one is deaf and the other hearing. Maternal sensitivity and, apparently as a result, the mother and child's ability to achieve mutually responsive, reciprocal interactions, are less likely when the mother is hearing and the child is deaf, or vice versa. The phenomenon of intuitive parenting, or unconscious adaptations by parents to produce interactive behaviors that meet their children's attention and other communication needs, seems to be stressed and even sometimes disrupted when mother and child do not share the same hearing status.

However, even in situations in which mother and infant hearing status differ, some apparently intuitive maternal adaptations have been noted. For example, deaf mothers have been found to vocalize more often during interactions with hearing toddlers and infants than with infants and toddlers who are deaf (Koester, Brooks, & Karkowski, 1998; Rea, Bonvillian, & Richards, 1988), and hearing mothers have been found to use more routine rhythmical games incorporating gestures with infants who are deaf or hard of hearing than with hearing infants (Koester, Papousek, & Smith-Gray, 2000). However, there seem to be limits to the accommodations that are made intuitively.

Some researchers and educators believe that intuitive parenting behaviors can be disrupted when parents or caregivers feel confused, worried, or have doubts about their ability to provide the "best" experiences for their children (Koester, 1992; Schlesinger, 1987). Mothers whose children's hearing status is different from their own may find themselves at a loss to know how to best communicate with their children and can question their own abilities to be effective parents. For example, a deaf mother may initially question how often and in what way to use voice with her hearing child (Waxman & Spencer, 1997). Hearing mothers, although recognizing their deaf children's need for visual communication, may not have the skills to communicate visually. Even after hearing parents begin to learn sign language, they usually do not use it as much as their own habitual spoken language (Spencer, 1993a, 1993b). Hearing parents also have to consciously think about translating their messages into sign language. Such concerns and ambiguities can cause naturally intuitive, unconscious processes to be brought into active consciousness and actually decrease parents' abilities to interact naturally and comfortably with their children. In addition, hearing parents may be generally fearful about their deaf or hard of hearing child's developmental potential and may tend to become more directive and "teacher-like" in an attempt to give their children extra opportunities to learn language (Wood, Wood, Griffiths, & Howarth, 1986). This kind of modification in parenting behaviors unfortunately works against the caregiver and child engaging in the kind of responsive, mutually reinforcing interaction that best supports development.

How can parents' tendencies to be sensitive and responsive to their children be reinforced? Early intervention and support from professionals seem to be helpful. For example, Meadow-Orlans and Steinberg (1993) found that mothers of deaf children who perceived high levels of support from professionals were as responsive and sensitive to their children as were mothers of hearing children. This is consistent with earlier reports by Greenberg and his colleagues that provision of counseling to hearing mothers increases their level of sensitive responding to children who are deaf (Greenberg, 1983; Greenberg, Calderon, & Kusche, 1984). In addition, Meadow-Orlans and Steinberg (1993) reported that receiving support soon after the diagnosis of hearing loss had the strongest association with the quality of mothers' interactive behaviors. These findings indicate that differences in access to intervention services, and perhaps in the timing and quality of those services, can affect the degree to which parents participate in interactions that optimally support the development of their children who are deaf and hard of hearing.

It is important to remember, however, that interaction is not unidirectional. Children's participation is influenced by their adult partners' behaviors, just as the adults' interactive behaviors are influenced by those of the children. Although there are more similarities than differences in the interactive behaviors of infants with and without hearing loss, even subtle differences may alter the flow of interactions, especially when those differences are perceived by parents as problematic.

Koester and colleagues have documented differences in behaviors of infants who are deaf and hard of hearing and hearing as early as 6–9 months of age when observed during interactions with their mothers (Koester, 1995; Koester, Papousek, & Smith-Gray, 2000). For example, deaf infants engaged in more repetitive, cycling-type movements with arms and legs than hearing infants. Patterns of eye gaze also differed; hearing infants tended to look back and forth between their mothers and their surroundings more often than infants with hearing loss, while infants with hearing loss tended to maintain gaze on their mothers. Finally, Koester (1995) reported that hearing infants made more easily identified attempts than deaf infants to restart interaction with their mothers when mothers were asked to be intentionally nonresponsive (in an experimental situation). The hearing infants were more likely than deaf infants to lean or reach toward their mothers and to smile at them, apparently trying to prompt a response.

Differences have also been reported among infants who are deaf and hearing at 12 months in the frequency of symbolic (pretend) play behaviors and of prelinguistic and linguistic communications judged to be intentional (e.g., pointing or reaching to direct attention to an object, vocalizing to attract parent's attention), with these behaviors being produced more often by hearing infants (Spencer, 1993a; Spencer & Meadow-Orlans, 1996). Eye gaze (visual attention) patterns during interactions with hearing parents at 12 and 18 months were also slightly different for deaf and hard of hearing infants with hearing parents compared with hearing infants. Hearing infants were somewhat more likely than deaf and hard of hearing infants to switch their visual attention back and forth between mother and an object, therefore including a social or conversational invitation to mother while also showing interest in the object (Spencer, 2000; Waxman & Spencer, 1997). However, the tendency on the part of the hearing children to display this developmentally more advanced eye gaze pattern was matched by deaf children whose parents were deaf. This similarity indicates once again that infant hearing status itself may not determine behavioral patterns during interactions. Instead, the pattern of differences shown across mothers and children is undoubtedly mutually influenced, and it is impossible in most situations to differentiate a cause from an effect.

It may be critical, however, to help hearing parents and caregivers apply positive interpretations to some of the behavioral differences they note in interactive behaviors of their infants and toddlers who are deaf or hard of hearing. Koester and Meadow-Orlans (1999) reported that this does not always happen. For example, although there were children in each group who were more active than others, hearing and deaf parents tended to interpret their deaf children's activity differently; hearing parents whose deaf or hard of hearing infants were highly active (waving their hands, kicking their feet, moving their bodies while in the infant seat) tended to rate them as more "difficult" than did deaf mothers whose children were similarly active. Koester (personal communication, March, 2001) reported that some hearing mothers were concerned that high activity levels indicated hyperactivity, in contrast to deaf mothers who perceived their children's similar repetitious limb movements as being early attempts to communicate. Clearly these different interpretations would influence parents' reactions to the children's behaviors, with negative interpretations perhaps leading to efforts to decrease the behaviors and positive interpretations leading to attempts to respond and shape those behaviors into more clearly communicative ones. Such differences in interpretation demonstrate the critical role of parental expectations, and perhaps their attitudes about hearing loss, in setting the tone and guiding behaviors during interactions.

Attachment

Just as engines are powered by gasoline or electricity, interactions are powered by emotions and relationships. When two people have a weak or insignificant relationship, their interactions will tend to be superficial, probably brief, and relatively unsatisfying. In contrast, people with strong, positive emotional relationships tend to spend much time in pleasurable interactions. Parents and infants typically begin to establish strong emotional bonds in their earliest interactions, as parents stimulate and care for the infant's needs, and as the infants' eye gaze, actions, and vocalizations reinforce the parents' behaviors (Rossetti, 1996). In a spiral fashion, experiences in which parents nurture and care for their infants during pleasurable interactions increase emotional bonding, which in turn tends to increase the frequency and positive tone of future interactions. Secure, positive attachment with caregivers during infancy promotes positive self-esteem as well as strong social, cognitive, and language skills at later ages (Lederberg & Mobley, 1990; Slade, 1987b; Thompson, 1998; Vondra & Barnett, 1999). The quality of infant–caregiver attachment is, therefore, a matter of concern to interventionists as well as to parents and other caregivers. Infants and toddlers who are securely attached to their caregivers turn to them for help and are comforted by their presence. Securely attached toddlers tend to exhibit more exploratory behavior and to be less generally fearful than those whose attachment is less secure. This security can increase their potential for acquiring knowledge about their social and physical environment.

The phenomenon of maternal sensitivity described in the previous section is expected to impact an infant's development of attachment, with more sensitive parenting leading to secure, positive attachment and less sensitive parenting leading to less secure patterns of attachment (Ainsworth, Blehar, Waters, & Wall, 1978). Thus, the frequency of disruptions in sensitive and reciprocal interactions among hearing mothers and deaf infants and toddlers might be expected to interfere with development of secure attachment by many infants who are deaf or hard of hearing. In addition, some professionals (Lang, 1996; Luterman, 1999) have suggested that the process of early attachment can be negatively influenced for children who are deaf with hearing parents because of the initial despair and even depression expressed by many of those parents in reaction to the diagnosis of their infant's hearing loss. Luterman (1999) has even suggested that very early identification of hearing loss can have especially negative effects on attachment. His argument is that, when the diagnosis occurs very early, the expected intuitive parenting behaviors and active caregiving that provide the basis for the emergence of secure attachment can be disrupted. This concern is based in part on studies of hearing mothers with hearing children who have experienced depression. In general, maternal depression puts young children at risk for attachment difficulties (Vondra & Barnett, 1999).

Additional concern about initial attachment between infants who are deaf or hard of hearing and their hearing caregivers has been based on the infants' lack of awareness of caregiver vocalizations, thus decreased lack of reaction to them (see Lederberg & Mobley, 1990, for a review). Lack of intuitively expected responses from an infant can disrupt parenting behaviors, result in a loss of reciprocity, and lessen mutual reinforcement. With interactions so altered, caregiver–infant interactions might be less mutually reinforcing than usual, putting emotional bonding at risk.

Fortunately, existing empirical research fails to support these fears. First, Meadow, Greenberg, and Erting (1983) found that patterns of attachment for deaf children with deaf parents matched those expected for hearing children with hearing parents. Therefore, a child's hearing loss itself does not seem to predispose the child toward difficulties with attachment. Second, studies of deaf children ages 18 months through preschool years with hearing parents have failed to find any significantly increased incidence of disordered attachment, even when the child's hearing loss was identified fairly early in the first year of life (Hadadian, 1995; Koester & MacTurk, 1991; Lederberg & Mobley, 1990).

Why do the available data fail to show the increased incidence of disruptions in attachment that were predicted by some theorists? The infants and parents in the studies mentioned above had specific advantages that may have served as protective factors. For example, the deaf parents in the Meadow et al. (1983) study tended to have positive attitudes about their children's abilities and felt competent communicating and interacting with young deaf children. These parents, therefore, may have been able to intuitively meet their children's interaction needs without any special intervention. Also, many of the children in the other studies, in addition to having hearing loss identified relatively early, had early intervention services provided soon after identification. This was especially true for the families in the sample studied by Koester and MacTurk (1991). Thus, any potential disadvantage implied by parents' learning about their infants' hearing loss very early may have been more than outweighed by the early provision of support services. Meadow-Orlans and Steinberg (1993) found that mothers who indicated that they had good support, especially from professionals involved in intervention, had both decreased stress and higher quality interactions with their infants than mothers who felt they had less support. Early intervention may have increased parents' tendencies to interact appropriately with their infants by providing more positive information about the children's potential for development and by preventing parents from feeling powerless to help their children (Schlesinger, 1987). Given Hadadian's (1995) finding that parents' attitudes about deafness correlate with the quality of parent–child attachment, such early assistance could be critical.

Additional factors may protect against negative effects of infant hearing loss on early attachment. Hearing and deaf parents intuitively communicate and interact with their infants using multiple sensory modalities. For example, the high-pitched, rhythmic spoken language that hearing parents often direct toward infants is almost always accompanied by rhythmic touch and by bright and positive facial expressions, regardless of infant hearing status. This typical "packaging" of interactive behaviors can allow an infant to be aware of parent interaction even without having access to sound, and a system of reciprocal parent–infant interactive behaviors may be supported. In addition, Rossetti (1996) indicated that early attachment is influenced more by sensitive, nurturing caring for infants' basic needs than by parents' language or effective use of oral communications. This suggests that the initial lack of sharing of a primary communication modality that is faced by hearing parents and deaf infants need not interfere with the development of secure, positive attachment during the early months.

These research findings indicate that parents, hearing or deaf, can be reassured that infant hearing loss in itself presents no significant barrier to forming close and positive primary attachments. However, children's feelings of security and attachment continue to develop and can change with age (Hamilton, 2000; Waters, Hamilton, & Weinfield, 2000; Waters, Merrick, Treboux, Crowell, & Albersheim, 2000). Parents should be aware that the degree to which they share a language system with their child who is deaf or hard of hearing can affect their ongoing relationship and the degree of secure attachment that is maintained during the preschool years and later (Greenberg & Marvin, 1979; Hadadian, 1995; Meadow et al., 1983).

Special Needs

At least one third of children who are deaf and hard of hearing have some additional health problem or disability (Moores, 2001). These children are at a higher risk than other children with hearing loss for difficulties in interactions and in establishing secure attachments with their caregivers. First, there may be increased prevalence of parental depression and grief when infants have multiple and even life-threatening illnesses or disabilities. Second, infants with multiple disabilities may exhibit behaviors that differ from those parents intuitively expect from children with hearing loss only. For example, premature infants and those with disabilities may display more subtle clues to their needs and interests than caregivers expect. This characteristic can make it difficult for a caregiver to "read" prelanguage communication and know when to respond (Barnard & Kelly, 1990; Gleason, 1999). Similarly, children who have visual impairments, especially when hearing sensitivity is also decreased, may be less likely to establish mutual gaze with their parents, less likely to vocalize, and may be relatively unresponsive to caregivers' attempts to interact (Fraiberg, 1977). In this situation, or one in which motor abilities are significantly compromised, it can be important to assist parents in identifying their child's unique behaviors that indicate awareness of parents' behaviors and that provide opportunities for parental responses. Infants with visual impairment, for example, may become completely still when perceiving a communication. (See Gleason, 1999, for an in-depth discussion of interactions with infants who are blind or visually impaired.) Infants with limited motor skills may indicate interest by eye movements or generalized physical activity.

Finally, infants with multiple disabilities and health problems can experience difficulty establishing secure attachment with caregivers because the circumstances of their early weeks and months interfere with active parenting. For example, children who are significantly premature or who spend much time in a hospital Neonatal Intensive Care Unit (NICU) before going home with their parents because of health problems (e.g., active cytomegalovirus, other viral or bacterial illness) can have decreased opportunities for early interactions and parental caregiving. When accommodations are not made to encourage early parent–infant interactions during the time in the hospital, bonding can be disrupted (Rossetti, 1996). In recognition of this possibility, parents' access to and contact with infants in NICUs is generally encouraged.

Unfortunately, there has been little research on interactions or on early attachment of infants with hearing loss plus other disabilities. Available information fails to provide a definitive picture of their prospects for positive interactions and secure attachment. One study illustrates the variability across families with infants who are deaf or hard of hearing and have cognitive or motor disabilities. Focusing on maternal stress, which is related to interactive behaviors, Meadow-Orlans, Smith-Gray, and Dyssegaard (1995) found that mothers reported levels ranging from extremely high (indicating a need for referral for clinical services) to extremely low (suggesting denial of actual stress level). In some cases, it appeared that the mothers thought of the child's hearing loss as a secondary issue, and, at least during the child's first 2 years, relief that the child had survived lessened their reactions to the child's hearing loss. Given these findings of individual differences across families, and the general lack of information available, interventionists should be ready to provide increased support (especially related to emotional needs and reactions) for families of infants with hearing loss plus other risk factors or disabilities. However, as in other cases, each family should be seen as unique, and needs should be assessed with sensitivity to individual, family, and cultural characteristics.

Enhancing the Visual Aspects of Interactions

The general characteristics of positive interactions among caregivers and young children tend to be similar whether the children are deaf, hard of hearing, or hearing. In addition, most infants and young children with hearing loss, like those who are hearing, benefit from auditory stimulation. Now that hearing loss can be identified at birth or soon after, amplification can be provided during the early months of life. Exposure to sound during these months is important for supporting later auditory skills development using traditional amplification or cochlear implants. Hearing parents can, therefore, feel comfortable continuing to talk to their infants who are deaf and hard of hearing. And the common repetitive and melodic speech patterns intuitively employed by hearing parents may be especially helpful because the "melody" may be perceived by infants with some residual hearing (or benefits from amplification) in the speech range.

Despite these similarities between the needs of young children with and without hearing loss, there is one important difference: Children with hearing loss depend more on visual and tactile cues for turn taking and for sharing information. This is the case whether the children are being exposed to signed language or are in an oral language environment in which speechreading is encouraged. Even children who are receiving auditory–verbal programming, in which visual information is intentionally de-emphasized, can benefit from the addition of visual information during informal communicative interactions with peers and with caregivers. The following excerpt is from a transcript of an interaction between a deaf mother and her 4-month-old deaf infant. In this interaction, the mother demonstrates a number of communicative strategies and behaviors that are especially sensitive to the needs of an infant with hearing loss.

Mother makes large signs—producing them a bit slowly—with a rhythmic, dance-like quality. She turns her head from side to side in an exaggerated way while signing "looking for." Baby Joseph watches his mother's face, then looks back toward his own feet. Mother taps Joseph gently on the right arm (to attract his attention). Getting no response, she rubs gently on his leg. Mother then leans her head lower so that he can see her while still looking at his own feet. When mother's face comes into view, Joseph smiles and looks up. Mother smiles brightly. Holding up one of the baby's feet, she points to the foot and signs, "Pretty foot. Pretty foot. You have a pretty foot." Joseph can see his foot, mother's face, and mother's signing at the same time. He smiles again and kicks his foot up and down while Mother continues to hold it gently and smile.

In the preceding interaction, the mother demonstrates several modifications in her communications that seem intuitively tailored to attract or respond to her child's visual attention focus. She enlarges and slows her signs, generally exaggerating them; she contacts the infant in an effort to obtain his visual attention; she even moves her head and hands so that the infant can see her while continuing to focus on his own feet. Researchers have documented a set of special modifications made by deaf mothers by analyzing the interactive behaviors of deaf mothers who are experienced visual communicators (Harris, Clibbens, Chasin, & Tibbitts, 1989; Kantor, 1982; Maestas y Moores, 1980; Masataka, 1992, 1996; Mohay, 2000; Mohay, Milton, Hindmarsh, & Ganley, 1998; Prendergast & McCollum, 1996; Spencer et al., 1992; Waxman & Spencer, 1997). They have identified an apparently universal set of modifications in interactive and communicative behaviors that promote smooth visually sensitive interactions with infants and young children with hearing loss. These visually sensitive strategies, although used less consistently by hearing parents without special training (Waxman & Spencer, 1997), can in most cases be built from the foundation of intuitive use of responsive and multimodal interactive behaviors (sometimes called "baby talk" or "motherese") typical for hearing as well as deaf parents. (See Table 8.1 in Chapter 8 for an overview of similarities in the communication modifications typically used by hearing and deaf mothers while interacting with their infants. Different modifications are emphasized as infants mature.)

The Early Months

Visual contact, or face-to-face eye gaze, is frequent during the earliest months of life, when infants will look for extended periods at their caregivers' faces. This is the time when hearing mothers tend to use rhythmic, fairly extended language with their infants. These language productions are often characterized by repetition of phrases and rhythmic changes in intonation that are sometimes described as being almost like singing. In fact, the characteristic of rhythm seems to readily attract infants' attention regardless of modality (Adamson, 1995). For example, the slowed, larger, almost "dance-like" rhythmic signing that is often produced by deaf mothers interacting with their infants attracts and tends to hold their attention (Erting, Prezioso, & Hynes, 1994; Masataka, 1996).

Again similar to the behaviors of hearing mothers, deaf mothers have been noted to use increased amounts of touch to communicate with their infants. The touches are often soft strokes of the body or limbs. In addition, deaf mothers have been noticed to occasionally move their children's hands to make simple sign-like motions, and the mothers also sometimes produce signs directly on their children's bodies. For example, one mother was observed to sign "pretty baby" by making the sign for "pretty" on the infant's own face, then leaning back a bit and signing "baby" while the infant looked at her. Increased touch during communicating may help to attract infants' attention to the communication, especially when their ability to receive auditory communication is limited.

Bright but strong facial expressions also seem to be used intuitively by mothers interacting with infants. Deaf mothers tend to use especially strong, positive facial expressions (Meadow-Orlans, MacTurk, Prezioso, Erting, & Day, 1987). This may result in their infants learning quickly that it is interesting to watch their mothers. And, deaf mothers' intuitive understanding of the importance of the affective (or emotional) tone of interactions leads to another special modification in their communications with infants: Certain signed expressions, such as "what" or "where" questions, that are accompanied by a facial expression of lowered brows when signed to older children or adults, are produced instead with positive, lifted brow facial expressions when signed to infants (Reilly & Bellugi, 1996). This modification, in which a grammatically correct adult facial expression is changed to look more positive emotionally, is an especially striking instance of the relative potency of the affective or emotional component of interactions with infants.

Another way that deaf mothers accommodate their infants' immature patterns of visual attention is to displace signs. That is, the mothers move their hands or bodies so as to make signs where their infants are already looking instead of trying to prompt the infants to look back at them. Some prompting does occur, and even during early months, deaf mothers use stroking or tapping on the child's body in an attempt to regain attention. However, these signals are neither persistent nor demanding and, instead, seem to serve as the introduction of signals that will be developed further as the infants mature.

The Challenge as Infants Mature

After 5 or 6 months of age, it becomes more difficult for parents' communicative behaviors to attract and maintain the attention of their infants. In place of the earlier fascination with people and faces, the maturing infant becomes attracted to objects and the activities occurring around him or her. This is, of course, a welcome indication of cognitive growth. But it also complicates the role of caregivers who are sensitive to visual communication needs. The challenge is in finding ways to accommodate those needs while remaining actively engaged with and sensitive to the infant. Also, during this general period, infants begin to indicate understanding of some language, and caregivers tend to modify their interactive behaviors again as they become more aware of their role as models for the child's developing language.

A typical parental reaction during this period of an infants' development is for parents to try to clarify the referents of the language they produce. That is, parents aim to assist the infant in matching a word or phrase with the person, object, or action to which it refers. This may be done by pointing to or holding up the referent or otherwise attracting attention to it. A second supportive parental tendency is that of "topic responsiveness" (Spencer & Gutfreund, 1990; Tannock, 1988). When parents are topic responsive, they talk about something in which the child has already shown or expressed interest. That is, they follow the child's lead in the interaction or communication topic. Joseph's mother, in the preceding vignette, demonstrated topic responsiveness by holding up and signing about the infant's "pretty foot" after the child had looked at his feet. Topic responsiveness is especially supportive of language development of hearing children (Tomasello & Farrar, 1986), and researchers have shown maternal topic responsiveness to be positively related to language development in deaf as well as hearing children (Spencer & Lederberg, 1997; Wilson & Spencer, 1997).

Parents of children with hearing loss, however, tend to face more challenges than parents of hearing children both in demonstrating the referent of language and in providing topic responsive language. For example, as infants become more independent, mobile, and less likely to gaze for long periods at their caregivers, it becomes difficult to make sure that they can view communication directed toward them (signs, gestures, or information from the speakers' face) while also attending to the referent. Hearing children can, of course, clearly hear a complete vocal message about a referent while looking away from the speaker. Although children eventually become adept at switching visual attention back and forth between a person and an object or other referent, that skill does not usually develop until after about 1 year of age for hearing infants (Bakeman & Adamson, 1984) or for deaf infants (Spencer, 2000). In the meantime, how do parents manage to make referents explicit and provide topic responsive language to infants who are deaf? During this stage, deaf parents continue to use the strategies of signing on or near an object to which the infant is attending, although incidences of signing directly on the child's body decrease. They also continue to use strongly positive facial expressions and to modify the speed and size of their signs.

Researchers in various locations have documented a number of other strategies that enrich interactions among deaf parents and older infants. These strategies include

- *Waiting for the infant to look up:* As simple as this strategy may seem, it requires considerable patience from a parent. However, it is an outstanding characteristic of interactions among deaf parents and their infants. While "waiting," a deaf mother tends to be completely focused on her child, watching his or her moves and behaviors and eye gaze. As soon as the child looks up from play or some other activity, the mother immediately signs about that activity or the object(s) involved. Having to wait for attention before expressing communication leads to interactions that seem to have a slower pace than those typical of hearing mothers and hearing infants, but the slower pace seems ideally matched for visual communication exchanges with a young child. Perhaps because the pace is different from their expectations, or perhaps because they are intent on "teaching" their children who are deaf and hard of hearing, hearing mothers have not been found to use the strategy of waiting very often, unless specific intervention has been provided (Spencer, Bodner-Johnson, & Gutfreund, 1992; Waxman & Spencer, 1997).

- *Pointing to or tapping on objects being named or discussed:* Deaf mothers often tap directly on an object before and then after naming it, making the referent explicit. This pattern of tap-name-tap (or name-tap-name) has been called "bracketing" (Mohay, 2000). As with the waiting strategy, hearing mothers also tap on or point to objects they are naming; however, they rarely tap as many times as deaf mothers. Hearing mothers also frequently omit the bracketing taps after the object name is given (Waxman & Spencer, 1997).

- *Producing short utterances with much repetition of single signs or words:* In conjunction with tapping on objects to identify the referent, deaf mothers frequently repeat the sign, labeling the object multiple times. The repetition extends the time available for the child to see the sign, even if it is seen only accidentally as attention drifts past mother and back to the object. The language hearing parents use to address hearing infants and toddlers is also characterized by much repetition. However, hearing parents tend to repeat phrases instead of the single-word/sign repetition pattern shown by deaf mothers (Ehrhardt, 1998).

- *Moving an object up to face:* Moving an object through an infant's field of vision almost always attracts the infant's attention to the object. When caregivers move objects near their faces, it usually attracts an infant's attention to the caregiver's face. Deaf mothers commonly move objects in this trajectory and then use multiple taps on the object plus repeated signs to label the object. This not only connects the label with the object, but it includes the mother and her expressions in the message. Hearing mothers of infants who are deaf and hard of hearing have also been found to move objects frequently during interactions and to successfully direct the infants' attention to the object. Without specific instruction, however, hearing mothers often move an object away from their face, holding it out while speaking its name or talking about it (Waxman & Spencer, 1997). This pattern can interfere with the child's ability to see his or her mother and the object at the same time.

- *Tapping on the child to signal "look at me":* From the earliest months, deaf mothers use touch (stroking, gently rubbing) to obtain or keep their infants' attention. One signal, that of tapping on the child's shoulder or arm to signal "look at me," becomes more standardized with time. Infants do not understand the meaning of this signal initially, however, and deaf mothers seem to actively (even if not consciously) teach the meaning of the signal (Kyle, Woll, & Ackerman, 1989; Swisher, 1992, 2000). Despite initial inconsistent responses, deaf children learn how to respond to this signal eventually, and it becomes incorporated into the system of signed communication that develops.

Because this signal's meaning must be learned, deaf mothers tend to combine it at first with other stimuli that provoke visual attention. For example, a mother may tap on her child's shoulder but not successfully prompt the child to look up at her. The mother may follow this immediately (perhaps even while continuing to tap) by moving an object through the child's visual field and up to her face. Thus, by pairing the tapping signal with other reliable attention-getting strategies, the mother helps her child learn the meaning of the tapping signal.

Hearing mothers, even when they have children who are deaf or hard of hearing, do not often spontaneously use the tapping-for-attention strategy. Waxman and Spencer (1997) proposed several reasons for this. First, it is rarely used in communication among hearing people and therefore is unlikely to be part of a hearing person's typical communication repertoire. Second, tapping to get attention may seem intrusive to hearing people, who are used to calling a person's name to attract attention. Third, hearing parents may be discouraged by the fact that infants do not initially respond reliably to the signal. However, use of this signal is associated with smooth communicative turn taking between mothers and deaf children in the second year of life (Spencer, 2000; Waxman & Spencer, 1997), so it can be a beneficial addition to the communicative strategy repertoire of hearing parents with infants who are deaf or hard of hearing.

Deaf parents' use of communicative strategies described results in interactions that tend to include fewer signed utterances and fewer different sign meanings than is typical of the vocal utterances of hearing parents with hearing children in this developmental stage (Harris et al. 1989; Mohay, 2000; Spencer & Lederberg, 1997). Deaf parents' relatively lower frequency of utterances is a natural outcome of their use of the strategy of waiting for visual attention as well as the strategies of repetition of signs, tapping on objects, and other strategies that clearly establish the association among signs and objects. These characteristics of deaf parents' language do not slow their children's initial development of language. If anything, they tend to accelerate it, and there are a number of reports of deaf children with deaf parents signing before ages typical for hearing children's first words (Meier & Newport, 1990). Spencer and Lederberg (1997) noted, however, that the turn taking pace in a signed interaction with a deaf child (of hearing parents) whose visual turn taking skills are still developing is slower than that with a hearing child at a similar language level.

Hearing parents of hearing children (like deaf parents) tend to simplify language directed to infants and toddlers. This simplification results in somewhat shortened productions that tend to be "well formed." That is, they provide a model of spoken English that tends to follow basic grammatical rules and subject–verb–object word order. Parents continue to talk mostly about the "here and now" and often follow their children's indications of interest in the topics of their language productions. Thus, both deaf and hearing parents tend to model language that is more readily perceived and more easily understood when their children begin to demonstrate that they understand and are beginning to produce single sign or single-word utterances.

The Next 2 Years

Infants typically demonstrate a number of developmental changes as they pass their first birthday that impact the interactions in which they participate. Expressive language in the form of one-word or single-sign utterances emerges, symbolically meaningful play behaviors emerge, and (by about 15 months of age) a pattern of visual attention that incorporates attention to people as well as objects in the same episode is in place (Bakeman & Adamson, 1984; Spencer, 2000). These emerging abilities influence both the content of interactions and the rate and ease of turn taking.

In addition, interactions increasingly become venues for the acquisition of language and cognitive skills. When early experiences have been positive and secure attachment is achieved, children are able to perform during interactions with a significant adult at a level somewhat higher than when playing alone. Parents or other caregivers who are familiar with the child provide a secure, encouraging atmosphere that promotes this advanced performance and prompts further growth in play, language, and attention skills by building on or expanding those produced by their children (Jamieson, 1994a, 1994b; Vygotsky, 1978).

Parents' language during interactions with toddlers gradually becomes more complex as the children demonstrate a readiness to increase their own language skills. Thus, hearing parents increase the number of different words they use during interactions, and they tend to expand on their hearing children's utterances (i.e., Child: "baw"; Parent: "Yes, that's a big red ball"). In this way, parents respond to their child's choice of communication topic while giving a model of more advanced grammar and a wider variety of word meanings. Similarly, deaf parents gradually increase the length and complexity of the signed utterances they direct toward their toddlers. These increases seem to be related as much to the children's advances in visual attention skills (i.e., spontaneously switching gaze back and forth between the communication partner and the object or event that is the topic of the communication) as to their language growth. But special linguistic modifications continue to be used by deaf parents. The most notable is that, until the children reach about $2^{1}/_{2}$ years of age and are producing multisign utterances routinely, deaf parents tend to use a simple subject–verb–object sign order and tend to produce signs in their simplest form. For example, deaf parents signing to infants and young children very rarely combine movements showing direction or the manner with a sign for a verb, as in adult ASL (Kantor, 1982). A simplified and easier-to-process form of the language is modeled until the children show awareness and emerging abilities to process the more complex forms.

By the age of 3 years, hearing children and deaf children with typical rates of development have quite sophisticated abilities. They generally demonstrate many of the grammatical niceties of their respective languages (e.g., spoken English, ASL). They also give evidence of advanced cognitive abilities in their play, demonstrating integrated sequences of pretend (or symbolic) play in which they mimic and elaborate on the experiences of their daily life (Lederberg, Love, & Yebra, 1997; Spencer, 1996a). Three-year-olds also have well-developed attention skills and can participate in interactions in which turn taking is smooth and exchanges are reciprocal. (Of course, children at this age may choose not to interact in this way, but they have the ability to do so.) Their abilities to play with other children and to participate in interactions with multiple partners are developing.

It should be noted, however, that a significant proportion of children who are deaf or severely hard of hearing and have no additional disabilities progress more slowly through the stages discussed above. For example, deaf toddlers with hearing parents often have less advanced visual attention skills during the second year of life than those with deaf parents who routinely employ the visual attention scaffolding strategies outlined previously (Spencer, 2000). Children with hearing loss who have fairly late access to intervention services and limited access to language models that they can perceive will often show delays in the language area and some higher level play skills (Schirmer, 1989; Spencer, 1996a). These delays can be further exacerbated if other aspects of interactions, such as parents' sensitivity and ability to respond to the child's interests, have been problematic (Spencer & Meadow-Orlans, 1996). Fortunately, early intervention seems to promote improved and faster development across developmental domains, regardless of the language mode or type of programming that has been chosen by the families (Yoshinaga-Itano & Apuzzo, 1998; Yoshinaga-Itano, Sedey, Coulter, & Mehl, 1998).

Children with Special Needs

Children who have sensory, motor, cognitive, or other disabilities in addition to hearing loss will often show slowed development of the communicative and cognitive skills addressed above. Some with physical disabilities will continue to require special positioning or supports to facilitate arm and hand movement or control of gaze. Children with visual impairment may be somewhat slowed in initial language development and may benefit from modifications in the characteristics of toys or other objects around which interactions are based (e.g., toys that have interesting tactile characteristics or that produce sounds when moved will be especially salient for these children). Caregivers should be especially aware of the importance of tactile stimulation and keeping physical contact during interactions with children with vision loss as well as hearing loss (Gleason, 1999). Children who have generally slowed development may pass through the stages outlined previously at later than typical ages. It is important, therefore, for parents and other caregivers to remain alert and responsive to their own child's emerging skills and base their interactive behaviors around them, rather than age norms provided by others.

Summary

The information in this chapter leads to four conclusions about interactions among caregivers and children who are deaf and hard of hearing from infancy through the toddler years:

1. The ability of caregivers and their children to establish reciprocal, mutually contingent communicative interactions is critical for development. These interactions are more at risk when the children are deaf or hard of hearing and their caregivers are hearing than when hearing status is the same for both children and caregivers.

2. Despite the prevalence of difficulties in establishing reciprocal, mutually contingent interactions, the formation of positive, secure attachment between infant and parent is not necessarily compromised when parent and child have a different hearing status.

3. Accomplishing mutually reinforcing and supportive interactions with a child with hearing loss is usually dependent on effective use of visual communication behaviors, such as gestures, facial expressions, body postures, and use of objects, as well as signed language if caregivers choose to use such a system.

4. The range of interactive styles and strengths varies at least as much for infants with hearing loss as for those who are hearing; therefore, intervention efforts must focus on assessment and response to the abilities and needs of each individual child.

RECOMMENDATIONS AND RESOURCES

The following sections of this chapter consider intervention efforts related to characteristics of early interactions. Both caregiver sensitivity (or responsiveness) and caregiver–child attachment are equally important for children with and without hearing loss. Therefore, with some modifications, procedures used by interventionists who work with hearing children are relevant to those working with children who are deaf and hard of hearing. However, in the area of visual communication strategies, specialized information and techniques are necessary. How is an interventionist to proceed?

Assessing for Intervention

Intervention efforts should begin by establishing a positive relationship between interventionist and family. It is then appropriate to initiate assessment of needs with the participation of family members. A common goal of assessment is to support the need for special services; use of formal or standardized instruments is sometimes required to achieve this goal. A second, equally important goal for assessment is to provide an evaluation of the specific kinds of intervention efforts to be given priority for an individual child and family. A variety of formal and informal instruments and approaches are available to assess characteristics of caregiver–child interaction. A few of these are discussed below, and some suggestions are provided about intervention approaches.

Formal Assessment Instruments Interventionists can use a number of scales to organize and systematize assessments of the sensitivity, responsiveness, and reciprocity of interactions among caregivers and children. These scales can also identify areas that require intervention. For example, Barnard and colleagues (Barnard, 1979; Barnard & Kelly, 1990) reported on the Nursing Child Assessment Satellite Training (NCAST) Teaching and Feeding Scales, in which child and caregiver behaviors are observed and rated in two different situations: a novel situation, in which the caregiver is to teach a new behavior to the child, and a routine feeding situation. The scales allow an observer to record information about caregivers' sensitivity to children's communicative cues, responsiveness to indications of distress, and techniques for promoting social-emotional and cognitive growth. Children's responsiveness to caregiver behaviors and the clarity of their communication attempts are also rated. Interventionists must be trained by a certified instructor before using the NCAST scales.

A similar approach to assessment of caregiver–child interaction is provided by Linder (1993) (see Chapter 5). This in-depth approach involves observing the child and his or her caregiver in a variety of contexts. Both child and caregiver behaviors, as well as the interaction between the child and caregiver, are rated. The assessment identifies behaviors and developmental skills that should be addressed in intervention. Again, use of this approach for assessment and intervention requires considerable training.

There are other assessment scales that focus only on caregiver interactive behaviors. For example, Klein and Briggs (1987a, 1987b) developed a scale that focuses on aspects of caregivers' provision of tactile stimulation, affective displays, response to child distress, conversational or turn taking patterns, and contingency of caregiver behaviors on those of the infant. Mahoney and colleagues (Mahoney, 1992; Mahoney, Powell, & Finger, 1986) developed the Maternal Behavior Rating Scale to rate behaviors demonstrated during a 10-minute interaction. This scale includes items that have been found across research studies to relate to children's development. This scale was developed specifically to assess caregiver interactive behaviors when the child has a disability. It may, therefore, be especially useful for children who have disabilities in addition to having a hearing loss.

Formally developed checklists and scales are helpful for organizing observations and for providing a way to make observations of interactive behaviors more objective. However, two dangers must be avoided. First, it is important to avoid a situation in which it appears that the interventionist is the "expert" who "judges" the caregiver. It is important to recognize that even when caregivers do not feel confident about their abilities to interact with a child, they are in fact the real experts on the child because of their relationship and extended experiences with that child. An important role for the interventionist is to identify and reinforce the beneficial things that are happening during an interaction. A second danger lies in using assessment instruments without actually using resulting information as a basis for interventions. Except in some situations in which specific assessments must be provided to justify intervention services, the outcome of assessment should always be to guide the kind of intervention implemented.

One respected instrument that accomplishes the dual goals of including the parent in the assessment process and providing a guide for intervention is the SKI-HI curriculum (SKI-HI Institute, 1993). This curriculum was developed especially for children with a hearing loss and their families. It provides interventionists with information about working with families in a collaborative manner and provides emotional support to encourage caregivers to respond in a confident and intuitive manner to their children. Assessment and intervention activities are provided that focus on interaction as well as on the child's development of auditory, language, and cognitive skills. Associated materials are available for children with dual sensory loss (Alsop, 1993).

Informal Assessments   Informal assessments of caregiver–child interaction, if they are based on discussions with caregivers to identify their concerns and needs, can fulfill both the goal of equal participation of interventionist and caregiver and the goal of providing a guide for immediate intervention activities. Of course, this requires that the interventionist be well trained in child development and highly knowledgeable about hearing loss, including ways a hearing loss does and does not affect interaction. In addition, the interventionist must be sensitive to differences in parents' interactive styles due to differences in personality and/or in cultural experiences. Most important, the interventionist must be prepared to listen to the caregiver's ideas but have a store of intervention activities available to suggest.

After parents and interventionists have identified a particular goal for an assessment, contexts can be identified in which interaction can be recorded for later observation. For young infants, face-to-face interaction with an infant in arms or sitting in an infant chair can be used. For older infants, toddlers, and preschool children, the best context is more likely to be one involving toys or daily routine activities. It is important that the context be one that occurs naturally for specific caregivers and children and that both caregiver and child are relaxed when the interaction is recorded.

Suppose, for example, that a caregiver wants to more easily identify child behaviors that have potential communicative meaning. The assessment process can begin with the caregiver–interventionist team reviewing a recorded interaction between the child and caregiver. A record sheet, such as the one found in Figure 11.1, can be used to document the child's behaviors during the recorded interaction. For each child behavior noted, caregiver behaviors or other environmental events that precede and follow such behaviors should also be recorded.

It is important that adults be willing to assume communicative potential in even subtle changes in the child's behavior. That is, the adults need to be alert to any potential signal from the child, such as a change in activity level or a change in direction of gaze, that can indicate an interest or need. For example, directing gaze at an object or activity can indicate interest in that object or activity. Looking at the caregiver can be assumed to indicate interest in play, a request for simple communication such as a smile, or some other need. Averting gaze from the caregiver when interaction is in progress can indicate a need for a moment of self-calming and respite from stimulation that might be acceptable to one infant but too strong for another. Of course, no assumption should be made that behaviors such as these, especially from young infants, are intentional expressions of communicative messages. Instead, the interventionist and caregiver are playing a game of "mind reading." The primary goal is to sensitize both caregiver and interventionist to the behaviors of a particular infant or child that provide opportunities for building communication and interaction. The interventionist can assist by "reframing" the caregiver's impression of the child's behaviors when necessary—that is, by applying meaning to behaviors that are not initially seen to be meaningful by the caregiver. Reframing also occurs when alternative, more positive interpretations of behaviors are suggested. (An example would be interpreting child hand and arm movements as

Goal of assessment: to assess child's visual attention to parent and reactions to type of parent's responses.

Date/child age: 6/8/01; 10.5 months

Persons present: mom, visiting teacher, child

Activity/setting: Child is in high chair in kitchen. Two wooden spoons are on tray of high chair; plastic stacking cups are on table within reach of mom. Mom is sitting in kitchen chair directly across from child. Child has just finished snack and is in good, attentive mood. (Teacher is videotaping activity.)

What happened before?	Child Action	"Guess" at child's meaning, interest, need	Adult reaction/ response	What does child do next?
Mom put spoons on chair tray	Looks at toys; looks up at mom briefly	"Can I play with these?"	Mom nods, smiles, says "Yeah, we can play."	Looks down at spoon while mom still talking; picks up spoon and looks at it
(See last column above)	Hits spoon on tray several times; looks only at spoon	Interest in spoon, maybe sound or vibration	Watches child at first. Says, "hey!" and taps on child's leg	Looks only at spoon, keeps hitting it on tray
(See last column above)	Same as above	Same as above	Picks up other spoon and hits it on tray, imitating child	Looks at mom's spoon, looks up at mom and smiles
(See last column above)	Looks at mom's spoon, reaches, looks at mom and smiles	Notices/interest in mom's action	Smiles and signs "spoon"; gives her spoon to child	Sees signs; holds both spoons, looks back at spoons and hits both on tray, looks back at mom and smiles

Figure 11.1. Informal record for assessing parent–child interaction.

evidence of children's interest in communicating instead of being an indication of overactivity.) Of course, it is important to acknowledge the caregiver's role in reframing some behaviors for the interventionist. Through such mutual encouragement and discussion, both caregiver and interventionist may see meaning in increasing numbers of child behaviors, thus providing more targets for responding to the child.

An identification activity such as this should merge naturally into one in which potential caregiver responses to child behaviors, as well as "topic responsiveness," are discussed. The interventionist and caregiver, using a format much like "brainstorming," can address different kinds of responses an adult could provide to specific child behaviors. In addition, providing responses in multiple modalities (i.e., vocal, gestural or signed, tactile) can be demonstrated and discussed. In follow-up sessions, specific kinds of responses can be tried by the caregiver and interventionist, and the child's reactions can be noted. Over time, caregiver topic responsiveness, the caregiver's tendency to send messages in modalities functional for the child, and mutually responsive interactions between caregiver and child can be expected to increase. In the rare situation in which contingency or mutual responsiveness does not increase with sensitive intervention, other difficulties, such as additional child disabilities or even a problem related to child–caregiver attachment, should be considered.

Assessing Attachment

Although attachment is a critical area for interventionists to consider, assessing attachment during infancy and toddler years requires specialized training and procedures. A situation called the "strange situation" is often employed (Ainsworth, 1973; Ainsworth et al., 1978). In this situation, caregiver and child participate in a series of separation and reunion activities, and a previously unknown person also interacts with the child. Although the procedure for obtaining data is relatively simple, the assessment and interpretation of the child's responses to these situations is complex and requires special certification. Hadadian (1995) used a "Q-sort" method for assessing attachment of young deaf children. In this method, parents identify behaviors most typical of their child in real-life situations, and these responses provide attachment information. Again, administration and interpretation should not be attempted without special training. The Rossetti Infant-Toddler Language Scale (Rossetti, 1990) also includes questions for parent response that can identify children for whom attachment seems to be at risk and who can benefit from referral for further assessment.

In addition to these more prescribed methods, interventionists should be alert for evidence of a lack of mutual responsiveness between child and caregiver or for evidence that the child is not comforted by the caregiver's presence. The possibility of attachment difficulties should be considered if a child consistently fails to seek contact with a caregiver in times of stress or fear, consistently pushes the caregiver away, or seems to relate no differently to the caregiver compared with other people. Of course, differences in children's temperament, as well as specific experiences, can influence children's behaviors in fearful or stressful situations regardless of their attachment status. However, interventionists who have concerns about a specific child–caregiver relationship should make a referral for further investigation of attachment difficulties to a social worker, counselor, psychologist, or other professional who specializes in this area.

There are some other steps to take in an intervention when attachment difficulties are suspected. For example, Rossetti (1996) stressed that involving parents in the care, record keeping, and decision making about their infants is critical for supporting attachment and parental feelings of competency. These suggestions are consistent with Schlesinger's (1987) hypothesis that promoting feelings of efficacy and a sense of control in parents of children who are deaf and hard of hearing can result in their being more responsive and less controlling during interactions with their children. In addition, parents can benefit from receiving information about their infants' abilities and strengths—especially with a focus on explaining the behaviors they see their infants produce. Therefore, efforts to increase parental sensitivity and responsiveness to their child's behaviors can provide support to the development of attachment.

Emphasizing Visual Information

Even when caregivers are alert to the interactive potential of a deaf or hard of hearing child's behaviors and respond contingently to them, the responses may not be salient or accessible to the child. Thus, in order to provide topic-responsive information to a child who is deaf or hard of hearing, parents must also employ visually sensitive communication strategies.

Information is available, primarily based on studies of the interactive behaviors of mothers who are deaf (Harris et al., 1989; Mohay, 2000; Waxman & Spencer, 1997), on ways to increase the visual salience of communications with infants and young children and thus make those communications more accessible. Guidance on visual communication techniques can also be obtained in publications from a number of centers including, but not limited to, the SKI-HI curriculum and video, as well as print publications available from the Boys Town National Research Hospital's Center for Hearing Loss in Children. In addition, Spencer (2001) provided an outline and examples of visual communication strategies in an on-line format that is accessible to interventionists and many caregivers. (See the Resources section at the end of this book for additional references.)

Perhaps the most comprehensive approach to providing information about visual communication strategies for communicating with young deaf children can be found in a curriculum developed by Mohay and her colleagues (Mohay, 2000; Mohay et al., 1998; Mohay, Milton, Hindmarsh, & Ganley, n.d.). Modules in this curriculum include written material explaining each strategy or topic, video clips illustrating the target behavior, and suggested activities for practice. The modules begin by directing attention to nonverbal aspects of parent and child interaction, including activities and information about using strong, positive facial expressions, gestures, and "body language" in interactions with young children with hearing loss. Other modules in the curriculum provide direct guidance on the use of strategies for obtaining and maintaining children's visual attention, including strategies discussed previously, such as moving hands to sign in the child's visual field, tapping on the child to redirect attention, and "bracketing" by interspersing labels for objects and events with points to indicate the referent. Strategies of waiting for visual attention, displacing, and repeating signs are also addressed in detail. Finally, this curriculum addresses the transition to literacy skills by demonstrating effective strategies for reading or telling stories to children who depend primarily on visual communication. (See Chapter 2 for related information.)

The following are examples of activities developed by Spencer (1996b) to help caregivers become more sensitive to the demands of visual communication and promote visual aspects of interaction. The activities described are designed for older infants or toddlers; however, they could be modified to suit the interests and motor skills of older children.

Caregiver and interventionist should have already discussed and looked at videotapes of other caregiver–child interactions and noted visual attention strategies. Then activities like the following can be used to practice and/or reinforce attention-related strategies as well as to give caregivers practice in topic responsiveness during interactions.

- *The waiting game:* A caregiver sits across from the child who is in a high chair and has been given an object with which to play. The caregiver's task is to wait until the child looks up, then to quickly smile and say or sign "hello" or something about the object. (Although labeling the object provides a better language-learning experience for the child, the caregiver can focus more on responding to the child's glances if asked to produce the same word or sign, like "hello," each time.) Alternatively, toddlers or preschoolers may be seated on the floor and engaged in playing "tea party" or caring for a baby doll, for example. With these slightly older children, it is more appropriate for the caregiver to label or say something about the child's action or the object manipulated when the child looks up. Therefore, the caregiver (if using signs) should learn signs for the objects and probable actions

---

Further information about the curriculum for promoting visual communication with deaf children that is mentioned in this chapter can be obtained from Heather Mohay, Ph.D., Associate Professor, Centre for Applied Studies in Early Childhood, Queensland University of Technology, Victoria Park Road, Kelvin Grove (Brisbane), Queensland 4059, Australia.

before engaging in this activity. The interventionist should record in some form the child's reaction to the caregiver's behaviors. The caregiver should be praised for waiting for the child to look up, and indications of child attention should be discussed in a "debriefing" session between caregiver and interventionist.

- *Including objects:* Caregiver and child can be seated on the floor or at a child-sized table, playing freely with a small set of toys. The adult can practice making signs near the toys on which the child is focused and moving related toys through the child's visual field to direct attention near the adult's face. When attention is obtained, the adult should gesture, speak, and/or sign briefly about the toy. This activity can also be done as a "role play" in which caregiver and interventionist participate. For the role play, each adult can take a turn being the "baby." "Baby" should create challenges for the adult by looking at toys instead of the adult. "Baby" should provide a variety of responses to the adult and make sure to look up occasionally to give the adult an opportunity to sign or say a quick word or short phrase. Of course, this activity should proceed like a game, in a light-hearted way.

- *Combining tapping with other signals:* (This activity is a modification of one found in Mohay et al., n.d.) After watching a videotape and demonstrations by the interventionist, the caregiver engages in play with the child. The child is given an interesting toy that has several constituent parts, such as a toy airport or dollhouse set. One or two parts of the array of toys in the set is given to the child, with the other related toys hidden where the caregiver can easily reach them but the child does not see them. When the child is focused on available toys, the caregiver gently taps on the child's leg, arm, or shoulder and then waits for the child to look up. This first signal may consist of two or three taps in rhythmic sequence, but the tap sequence should be repeated only once if the child fails to look up. In the case of nonresponse, the caregiver should move a new related toy from its hiding place into the child's visual field while tapping again with the free hand. The object should be moved toward the adult's face. When the child looks up, the caregiver should make a strongly positive facial expression, sign or speak a brief label for the object, then give the toy to the child. After the child incorporates this new object into play, the sequence should be repeated with another of the hidden toys.

The previous examples are just a few ideas of the kinds of activities that can be generated informally to meet the needs of individual families who want to increase the visual salience of interactions with infants, toddlers, or young children who are deaf or hard of hearing. Caregivers and interventionists working together to meet the strengths and needs of individual children and families can develop additional activities.

Summary

Early interactions between caregivers and children provide important bases for children's social-emotional, linguistic, and cognitive development. Parents bring a set of intuitive skills for altering habitual communications to interactions in order to attract the attention and meet the needs of infants. Use of these intuitive skills may be complicated with a child who has a hearing loss because the child's responses may not always match those that a parent unconsciously expects. Hearing parents may lack confidence in their ability to interact successfully with a child who is deaf or hard of hearing, and this lack of confidence itself can interfere with optimal interactions. This can be further complicated when a child has conditions such as prematurity, health problems, or developmental disabilities in addition to hearing loss.

Spencer (1998) found that deaf children's play, language, and visual attention skills at 18 months were related to both the responsiveness and the visual salience of their mothers' interactive behaviors. Therefore, both aspects of communication are worthy of attention during intervention efforts. It is important, however, to acknowledge that such behaviors already exist in the communication repertoires of most hearing parents. Thus, the role of the interventionist is to identify existing interaction strengths in the caregiver and child, then help to enhance and increase those behaviors through providing models, information, and sensitive support.

CHALLENGES AND PREDICTIONS

Information about the pattern and importance of early interactions with infants and young children who are deaf and hard of hearing began to emerge in the 1970s (Schlesinger & Meadow, 1972) and has become increasingly available due to increasing research. Until the late 1990s, much of this research took place in a context in which identification of hearing loss was delayed until at least the second year of a child's life. As age of identification has continued to decrease, interventionists have had access to more information about the experiences of children who are deaf and hard of hearing during the first 2 years of life (Meadow-Orlans, 1997; Meadow-Orlans, MacTurk, Spencer, & Koester, 1991; Yoshinaga-Itano & Apuzzo, 1998; Yoshinaga-Itano et al., 1998).

The advent of universal newborn hearing screening protocols in the United States and other advantaged countries will provide even earlier opportunities for intervention and support of families and young children with hearing loss. These opportunities will be accompanied by the availability of increasingly sophisticated technology (such as digitally programmed hearing aids and cochlear implants) to enhance the children's access to sound, including spoken language, during the early years (Niparko et al., 2000; Spencer, 2002). At the same time, the value of early access to naturally developed sign language (such as ASL and Auslan) is being increasingly recognized (Chamberlain, Morford, & Mayberry, 2000). A major challenge for interventionists will be to incorporate continually new information into their procedures for supporting early interactions, and supporting interaction strategies that promote optimal development of individual children in interactive contexts.

In spite of the advances in information, many issues still need more intensive research. For example, what is the role of visual and tactile communication strategies (as described in this chapter) with children who have hearing loss but some access to auditory information? These might be children who are audiologically hard of hearing or who, although audiologically deaf, benefit from amplification or cochlear implants. It is important to determine to what degree interactive and communicative information from multiple modalities, perhaps simultaneously, promotes or complicates their development.

Research is also needed to determine the degree to which available information about patterns of early interaction can be applied across various cultures. Most available information about early interactions with infants and young children who are deaf and hard of hearing has been obtained in developed countries and from advantaged groups within those countries. Some more diverse information is becoming available, such as Chiswanda's (1999) documentation of positive effects of intervention with hearing mothers and deaf infants and young children in Zimbabwe. Much more information of this kind is needed. It will be increasingly important to ensure that gains made in the world's more affluent countries are extended in culturally sensitive ways to inform intervention approaches across cultural groups, both within and among countries.

Additional information is also critically needed regarding early interactions of caregivers with infants and young children who have multiple disabilities that include a hearing loss. The multiple and often unique needs of such children require interdisciplinary knowledge and interactions among intervention specialists. Given the increasing proportion of children with hearing loss who have multiple disabilities, interventionists working with children who are deaf and hard of hearing will need to be increasingly knowledgeable about effects of a variety of disabilities in cognitive, motor, and social-emotional areas as well as interactions among hearing loss and other disabilities.

Much information now exists to assist families in their efforts to support the development of their young deaf and hard of hearing children through natural and positive interactions. As diagnosis of hearing loss occurs at ever earlier ages, and the natural strengths that families bring to parenting are increasingly recognized, opportunities for effectively promoting children's growth in cognitive, social, and language domains will continue to increase.

REFERENCES

Adamson, L. (1995). *Communication development in infancy.* Madison, WI: Brown and Benchmark.

Ainsworth, M. (1973). The development of infant-mother attachment. In B. Caldwell & H. Ricciuti (Eds.), *Review of child development research* (Vol. 1, pp. 1–95). Chicago: University of Chicago Press.

Ainsworth, M., Blehar, M., Waters, E., & Wall, S. (1978). *Patterns of attachment: A psychological study of the strange situation.* Mahwah, NJ: Lawrence Erlbaum Associates.

Alsop, L. (Ed.). (1993). *A resource manual for understanding and interacting with infants, toddlers, and pre-school age children with deaf-blindness.* Logan, UT: SKI-HI Institute.

Bakeman, R., & Adamson, L. (1984). Coordinating attention to people and objects in mother-infant and peer-infant interaction. *Child Development, 55,* 1278–1289.

Barnard, K. (1979). *Instructor's learning resource manual.* Seattle: NCAST Publications, University of Washington.

Barnard, K., & Kelly, J. (1990). Assessment of parent-child interaction. In S. Meisels & J. Shonkoff (Eds.), *Handbook of early childhood intervention* (pp. 278–297). Cambridge, England: Cambridge University Press.

Baumwell, L., Tamis-LeMonda, C., & Bornstein, M. (1997). Maternal verbal sensitivity and child language comprehension. *Infant Behavior and Development, 20,* 247–258.

Chamberlain, C., Morford, J., & Mayberry, R. (Eds.). (2000). *Language acquisition by eye.* Mahwah, NJ: Lawrence Erlbaum Associates.

Chiswanda, M. (1999). Hearing mothers and their deaf children in Zimbabwe: Mediated learning experiences. *Infant-Toddler Intervention, 9*(4), 391–406.

Dunham, P., & Dunham, F. (1992). Lexical development during middle infancy: A mutually driven infant-caregiver process. *Developmental Psychology, 28,* 414–420.

Ehrhardt, G. (1998, November). *Use of repetition in the "motherese" of hearing mothers.* Poster session presented at the conference of the American Speech-Language-Hearing Association, San Antonio, TX.

Erting, C., Prezioso, C., & Hynes, M. (1990). The interactional context of deaf mother-infant communication. In V. Volterra & C. Erting (Eds.), *From gesture to language in hearing and deaf children* (pp. 97–106). Washington, DC: Gallaudet University Press.

Fraiberg, S. (1977). *Insights from the blind.* Ann Arbor: University of Michigan Press.

Gleason, D. (1999). Early interactions with children who are deaf-blind. Retrieved January 10, 2000, from http://www.tr.wou.edu/dblink/early.htm

Greenberg, M. (1983). Family stress and child competence: The effects of early intervention for families with deaf infants. *American Annals of the Deaf, 128,* 407–417.

Greenberg, M., Calderon, R., & Kusche, C. (1984). Early intervention using simultaneous communication with deaf infants: The effects on communication development. *Child Development, 55,* 607–616.

Greenberg, M., & Marvin, R. (1979). Attachment patterns in profoundly deaf preschool children. *Merrill-Palmer Quarterly, 25,* 265–279.

Hadadian, A. (1995). Attitudes toward deafness and security of attachment relationships among young deaf children and their parents. *Early Education and Development, 6*(2), 181–191.

Hamilton, C. (2000). Continuity and discontinuity of attachment from infancy through adolescence. *Child Development, 71*(3), 690–694.

Harris, M., Clibbens, J., Chasin, J., & Tibbitts, R. (1989). The social context of early sign language development. *First Language, 9,* 81–97.

Jamieson, J. (1994a). Instructional discourse strategies: Differences between hearing and deaf mothers of deaf children. *First Language, 14,* 153–171.

Jamieson, J. (1994b). Teaching as transaction: Vygotskian perspectives on deafness and mother-child interaction. *Exceptional Children, 60*(5), 434–449.

Kantor, R. (1982). Communicative interaction: Mother modification and child acquisition of American Sign Language. *Sign Language Studies, 38,* 233–282.

Klein, M., & Briggs, M. (1987a). Facilitating mother–infant communicative interaction in mothers of high risk infants. *Journal of Childhood Communication Disorders, 10,* 95–106.

Klein, M., & Briggs, M. (1987b). *Observation of Communicative Interaction (OCI).* (Available from California State University, Division of Special Education, 5151 State University Drive, Los Angeles, CA 90032)

Koester, L. (1992). Intuitive parenting as a model for understanding parent–infant interactions when one partner is deaf. *American Annals of the Deaf, 137*(4), 362–369.

Koester, L. (1995). Face-to-face interactions between hearing mothers and their deaf or hearing infants. *Infant Behavior and Development, 18,* 145–153.

Koester, L., Brooks, L., & Karkowski, L. (1998). A comparison of the vocal patterns of deaf and hearing mother-infant dyads during face to face interaction. *Journal of Deaf Studies and Deaf Education, 3*(4), 290–301.

Koester, L., & MacTurk, R. (1991). Attachment behaviors in deaf and hearing infants. In *Interaction and support: Mothers and deaf infants* (Final Report, Grant No. MCJ-110563). Washington, DC: Gallaudet Research Institute.

Koester, L., & Meadow-Orlans, K. (1999). Responses to interactive stress: Infants who are deaf or hearing. *American Annals of the Deaf, 144*(5), 395–403.

Koester, L., Papousek, H., & Smith-Gray, S. (2000). Intuitive parenting, communication, and interaction with deaf infants. In P. Spencer, C. Erting, & M. Marschark (Eds.), *The deaf child in the family and at school: Essays in honor of Kathryn P. Meadow-Orlans* (pp. 55–71). Mahwah, NJ: Lawrence Erlbaum Associates.

Kyle, J., Woll, B., & Ackerman, J. (1989). *Gesture to sign and speech: Final report to ESRC* (Project No. C 00 23 2327). Bristol: Centre for Deaf Studies, University of Bristol, England.

Lang, D. (1996). Neonatal otoacoustic emission screening (OAE) for deafness: Psychological costs. *Archives of Disease in Childhood, Fetal & Neonatal Edition, 75,* 143F.

Lederberg, A., Love, A., & Yebra, M. (1997, April). *The use of scripts in pretend play: A comparison of deaf and hearing children.* Paper presented at the biennial meeting of the Society for Research in Child Development, Washington, DC.

Lederberg, A., & Mobley, C. (1990). The effect of hearing impairment on the quality of attachment and mother–toddler interaction. *Child Development, 61,* 1596–1604.

Lederberg, A., & Prezbindowski, A. (2000). Impact of child deafness on mother-toddler interaction: Strengths and weaknesses. In P. Spencer, C. Erting, & M. Marschark (Eds.), *The deaf child in the family and at school: Essays in honor of Kathryn P. Meadow-Orlans* (pp. 73–92). Mahwah, NJ: Lawrence Erlbaum Associates.

Linder, T.W. (1993). *Transdisciplinary play-based intervention: Guidelines for developing a meaningful curriculum for young children.* Baltimore: Paul H. Brookes Publishing Co.

Luterman, D. (1999). *The young deaf child.* Baltimore: York Press.

Maestas y Moores, J. (1980). Early linguistic environment: Interactions of deaf parents with their infants. *Sign Language Studies, 26,* 1–13.

Mahoney, G. (1992). *Maternal behavior rating scale (MBRS)* (Rev. ed.). (Available from Family Child Learning Center, 90 W. Overale Drive, Tallmadge, OH 44278)

Mahoney, G., Powell, A., & Finger, I. (1986). The Maternal Behavior Rating Scale. *Topics in Early Childhood Special Education, 6,* 44–56.

Masataka, N. (1992). Motherese in a signed language. *Infant Behavior and Development, 15,* 453–460.

Masataka, N. (1996). Perception of motherese in a signed language by 6-month-old deaf infants. *Developmental Psychology, 32*(5), 874–879.

Meadow, K., Greenberg, M., & Erting, C. (1983). Attachment behavior of deaf children with deaf parents. *Journal of the American Academy of Child Psychiatry, 22*(1), 23–28.

Meadow-Orlans, K. (1997). Effects of mother and infant hearing status on interactions at twelve and eighteen months. *Journal of Deaf Studies and Deaf Education, 2*(1), 26–36.

Meadow-Orlans, K., MacTurk, R., Prezioso, C., Erting, C., & Day, P. (1987, April). *Interactions of deaf and hearing mothers with 3- and 6-month-old infants.* Paper presented at the biennial meeting of the Society for Research in Child Development, Baltimore, MD.

Meadow-Orlans, K., MacTurk, R., Spencer, P., & Koester, L. (1991). *Interaction and support: Mothers and deaf infants* (Final Report, Grant No. MCJ-110563). Washington, DC: Gallaudet Research Institute.

Meadow-Orlans, K., Smith-Gray, S., & Dyssegaard, B. (1995). Infants who are deaf or hard of hearing, with and without physical/cognitive disabilities. *American Annals of the Deaf, 140*(3), 279–286.

Meadow-Orlans, K., & Spencer, P. (1996). Maternal sensitivity and the visual attentiveness of children who are deaf. *Early Development and Parenting, 5,* 213–223.

Meadow-Orlans, K., & Steinberg, A. (1993). Effects of infant hearing loss and maternal support on mother-infant interactions at 18 months. *Journal of Applied Developmental Psychology, 14,* 407–426.

Meier, R., & Newport, E. (1990). Out of the hands of babes: On a possible sign advantage in language acquisition. *Language, 66,* 1–23.

Mohay, H. (2000). Language in sight: Mothers' strategies for making language visually accessible to deaf children. In P. Spencer, C. Erting, & M. Marschark (Eds.), *The deaf child in the family and at school: Essays in honor of Kathryn P. Meadow-Orlans* (pp. 151–166). Mahwah, NJ: Lawrence Erlbaum Associates.

Mohay, H., Milton, L., Hindmarsh, G., & Ganley, K. (1998). Deaf mothers as language models for hearing families with deaf children. In A. Weisel (Ed.), *Issues unresolved: New perspectives on language and deafness* (pp. 76–87). Washington, DC: Gallaudet University Press.

Mohay, H., Milton, L., Hindmarsh, G., & Ganley, K. (n.d.). *Communication with deaf children.* Unpublished paper, Centre for Applied Studies in Early Childhood. Brisbane, Australia: Queensland University of Technology.

Moores, D. (2001). *Educating the deaf: Psychology, principles, and practices* (5th ed.). Boston: Houghton Mifflin.

Niparko, J., Kirk, K., Mellon, N., Robbins, A., Tucci, D., & Wilson, B. (2000). *Cochlear implants: Principles & practices.* Baltimore: Lippincott Williams & Wilkins.

Papousek, H., & Papousek, M. (1987). Intuitive parenting: A dialectic counterpart to the infant's precocity in integrative capacities. In J. Osofsky (Ed.), *Handbook of infant development* (2nd ed., pp. 669–720). New York: Wiley.

Prendergast, S., & McCollum, J. (1996). Let's talk: The effect of maternal hearing status on interactions with toddlers who are deaf. *American Annals of the Deaf, 141,* 11–18.

Pressman, L., Pipp-Siegel, S., Yoshinaga-Itano, C., & Deas, A. (1999). Maternal sensitivity predicts language gain in preschool children who are deaf and hard of hearing. *Journal of Deaf Studies and Deaf Education, 4*(4), 294–303.

Rea, C., Bonvillian, J., & Richards, H. (1988). Mother-infant interactive behaviors: Impact of maternal deafness. *American Annals of the Deaf, 133,* 317–324.

Reilly, J., & Bellugi, U. (1996). Competition on the face: Affect and language in ASL motherese. *Journal of Child Language, 23*(1), 219–239.

Rossetti, L. (1990). *The Rossetti Infant-Toddler Language Scale—A measure of communication and interaction.* East Moline, IL: LinguiSystems.

Rossetti, L. (1996). *Communication intervention: Birth to three.* San Diego: Singular Publishing Group.

Schirmer, B. (1989). Relationships between imaginative play and language development in hearing-impaired children. *American Annals of the Deaf, 134,* 219–222.

Schlesinger, H. (1987). Effects of powerlessness on dialogue and development: Disability, poverty, and the human condition. In B. Heller, L. Flohr, & L. Zegans (Eds.), *Psychosocial interventions with sensorially disabled persons* (pp. 1–27). New York: Grune & Stratton.

Schlesinger, H., & Meadow, K. (1972). *Sound and sign: Childhood deafness and mental health.* Berkeley: University of California Press.

SKI-HI Institute. (1993). *The model: A resource manual for family-centered home-based programming for infants, toddlers, and pre-school-aged children with hearing impairments.* Logan, UT: Hope.

Slade, A. (1987a). A longitudinal study of maternal involvement and symbolic play during the toddler period. *Child Development, 58,* 367–375.

Slade, A. (1987b). Quality of attachment and early symbolic play. *Developmental Psychology, 23,* 78–85.

Smith, C., Adamson, L., & Bakeman, R. (1988). Interactional predictors of early language. *First Language, 8,* 143–156.

Spencer, P. (1993a). Communication behaviors of infants with hearing loss and their hearing mothers. *Journal of Speech and Hearing Research, 36,* 311–321.

Spencer, P. (1993b). The expressive communication of hearing mothers and deaf infants. *American Annals of the Deaf, 138*(3), 275–283.

Spencer, P. (1996a). The association between language and symbolic play at two years: Evidence from deaf toddlers. *Child Development, 67,* 867–876.

Spencer, P. (1996b). *Showing love, sharing meaning.* Unpublished manuscript, available from the author (Department of Social Work, Gallaudet University, 800 Florida Avenue NE, Washington, DC 20002).

Spencer, P. (1998, July). *Communication, attention, and symbolic development: Mothers and infants as an interactive system.* Poster session presented at the International Conference for the Study of Behavioral Development, Berne, Switzerland.

Spencer, P. (2000). Looking without listening: Is audition a prerequisite for normal development of visual attention during infancy? *Journal of Deaf Studies and Deaf Education, 5*(4), 291–302.

Spencer, P. (2001, January). *A good start: Suggestions for visual conversations with deaf and hard of hearing infants and toddlers.* Retrieved from Kids WorldDeafNet web site at http://clerccenter2.gallaudet.edu/KidsWorldDeaf Net/e-docs/visual-conversations/visual-conversations.pdf

Spencer, P. (2002). Language development of children with cochlear implants. In J. Christiansen & I. Leigh, *Cochlear implants in children: Ethics and choices* (pp. 222–249). Washington, DC: Gallaudet University Press.

Spencer, P., Bodner-Johnson, B., & Gutfreund, M. (1992). Interacting with infants with a hearing loss: What can we learn from mothers who are deaf? *Journal of Early Intervention, 16,* 64–78.

Spencer, P., & Gutfreund, M. (1990). Characteristics of "dialogues" between mothers and prelinguistic hearing-impaired and normally-hearing infants. *The Volta Review, 97,* 351–360.

Spencer, P.E., & Lederberg, A. (1997). Different modes, different models: Communication and language of young deaf children and their mothers. In L.B. Adamson & M.A. Romski (Eds.), *Communication and language acquisition: Discoveries from atypical development* (pp. 203–230). Baltimore: Paul H. Brookes Publishing Co.

Spencer, P., & Meadow-Orlans, K. (1996). Play, language, and maternal responsiveness: A longitudinal study of deaf and hearing infants. *Child Development, 67,* 3176–3191.

Swisher, M.V. (1992). The role of parents in developing visual turn-taking in their young deaf children. *American Annals of the Deaf, 137*(2), 92–100.

Swisher, M.V. (2000). Learning to converse: How deaf mothers support the development of attention and conversational skills in their young deaf children. In P. Spencer, C. Erting, & M. Marschark (Eds.), *The deaf child in the family and at school: Essays in honor of Kathryn P. Meadow-Orlans* (pp. 21–39). Mahwah, NJ: Lawrence Erlbaum Associates.

Tannock, R. (1988). Mothers' directiveness in their interactions with their children with and without Down Syndrome. *American Journal on Mental Retardation, 93,* 154–165.

Thompson, R. (1998). Early sociopersonality development. In W. Damon (Series Ed.) & N. Eisenberg (Vol. Ed.), *Handbook of child psychology: Vol. 3. Social, emotional, and personality development* (5th ed., pp. 25–104). New York: Wiley.

Tomasello, M., & Farrar, M. (1986). Joint attention and early language. *Child Development, 57,* 1454–1463.

Vondra, J., & Barnett, D. (1999). Atypical attachment in infancy and early childhood among children at developmental risk. *Monographs of the Society for Research in Child Development, 64*(3, Serial No. 258).

Vygotsky, L. (1978). *Mind in society.* Cambridge, MA: Harvard University Press.

Waters, E., Hamilton, C., & Weinfield, N. (2000). The stability of attachment security from infancy to adolescence and early adulthood: General discussion. *Child Development, 71*(3), 678–683.

Waters, E., Merrick, S., Treboux, D., Crowell, J., & Albersheim, L. (2000). Attachment security in infancy and early adulthood: A twenty-year longitudinal study. *Child Development, 71*(3), 684–689.

Waxman, R., & Spencer, P. (1997). What mothers do to support infant visual attention: Sensitivities to age and hearing status. *Journal of Deaf Studies and Deaf Education, 2,* 104–114.

Waxman, R., Spencer, P., & Poisson, S. (1996). Reciprocity, responsiveness, and timing in interactions between mothers and deaf and hearing children. *Journal of Early Intervention, 20*(4), 341–355.

Wilson, S., & Spencer, P. (1997, April). *Maternal topic responsiveness and child language: A cross-cultural, cross-modality replication.* Paper presented at the biennial conference of the Society for Research in Child Development, Washington, DC.

Wood, D., Wood, H., Griffiths, A., & Howarth, I. (1986). *Teaching and talking with deaf children.* New York: Wiley.

Yoshinaga-Itano, C., & Apuzzo, M. (1998). The development of deaf and hard of hearing children identified early through the high-risk registry. *American Annals of the Deaf, 143*(5), 416–424.

Yoshinaga-Itano, C., Sedey, A., Coulter, D., & Mehl, A. (1998). Language of early- and later-identified children with hearing loss. *Pediatrics, 102,* 1161–1171.

The Role of
the Early Interventionist

*Gail L. Strassel, Parent–Infant Program
Coordinator, Florida School for the Deaf
and the Blind; State Coordinator, SKI-HI*

"I can't wait to get started!" is a phrase uttered by many parents
and caregivers after their child's hearing loss has been confirmed
and they are having an initial conversation with an interventionist.
Parents and caregivers are sometimes all too eager to place their
child in the arms of the interventionist and sit back and watch "it"
happen. The key to responsible early intervention is to help parents
and caregivers realize that "it" happens with them during every interaction. In fact, caregivers started "it" the day that they first gazed at
their child and continue "it" each time they interact with their child
in every daily routine. Helping parents and caregivers to realize this
and to recognize the fact that they are already doing "it," is the primary job of the interventionist. The interventionist's role is not to try
to fix; the prevailing model of home intervention is for an early interventionist to provide 1 or 2 hours of intervention weekly. If the intervention is provided directly to a child in a teacher–pupil style, and
the caregivers are either included peripherally or not at all, little or
no lasting impact on the knowledge, skills, or development of the
child will occur. Why? Even if an interventionist has the best of

intentions and knowledge, intervention directed to the child instead of the caregivers is less than effective. Parents/caregivers interact with their child every day. They feed, clothe, diaper, and bathe their child on a daily basis. Routines-based intervention is the key to helping parents and caregivers recognize and build upon their natural daily interactions with their children. An interventionist should be a careful observer and note what the caregiver is doing. The interventionist is in a position in the natural environment to identify the strengths of the existing interaction and to enhance that behavior by providing information, reinforcement, and "sensitive support." Dr. Spencer states that the role of the interventionist is to "identify existing interaction strengths in the caregiver and child, then help to enhance and increase those behaviors through providing models, information, and sensitive support."

Dr. Spencer offers valuable, research-based insight into how an interventionist can interact with a family and help them to discover their strengths and to help their child grow and develop. The specific examples cited by Dr. Spencer are excellent and specifically identify areas that interventionists can focus on to help the family help their child. Most parents and caregivers interact with their children in albeit different manners, and it is of critical importance for the interventionist to help parents recognize what they are already doing.

As Dr. Spencer notes in her chapter, universal newborn hearing screening is providing opportunities for intervention for very young children with hearing loss and their families. The research suggests that the earlier hearing loss is identified and intervention begins, *the better the outcome for the child.* As Dr. Spencer states, quality intervention services "can affect the degree to which parents participate in interactions that optimally support the development of their children who are deaf and hard of hearing."

The burden on interventionist training programs becomes critical to appropriately train interventionists. Often, people drawn to the field of early intervention are teachers, and it can be a natural instinct to want to "teach" the child. While teaching the child may have short-term benefits, if the intervention is to have lasting impact, the focus needs to be on helping parents and caregivers learn to "tune in" to their child and their interactions. This includes helping parents and caregivers to understand and build on their "intuitive" parenting skills.

The suggestions that Dr. Spencer makes in her chapter are very practical and, if used, could help many families. As a SKI-HI Parent Advisor, Trainer, and State Coordinator, the responsibility to prepare interventionists to understand their role in working with a family with a young child with hearing loss is essential. Our program (The Parent–Infant Program at the Florida School for the Deaf and Blind) provides SKI-HI training to qualified professionals who are interested in working with families with young children with hearing loss. While the SKI-HI manuals are comprehensive and provide extensive support for the interventionist, the most critical aspect of the training is to help the interventionists understand their role as an interventionist. That includes the concepts so thoroughly researched and presented in Dr. Spencer's chapter. The Parent-Infant Program has trained many professionals in SKI-HI and not one has left the training with a magic wand. While the training is thorough and as complete as we can make it, the most vital aspect of the training is to help the interventionists understand that parents and caregivers have the "magic" and it is their interactions that will help the child grow and develop. Regardless of the number of therapies or interventions in which the child and family participate, when asked the question, "Who is responsible for your child's progress?" the parents should reply with confidence, "We are."

CHAPTER TWELVE

Language and Literacy Development in Deaf Children

Implications of a Sociocultural Perspective

CAROL J. ERTING

As they waited anxiously in the clinic waiting room for the audiologist to return with the results of the hearing test, Amy and Dan wondered what the future would hold for their infant daughter. They had suspected for the past several months that Jennifer could not hear and were finally about to find out if their fears would be confirmed. After what seemed like an eternity, the door opened and Dr. Montillo invited them into his office. When he told them that the hearing tests had confirmed that Jennifer was deaf, with profound hearing loss in both ears, they were at the same time relieved to know something definitive and overcome with emotion. Amy tried to listen carefully to what Dr. Montillo was telling them, the advice he was giving regarding hearing aids, cochlear implants, and therapy for Jennifer, but all she could think about was how she would communicate with her daughter. If Jennifer could not hear her mother's voice, how would Amy sing to her, read to her, play with her, talk to her about their daily routines? And how would Jennifer be able to talk to her parents and her grandparents? When Dr. Montillo paused and asked if they had any questions, Amy didn't hesitate to ask, "Will my child learn to talk?"

"Will my child learn to talk?" This question is often among the first asked by worried hearing parents after learning from a doctor or an audiologist that their child is deaf. The question focuses on speech, the form of language most people consider synonymous with underlying linguistic competence and through which most everyday human relationships are created and maintained. As a result of their own cultural and linguistic experiences, beliefs, and expectations as hearing/speaking individuals, most parents understandably seek to find ways to restore their child's hearing and establish early communication if at all possible through the auditory/vocal modality. Doctors and audiologists, who usually share this worldview, rarely inform parents about another perspective on deaf children, one held by a small percentage of parents who are themselves Deaf[1] and communicate using the visual/gestural modality in sign language. Although Deaf parents also are usually interested in whether their child will learn to speak, their first response after receiving confirmation that their child is deaf is often a confident, delighted one, such as "Our child will learn to sign, like we do." The contrast between these two parental responses could not be more striking, yet both hearing and Deaf parents care deeply about the welfare of their deaf children. Both hope their children will grow up in a happy family, attend school successfully, and fulfill their ambitions. But for hearing parents, the prospect that their child will not understand them when they use their own language and will not acquire and produce that language effortlessly, as they did when they were children, is almost impossible to imagine.

LINGUISTIC SOCIALIZATION IN EARLY CHILDHOOD

Although most of the messages that human beings convey to one another are nonverbal, language sets humans apart from other animals. Infants acquire the foundations of language during finely tuned, repetitive, emotionally salient social routines between caregiver and infant (Bruner, 1983; Locke, 1993; see Chapter 11). Nonverbal and linguistic messages are interwoven in a seamless tapestry as adult and child, each a contributor to the exchange, make meaning and create a relationship. Beginning in infancy, children the world over learn to understand significant others and make themselves understood, participate in and jointly construct the social worlds of family and community, and acquire the languages

---

[1]In this chapter I have adopted the D/d distinction that was first used by Woodward (1972) and has since become conventional to differentiate individuals with a hearing loss who consider themselves members of a cultural group (Deaf) from those who do not (deaf).

and cultures into which they were born. For most parents and caregivers, the successful linguistic socialization of their tiny new family member is taken for granted, and the intricacies of the process remain unanalyzed (Papousek & Papousek, 1987). Even as their infant's early vocalizations and prelinguistic gestures are celebrated, parents look forward to the inevitable first words between 12 and 18 months and the emergence of what is considered by most linguists to be true language, the first two-word combination at approximately 24 months. Adults in the child's environment provide the necessary communicative and linguistic input as well as the scaffolded interactions that assist the child's linguistic, cognitive, and social-emotional growth (Bruner, 1983; Rogoff, 1990).

During these first 2 years of life, language is the symbolic tool through which children accomplish the important developmental tasks of early childhood (Wertsch, 1985). Any natural language is appropriate, spoken or signed, as long as it is accessible to the child and used by the caregiver to engage the child in social interaction (Slobin, 1985). Signed languages can accomplish these linguistic, cognitive, and social-emotional tasks as satisfactorily as spoken languages, and, contrary to the experience of monolingual Americans, many children throughout the world grow up bilingually, with two or more languages fulfilling these functions (Grosjean, 1992). Whatever the particular circumstances, the languages acquired during these early years are integral to the children's personal, social, and cultural identities. They are perceived as part of the natural order, as are the cultural categories embedded within them. It is only later, when children or adults encounter other languages and worldviews that this ethnocentrism is challenged, and, intellectually at least, subject to revision. But emotional attachment to the language of early socialization remains strong so that when individuals have children of their own they expect and look forward to reenacting their own early interactions, this time as caregivers. When it comes to the language used between caregiver and child, in the view of most parents, no language is as beautiful, as expressive, as flexible, and as appropriate as their mother tongue.

Considered from this perspective, the problem nonsigning parents face when confronted with the question of how to communicate with their deaf child is not only intellectual and logistical, but also a highly charged emotional question. From the developing child's point of view, the need is for fully accessible communication with parents, caregivers, and peers. Unlike the adults surrounding them, young children are unconcerned with ideology, emotional ties to language and culture, and academic arguments for or against a particular pedagogical approach; rather, they act on their environment in order to make pleasurable and interesting things happen. Like an ethnographer attempting to understand a foreign culture, caregivers and teachers need to recognize and leave aside their own biases and attempt to see the world through the children's eyes (Taylor, 1993).

For the purposes of this discussion, deaf children are defined as children who, as a result of impaired hearing, process information primarily through vision rather than audition, regardless of audiological status with or without the use of assistive devices such as hearing aids or cochlear implants. In other words, using Bahan's terminology, deaf children are seeing people, that is, primarily visual human beings (1989). This definition is functional and contrasts with a definition of hard of hearing children as those children who, with or without the use of assistive devices, learn primarily through the auditory channel even though their hearing is impaired. Although no test will indicate with certainty how a particular child will function, if children are carefully observed and their perspectives taken seriously, parents and teachers will be able to discern the children's primary functional modality. This perspective does not deny the utility of auditory input the visual child may receive, especially with early amplification, but emphasizes the child's use of auditory or visual information for communication, language acquisition, and social interaction.

The majority of deaf children are born or adopted into hearing, speaking families but need a visually accessible communicative and linguistic environment if they are to develop to their full potential. During the preschool years they must progress developmentally at the same rate and achieve linguistic, cognitive, social, and emotional milestones along the same timelines typically achieved by hearing children if they are to be prepared for the academic challenges in their futures. At the beginning of the 21st century, most deaf children do not arrive at school ready to learn at grade level. And even for those who do—and these are typically the children of Deaf parents who are bilingual in American Sign Language (ASL) and English—most schools and teachers are not well prepared to provide them with the kind of education that builds on their visual strengths and the bilingual foundation they have acquired at home. The barriers to improvement are not insurmountable, but they are varied and numerous, including late identification of the majority of deaf children; negative attitudes and misinformation about Deaf people and their visual language and culture; lack of descriptive, longitudinal research on diverse deaf children, their families, and their school environments; and lack of knowledge about the nature of Deaf bilingualism in home, school, and community contexts, including the relationship of ASL and English literacy. Progress is occurring in each of these areas, but parents and educational programs are required to make decisions based on current knowledge.

Understanding the typical course of language development and the role of language in cognitive development and literacy learning can provide caregivers, teachers, and other professionals a framework for considering the needs of deaf children and their families. The remainder of this chapter briefly reviews research findings about language and literacy development in hearing and deaf children from a sociocultural perspective and the implications of this knowledge for schools and programs serving deaf children and their families. Then a model of deaf children, their families, and their schools as bilingual is suggested as a useful way of conceptualizing language development and Deaf life in a world in which the majority of people interact using spoken language. Finally, recommendations within the context of future perspectives are then presented.

LANGUAGE, LITERACY, AND COGNITIVE DEVELOPMENT IN THE FIRST 5 YEARS

What do we know about the typical course of language, literacy, and cognitive development during the preschool years, from birth to 5 years of age?[2] Perhaps the most important accomplishment of the last 2 decades of research in the United States has been to document how the early language experiences of children at home and at school relate to literacy development during the school years (Dickinson & Tabors, 2001; Hart & Risley, 1995, 1999; Heath, 1983; Snow, 1983; Snow, Barnes, Chandler, Goodman, & Hemphill, 1991). Hart and Risley (1995), in their $2^{1}/2$ year longitudinal study of 42 middle-class, working-class, and welfare families with 1- to 2-year-old children, found significant differences among families in the amount of interaction and language they provided for their young children. A follow-up study of 29 of the children showed that these differences were strongly associated with vocabulary at age 3 and with the children's performance on tests of language skills at the end of third grade.

After more than 10 years of painstaking analysis of 1,318 observations, Hart and Risley (1999) concluded that the first 3 years of children's lives were even more important than they had thought when they began

---

[2]Although there have been notable exceptions (Goodwin, 1991; Hart & Risley, 1995, 1999; Heath, 1983; Schieffelin & Gilmore, 1986; Scribner & Cole, 1978; Snow et al., 1991), Anglo-American, middle-class children learning the majority language have been studied far more frequently since Roger Brown's classic study of Adam and Eve in the early 1960s than children from other sociocultural, socioeconomic, and linguistic groups, including Deaf children acquiring sign language.

their landmark study. Furthermore, they were able to state with confidence that one aspect of family life, the amount of parent–child interaction per hour, was profoundly related to the children's cognitive development. They demonstrated that the children's accomplishments had less to do with material and educational advantages in the home and more to do with the kinds of experiences their parents had provided with language diversity (e.g., number of different nouns and modifiers the parents produced in an hour with the child), affirmative feedback, symbolic emphasis (language that refers to relations between things and events), gentle guidance (prompting and asking rather than telling the child what to do), and responsiveness (having the child rather than parent control the interaction). The parents who talked to their children the most were also the ones who provided more of the experiences thought to be so important to cognitive development and academic success—learning about words, symbolic relations, and self-competence.

When does this immersion in social discourse begin? Children are surrounded by talk from the moment they are born and even enter the world having heard the spoken language of their mother while in the womb (Mehler et al., 1988). In fact, in Hart and Risley's (1999) study, before saying their first words at an average age of 11 months, the children had been listening to a surprising amount of social discourse around them, an average of 700–800 utterances per hour spoken within their range of hearing. Only about half of the utterances were directed to the children, while the rest were the result of conversations among parents, siblings, grandparents, friends, and visitors. Hart and Risley found that the children's experiences with overheard words and discourse were richer and more varied than they expected. This finding lends support to Forrester's (1993) proposal that overhearing conversations provides children with an important developmental context through which they gain information and find opportunities to interact with others.

When Hart and Risley (1999) analyzed the talk between parent and child during these early years they concluded that conversational interaction was like a dance—a social dance—with three developmental stages. First, parents and children interacted together to become partners (11–19 months). During this stage, children vocalized and produced few words, but they actively engaged with their parents in routinized, reciprocal interactions.[3] Exposure to language far exceeded practice,

---

[3]Jerome Bruner has described early caregiver–child interaction in detail, emphasizing the importance of the dyadic exchanges that occur during idealized word games such as peek-a-boo during this period. He compared these game routines to protoconversations with their highly structured format and assignment of turn-taking roles (1983).

with children producing, on average, 300,000 words while the parents averaged 4 million words. Hart and Risley called the next stage "staying and playing" (20–28 months). In this stage intensive one-to-one conversations between toddler and parent were prevalent. By the end of this period, the children were perceived as competent speakers and their practice with talk was contributing as much to their cumulative language experience as did the exposure to their parents' talk. Finally, in the third period (29–36 months), the children were the primary speakers, practicing their talk and honing their skills, with parents listening and providing feedback and elaboration.

By age 3, all of the children were displaying increasing fluency in the language spoken by their parents. They produced an average of 413 utterances per hour and 1,041 words per hour (232 different words), and initiated conversations 55 times per hour on average. Parents, rather than acting as language teachers, were acting as social partners, arranging the social context of conversation so that the children could gain practice in talking about increasingly complex and varied topics in linguistically sophisticated ways. By the time the children were 36 months of age, opportunities to converse with partners other than their parents were more prevalent as parents invited other children over to play and left the children with relatives and other caregivers more often. These conversational contexts challenged the children to develop their narrative skills in order to communicate effectively with social partners less familiar and perhaps less accepting of ambiguity than their parents.

In addition to the importance of exposure to talk and practice with talk, Hart and Risley's (1999) research highlights the centrality of discourse between caregiver and developing child. Conversation is a social partnership that depends on reciprocity, and parents in this study seemed intent on creating this context for their children learning to talk from the earliest stages. Emphasis was on the social relationship rather than the language. When their children were infants, parents emphasized the affectionate engagement with people through face-to-face interaction instead of attending to the sounds their children made. Once children began to produce recognizable words, parents attended to their vocalizations and used them as an opportunity to recruit the children into reciprocal conversation-like interactions. In the beginning, parents did much of the work, making sense of children's utterances, however incomplete, tolerating mistakes, modeling, demonstrating, prompting, and encouraging. Hart and Risley concluded that the parents were not doing anything consciously aimed at encouraging language development or teaching; rather, their goal was to keep children engaged, to keep them practicing their conversational skills and exploring within the context of social interaction. Developing a relationship with the child and the amount of enjoyable conversational interaction they sustained together while learning about each other was of primary importance to the parents.

These researchers also were struck by how actively the children were influencing the behavior of their parents, especially once the children were producing utterances. When children imitated words their parents asked them to say, for example, the vocalization was a signal to the parent that the child was listening, and parents always appeared to be willing to continue interacting if they saw behaviors that indicated the child was listening. Once children were talking as much in an hour as their parents and were speaking fluently and grammatically, they no longer needed encouragement to practice, and parents responded to them as they would to any conversational partner in their culture. By the age of 3 years, these children had a "trajectory of vocabulary growth and the foundations of analytic and symbolic competencies" that would make a lasting difference to how the children performed in later years (Hart & Risley, 1999, p. 193). The children were also competent conversational partners who enjoyed interacting with others and who were likely to be invited to participate in social interactions within an ever-widening circle of significant others.

While Hart and Risley studied how children learned to talk at home during their first 3 years of life and how this early social partnership with their parents and significant others related to later academic achievement, another research team studied children beginning at 3 years of age. The Home–School Study of Language and Literacy Development focused on 74 young children from low-income families and demonstrated how conversational interactions made crucial contributions to their literacy achievement in kindergarten and beyond (Dickinson & Tabors, 2001). Researchers examined how adults and children as well as peers actually talked together in different activity settings at home and at preschool and how these extended conversations (e.g., explanations, narratives, pretend play) supported the development of the children as readers and writers. The researchers argued that because reading is ultimately a linguistic activity, it is important to examine discourse opportunities that replicated the demands of literacy—talk requiring interlocutors to develop understandings beyond the present using several utterances or turns to build a linguistic structure (Snow, Tabors, & Dickinson, 2001).

When the researchers examined different types of talk occurring in the home, they found four kinds of "Extended Discourse" occurring in three conversational settings: nonimmediate discourse during book reading, pretend talk during toy play, and narrative and explanatory conversation during mealtimes. They were able to gauge the quality of the vocabulary used in each conversational setting by measuring what they called "rare words," and they assessed home support for literacy by collecting information on the types of literacy activities mothers reported doing with their children. All three of these variables—"Extended Discourse," "Rare Word Density," and "Home Support for Literacy"—were significantly related to how well the children performed on literacy-related tasks administered when they were in kindergarten (a narrative production task, emergent literacy tasks measuring book concepts, phonological awareness and print skill, and a receptive vocabulary task measuring word knowledge). The researchers reported that

> The kinds of activities that the mothers and other family members engaged in around books with the children; the types of language that mothers used during book reading, toy and magnet play, and during mealtimes; and the level of vocabulary that the mothers used when they talked with their children during mealtimes and toy play were all crucial in helping the children develop certain language and literacy skills that are important in kindergarten. (Tabors, Roach, & Snow, 2001, p. 135)

When the focus turned to the preschool classroom, the researchers were interested in detailed examination of the children's conversations with their teachers and peers, as well as the teachers' pedagogy, revealed through interviews, cases studies, and observations of conversations, materials, displays, and classroom organization. Previous research had suggested that they would find the most useful information about factors relating to language and literacy development in the details of conversations between children and others in the classroom, especially the adults, rather than in more global assessments of teacher–child interactions (Dickinson & Smith, 2001). Furthermore, the researchers' theory of literacy development led them to expect that an important aspect of emergent literacy skill is the ability to engage in extended discourse, a skill likely to be acquired by children through participation in classroom conversations about topics other than those focused on immediate classroom experiences and involving a variety of words. Although the researchers expected that the adults in the classroom would be more likely than peers to extend a child's thinking about a topic and to supply appropriate new vocabulary, they also thought it likely that skill in extended discourse would be acquired during pretend play with peers.

Analysis of audio and video recordings of extended teacher discourse when the children were 4 years of age and measures of children's language and literacy development at the end of kindergarten show a strong correlation between teacher–child conversations in a variety of classroom contexts and kindergarten outcomes, especially in emergent literacy and receptive vocabulary (Dickinson, 2001). Because previous studies have demonstrated a significant relationship between achievement in kindergarten and later academic success, Dickinson concluded that these results "clearly [suggest] that the quality of teachers' extended conversations with children throughout the day has a significant bearing on the child's long-term language and literacy development" (p. 274). When the researchers examined the children's exposure to rare words during mealtime, large-group time and free play, their data suggested that vocabulary use by the teachers as well as the patterns of vocabulary use by the children during conversations with their teachers could contribute to children's vocabulary development. Finally, classroom curriculum variables, specifically the quality of the writing program and curriculum content, were related to the children's subsequent literacy skill, receptive vocabulary, and storytelling skill. Dickinson concluded,

> Our results indicate clear and consistent patterns of relationship between children's language and literacy development and opportunities for children to engage in extended conversations with their teachers and friends throughout the day, to write and learn about varied topics, and to engage in dramatic play with friends. (p. 284)

The overwhelming evidence from the Home–School Study of Language and Literacy Development is that the preschool teacher's role (and by extension, the child care professional's role) is critical in providing classroom language environments that foster long-term language and literacy development. Teachers who used varied vocabulary, challenged the children to think, and provided activities and opportunities to stimulate the children's curiosity and imagination were those who were most successful in supporting language and literacy development. However, only a few of the teachers provided optimal support for learning across all of the learning contexts studied, with low use of rare vocabulary overall and low frequency of intellectually challenging conversations. Furthermore, most of the teachers demonstrated little understanding of the developmental nature of literacy development, the place of conversation in supporting literacy, or the critical role teachers can play in fostering language and literacy development. Because Dickinson and his colleagues found strong evidence for the centrality of teacher–child conversations to this process, they concluded that teachers need to organize their classroom day so that they have time to create extended conversations with children individually as well as in small- and large-group contexts. They need to engage in intentional teaching; that is, they must have detailed knowledge of what children need and the ability and energy to provide the experiences throughout the day that support children's development. Especially critical is the teacher's ability to craft rich conversational interactions that push children to explore new ideas, clarify their thinking, and express themselves in increasingly sophisticated ways. Teachers, like all conversational partners, make unconscious decisions during interactions because of their sensitivity to contextual variables, including those related to children's cultural, linguistic, and social backgrounds as well as to more immediate environmental factors such as the size of the group or the activity setting. Dickinson argued that teachers must consciously attend to how such factors shape their use of language and their conversations with children throughout the school day and they need to be taught to do so through preservice and in-service training.

Finally, the Home–School Study of Language and Literacy Development researchers analyzed the relative contributions of the home and the school environments to children's language and literacy development. They concluded that although activities in the home make important contributions to success in literacy, home environments that were strong in their support for language and literacy did not counteract the negative effects of preschools that were weak, at least when the children's performance in kindergarten was measured. Excellent preschools, however, did make a difference in promoting language and literacy development for children who came from homes with low support. In both environments, the study found that a broad pattern of adult–child activities and interactions supported language and literacy development rather than the frequency of book reading or the quality of talk accompanying book reading alone. The classroom findings are particularly important because, in the authors' words, they reveal "with great clarity the power of preschool classrooms to contribute to children's language and literacy development" (Tabors, Snow, & Dickinson, 2001, p. 330). According to this study, access to specific kinds of language and literacy experiences in preschool affects child outcomes. Classrooms may appear welcoming, safe, friendly, and pleasant places for children, but they still might not provide the particular kinds of experiences children need to build their language and literacy capacity. In addition to the kind of teacher language use and curricular focus described previously, this study suggested that children benefit from overhearing conversations other children have with their teachers and professional child care providers. Children learn from each other, and teachers need to find ways to support peer learning.

Finally, for most children, home and school interact synergistically, especially when parents are involved with the school, and teachers encourage this involvement. Both environments are important for providing early experience with language and therefore literacy. However, if attempts to foster parent involvement and support children at home are unsuccessful, the good news from this study is that an excellent preschool can make a critical difference.

EARLY LANGUAGE, LITERACY, AND COGNITIVE DEVELOPMENT OF DEAF CHILDREN

> Our results demonstrate that children do begin literacy learning with language and that enhancing their language development by providing them with rich and engaging language environments during the first 5 years of life is the best way to ensure their success as readers. (Tabors et al., 2001, p. 334)

The two longitudinal studies in homes and preschools summarized have described these "rich and engaging language environments" in great detail, and with this knowledge it is not difficult to see the implications for deaf children. In the past, most deaf children in the United States have not been identified as deaf until, on average, the second year of life. Typically, the advice of doctors, audiologists, and educators has been to "fit" the child with hearing aids and enroll the child (and parents) in an educational or clinical program that will provide oral "training," with the caveat that progress in spoken language development will be painstakingly slow. Even those professionals who advocate sign language for deaf children often encourage parents to place greater emphasis on auditory training, speechreading, and speech development in the early years and only add signs later, once the child's progress with spoken language has been judged to be unsatisfactory. It is still relatively rare for parents who discover that their child is deaf in the earliest months of life to begin to learn sign language and immediately seek to surround their child with fully accessible visual language. Therefore, most deaf children are deprived of these "rich and engaging language environments" at home and in preschool during these critical years from birth to 5 years.

Deaf Children of Deaf Parents

When interactions between Deaf parents and their young Deaf children have been studied, a clearer picture has emerged of the developmental trajectory of visual children in the early years when the world around them, especially the linguistic world of their immediate family, is fully accessible to them. More than 20 years ago, a study of four groups of mothers and their children demonstrated that Deaf mothers and their 3- to 5-year-old Deaf children using American Sign Language, like hearing mothers and their hearing children using spoken English, were able to engage in conversations about each other and about immediate and nonimmediate objects and events (Meadow, Greenberg, Erting, & Carmichael, 1981). Their interactions were typically extended, complex, elaborated, and child initiated. However, deaf children whose mothers chose to interact with them only through spoken English ignored 40% of their mothers' requests and attempts to gain their attention. Rather than engaging in extended discourse with each other, these mothers and children spent significantly less time engaged in interaction, and when they did interact their conversations were simple, more frequently mother-initiated, object-focused, and not elaborated. Similarly, Jamieson and Pedersen (1993) reported that in research with 4- to 5-year-old deaf children engaged in a joint problem-solving task with their mothers, Deaf mothers, in contrast to hearing mothers, engaged in interactional patterns with their children that closely resembled those of hearing mothers with their hearing children. Their skillful scaffolding provided instruction and assistance through language and their interventions were contingent on their children's initiations and responses (Jamieson & Pedersen, 1993).

In the 1980s and 1990s, analyses of the early communicative and linguistic environments created by Deaf mothers and their Deaf children in the first 3 years of life showed patterns of face-to-face interactions similar to those of hearing pairs (Erting, Prezioso, & Hynes, 1990; Koester, Papousek, & Smith-Gray, 2000; Meadow-Orlans, MacTurk, Prezioso, Erting, & Day, 1987; Meadow-Orlans, MacTurk, Spencer, & Koester, 1991; Swisher, 2000). Qualitative analyses of these interactions have revealed the complexity of the conversations and extended dialogues in which Deaf/Deaf pairs engage. Notable is the extent to which Deaf mothers who are fluent in both ASL and English skillfully draw on the representational systems available to them, including child-directed ASL, fingerspelling, and spoken and written English to scaffold meaningful, comprehensible, and enjoyable interactions with their young children from the first year of life (Akamatsu & Andrews, 1993; Blumenthal-Kelly, 1995; Erting, 1982/ 1994; Erting, Thumann-Prezioso, & Benedict, 2000; Maxwell, 1980, 1984; Padden, 1996).

Research on the acquisition of natural sign languages by Deaf children of Deaf parents also adds clarity to the developmental picture. For 3 decades, beginning with the pioneering studies of Schlesinger and Meadow (1972), Boyes Braem (1973, 1990/1994), Newport and Ashbrook (1977), Hoffmeister (1978), and Newport and Meier (1985), evidence has continued to demonstrate that the developmental milestones of sign language acquisition are similar to those of spoken language acquisition and achieved by native signers and native speakers along fairly similar timelines (Chamberlain, Morford, & Mayberry, 2000). One exception is the appearance of first signs earlier than the appearance of first words

(Anderson & Reilly, 2002; Meier & Newport, 1990), possibly due to greater ease of production and perception in the visual/gestural modality as compared with the auditory/vocal one during infancy.

Data collected on 69 Deaf children of Deaf parents using the MacArthur Communicative Development Inventories for American Sign Language (ASL-CDI) showed that the early productive vocabularies of these Deaf children surpassed those reported for English-speaking children, but by 18–23 months median scores and ranges for children acquiring ASL were comparable to those of children acquiring spoken English. Further analyses indicated that although the sequence and developmental timeline for signs for emotion, cognitive verbs, and *wh*-forms were similar to those in English, and although the first 35 signs in both ASL and first 35 words in English were quite similar, children learning ASL produced more verbs in their early lexicon, a pattern evident throughout their first 3 years (Anderson & Reilly, 2002). These results taken together with findings of numerous case studies demonstrate that by the age of 3 years, native signing children, while continuing to acquire the more complex features of ASL grammar are, like the children studied by Hart and Risley, fluent in the language signed by their parents and engage as social partners in increasingly complex, extended conversations with adults and peers.

Deaf Children of Hearing Parents

Lederberg and Everhart's (2000) study of communication between Caucasian hearing mothers and their deaf or hearing children in their third year of life showed that these mothers' communication with their deaf children frequently did not provide access to language, and their deaf children were severely delayed linguistically. Seventeen of the twenty deaf children were enrolled in simultaneous communication (SC) classes, and three were in auditory verbal programs with the majority of parents learning to sign. Nevertheless, at 22 months, less than 15% of the SC mothers' communications contained signs, and by 3 years, that percentage had only increased to 30%. At 22 months, half of the deaf children produced no linguistic communication in 10 minutes of free play and 30% of them used fewer than nine single-word utterances. At 3 years, 70% of these deaf children were using only single-word utterances. When compared with hearing children at the same ages, these deaf children were less skilled at maintaining topics, less likely to be able to make the pragmatic function of their communication clear, and were less likely to ask questions. The researchers concluded that differences in communication by mothers of deaf and hearing children were attributable to deaf children's linguistic delays and the lack of success of intervention programs in improving the mothers' ability to sign. Support for these findings comes from Calderon's (2000) study that examined the relationship between school-based parental involvement and later child outcomes for deaf children of hearing parents. Maternal communication skill, rather than direct parental involvement in their child's education program, was significantly related to language development, early reading skills, and social-emotional development.

Research on language acquisition of children who are deaf with hearing parents is not encouraging within the context of the longitudinal studies of hearing children discussed previously. In a study of the vocabulary development of 113 24- to 37-month-old deaf and hard of hearing children of hearing parents using the ASL-CDI, Mayne and her colleagues found that even though cognitively typical children identified as deaf or hard of hearing prior to the age of 6 months demonstrated larger vocabularies than previous research had reported, these children were still delayed relative to hearing children (Mayne, Yoshinaga-Itano, Sedey, & Carey, 2000). Their scores fell below the 25th percentile for children with normal hearing at 30 months. Most of these children (95%) were enrolled in a family-focused early intervention program employing professionals with graduate degrees in audiology, speech-language pathology, or deaf education who delivered services to the home approximately 1 hour per week. Similarly, although Moeller (2000) found that deaf and hard of hearing children who were enrolled in intervention programs before the age of 11 months demonstrated significantly better vocabulary and verbal reasoning skills at 5 years of age, even these children achieved abstract reasoning scores in the low average range when compared with their hearing peers. Early identified children fared far better than their later identified counterparts, however. The children who were enrolled in intervention programs after the age of 24 months scored on average well below their hearing peers and had great difficulty responding to the reasoning-based questions, scoring well below hearing students' scores in this domain as well. These studies suggest that early identification is necessary but not sufficient for optimal developmental outcomes for deaf children. Unless nonsigning parents, family members, professional child care providers, and infant and preschool teachers become visually oriented, learn to sign proficiently, and understand how to create language and literacy rich interactional environments, deaf children will continue to arrive at kindergarten unprepared for school.

Deaf Children and Schooling

Data from the 2000–2001 Annual Survey of Deaf and Hard of Hearing Children and Youth conducted by the Gallaudet Research Institute indicate that the number of children younger than 3 years of age who are enrolled in educational programs of any kind in the United States is quite low. Of the 42,647 students for whom survey data were reported, only 1,205 younger than the age of 3 years were enrolled in educational programs. Those numbers increased to 4,061 for children 3–5 years of age, still only 41% of the 9,870 children between the ages of 6 and 9 years reported to be enrolled in education programs. Clearly, educational programs are not serving large numbers of children who are deaf and hard of hearing younger than 5 years.[4] Furthermore, when data on sign use in the home are examined, only 28.2% of the 37,943 children for whom data are available are reported to be from families in which members regularly sign. Because 73% of the 37,511 students for whom data are reported have moderate/severe to profound hearing losses in their better ears and may be primarily visual rather than auditory learners, it is clear that staggering numbers of children are without adequate access to communicative, linguistic, affective, and educational input in the home and, therefore, cannot acquire language, develop cognitively, and participate in the kinds of extended discourse shown to be related to literacy development. In this light, it is not surprising that in this same national survey, of the students for whom information was reported, 42.9% of them were judged to have disabilities other than a visual disability or cerebral palsy (e.g., learning disabilities, mental retardation, attention-deficit/hyperactivity disorder, serious emotional disturbance).

The data reported in the category of "functional assessment" are even more revealing and alarming. Of the 39,397 children for whom data were reported, 34.3% were judged to have a functional limitation in thinking/reasoning, 37.7% were reported to be deficient in maintaining attention, 51% were judged to be limited in expressive communication, 52.2% were seen as having a functional limitation in receptive communication, and 29.7% were judged to have problems in the area of social

---

[4]One can only guess at what percentage of the children enrolled are actually in fully accessible environments where their linguistic, emotional, and cognitive development can proceed unimpeded. Studies of deaf children interacting with their peers and teachers in preschool classrooms are almost nonexistent, especially classrooms where ASL is one of the languages shared by children and adults. In one classroom study of eight 4- and 5-year-old deaf children, four with Deaf parents and four with hearing parents, the children's discourse with the hearing teacher, a relatively new signer who communicated with the children by speaking and signing simultaneously, and the Deaf teacher's assistant, a member of the Deaf community who signed ASL and fluent English signing, was analyzed during one activity setting (Erting, 1980). Conversations averaged 3 turns in length when they involved the Deaf assistant, with several consisting of 5 and 6 turns, but only 1.6 turns when the children were communicating with the hearing teacher. The children who initiated more interaction and participated in extended conversations with the adults were the four children of Deaf parents and the one deaf child of hearing parents who had attended a residential school and acquired ASL. When peer interaction was examined among children proficient in ASL and those who were not, the fluent signers carried on extended conversations while the children who were less proficient linguistically were primarily passive (Johnson & Erting, 1989).

interaction/classroom behavior. Some of these disabilities, in fact, may be a result of society's failure to provide children who are deaf with accessible language and literacy environments in the earliest years of their lives.

Not surprisingly, academic achievement data indicate that the majority of children who are deaf and hard of hearing perform well below grade level on tests of reading comprehension upon leaving high school (Traxler, 2000). Even Deaf children who have Deaf parents, the majority of whom may have early and consistent access to sign language in the home, achieve on average well below grade level, despite attaining consistently higher scores than their peers with hearing parents, most of whom probably do not have families who sign at home. Depressed scores on tests of academic achievement are not puzzling when considered alongside the findings of the Home–School Study of Language and Literacy Development. In that study, as mentioned previously, even home environments that provided strong support for language and literacy could not counteract the negative effects of weak preschools in preparing children for literacy and academic achievement in kindergarten and beyond. Considering that the majority of children who are deaf do not have accessible linguistic input from birth onwards in the home, often are not identified and/or placed in a preschool program prior to age 3 and perhaps later, and once in an educational program usually do not have the opportunity to interact with caregivers and teachers who are proficient in a fully accessible natural sign language, it is not surprising, and in fact would be predicted from the results of the longitudinal studies described above, that deaf children on average do not achieve grade level performance on tests of academic achievement, especially English literacy-related measures. Although the preponderance of writings on deaf education insist that it is the child's inability to access and acquire the spoken language of the society that accounts for this deplorable educational record, it is likely that the blame should fall on the failure of society to give children who are deaf the means whereby they can easily engage in extended discourse from the earliest years of their lives in a variety of contexts, both in and out of school, with a variety of adults and peers. By adopting a model of deaf children living in the world bilingually and even multilingually, parents, educators, and society as a whole can begin to think and act differently with regard to meeting the needs of these children in the areas of early language and literacy.

Deaf Children Living Bilingually

Since the 1970s, the argument has been made that children who are deaf should be seen and treated as bilingual children who have the right to access and participate in both worlds into which they are born (Bouvet, 1982/1990; Erting, 1978; Hansen, 1994; Israelite, Ewoldt, & Hoffmeister,

1989; Johnson, Liddell, & Erting, 1989; Kannapell, 1974; Supalla, 1994; Wallin, 1994). Most children who are deaf are connected to generations of hearing relatives when they are born to or adopted by hearing parents. At the same time, by virtue of their hearing loss and the resulting experiences they will have throughout their lives, they are also part of the Deaf World (Erting, 1982/1994; Erting, Johnson, Smith, & Snider, 1994; Lane, Hoffmeister, & Bahan, 1996). Roberta Thomas, a hearing parent with a deaf son, has written eloquently about her realization of this truth about her son's identity and what it meant for her family:

> Having Jesse taught me that there are many ways of being human: a black way, a white way, a male way, a female way, a deaf way, a hearing way—and that all of these ways are human. Equality doesn't mean that all human beings must be the same. Equality means that we must respect differences among human beings. Deafness is a difference; it need not be an impairment. Once parents understand this, they can make the imaginative leap of understanding that will make it possible for them to let their child be deaf and at the same time make him or her a member of the family and the larger culture. (Thomas, Tillander, & Bergmann, 1994, p. 553)

For a small percentage of deaf children born or adopted into Deaf families, caregivers interact with the infant from the first hours of life by means of a signed language. These children often live in families with both deaf and hearing members, and therefore experience Deaf bilingual lives from birth within the home environment. Francois Grosjean, a well-known researcher in the area of bilingualism, has written about the right of all deaf children to grow up bilingually and biculturally (2001), and the World Federation of the Deaf has adopted his statement as a manifesto (F. Grosjean, personal communication, 2002).

In the United States, the view of children who are deaf and their families as bilingual or multilingual (families of deaf children may use two or more signed and/or spoken languages in their everyday lives) has not fit comfortably with the dominant English-only language ideology of the majority Anglo-American culture (Nover, 1993). Bilingual education for hearing children has been debated in the United States primarily with respect to Latino and Asian American children, with the emphasis on transitional models seeking to move children from the home language to English within 5 years. Large-scale, well-financed efforts are underway to eliminate even these transitional bilingual programs, as exemplified by the passage of Proposition 227 in California in 1998, aimed at eliminating bilingual education (Cummins, 2000). Bilingualism as a stable condition has tended to be valued primarily for affluent majority-language children who first acquire English and later learn other languages, usually as academic subjects or for personal enhancement. For children who are deaf, however, being deaf involves a physical difference that requires a different way of being in the world, in most cases permanently. Children who are deaf cannot choose, through hard work and determination, to shed their identity as seeing people and assimilate into the hearing-speaking mainstream even though the monolingual, spoken language approach known as oralism has promoted that position. In response to the dissatisfaction with the academic achievement of the majority of deaf children nationwide (Commission on Education of the Deaf, 1988; Johnson, Liddell, & Erting, 1989), the recognition that ASL is not only a sophisticated natural language but also contributes to the development of English literacy (Chamberlain et al., 2000; Prinz, 1998; Strong & Prinz, 1996) and the realization by parents and teachers that children who are deaf are different, not deficient (Raimondo, 2000; Thomas et al., 1994), bilingual education for deaf students is now being implemented for a small but growing number of students who are deaf nationwide (LaSasso, 1999; Strong, 1995). Parents who choose these programs for their children are also successfully creating bilingual family environments with hearing and deaf members who use ASL and spoken and written English (Blackburn, 2000).

Another trend, gaining in popularity, is the promotion of signing with hearing infants. Proponents argue that by signing with their infants and toddlers, hearing parents can communicate with their infants earlier, lessen young children's frustration by giving them a means to express themselves, and increase joyful, meaningful interactions with their children. Others argue that using sign language with young hearing children may provide them with a cognitive or linguistic advantage (Capirci, Cattani, Rossini, & Volterra, 1998; Daniels, 1996a, 1996b). It has been recognized in both popular and scientific literature that infants who have been exposed to signing are seen as communicating intentionally and meaningfully at a younger age than children who have not been exposed to signing. Yet, for children born deaf, parents are encouraged to try hearing aids or consider a cochlear implant and avoid signing even while they are also told that it will take years of regular and arduous practice for the infant or toddler to learn to use the implant to "hear" and that the child will always be a deaf person. The fear is that if allowed to sign, the children will never develop fluency in spoken language. To this end, professionals are willing to sacrifice deaf children's access to a natural language that will allow typical language development and participation in the kinds of extended discourse described above, so important for social-emotional, cognitive, and literacy development.

It is clear from the literature on bilingualism that children worldwide commonly acquire two languages simultaneously if given the opportunity, including hearing children of deaf parents who acquire ASL and spoken English. If a deaf child's assisted auditory access to language is sufficient for spoken language development to occur, it will, and early and continuing interaction in sign language will not harm that process (Spencer, 2000). In fact, when children who are deaf are given the opportunity to develop to their maximum potential through the visual channel while their auditory potential is being explored, parents and teachers are ensuring that they are not deprived of those critical early social interactions that create the foundation for later academic success.

ENVISIONING THE FUTURE

Deaf children, like all children, need to be surrounded by fully accessible natural language from the moment they are born. With the advent of widespread newborn hearing screening, there is a greater chance than ever before that infants who are deaf will be identified in the first months of life. But identification will only be effective in meeting the needs of these infants and families if appropriate educational programs are available to provide the infants with a linguistic and sociocultural environment for which they are biologically prepared and to which they have an inalienable right. These educational programs, however, are currently unavailable in the United States. At present, if hearing parents seek to place their infant in a center several hours a day where their visual child will be surrounded by fluent signers who can foster their linguistic and cognitive development barrier-free, they will not find such a center. The burden instead will be on the parents to organize such an environment using their own private resources; this is a formidable task.

If children who are deaf are to be given the same opportunities to develop linguistically, cognitively, socially, and emotionally as hearing children, centers should be established in which children who are deaf and their families can learn to be visual communicators (Erting, 1992). These bilingual early education centers would include deaf and hearing children and adults in which all are provided with opportunities to acquire ASL and English in a supportive environment. They would be exciting, lively centers of living and learning, offering deaf children opportunities for multiple interactional partners—adults and peers—with whom they would develop social partnerships and practice their conversational skills, building a foundation for literacy and academic achievement.

By 3 years of age, these deaf children, like children who are deaf with Deaf parents, would be cognitively and linguistically prepared to interact with teachers who would engage them in extended discourse about topics other than those in the immediate context and involving varied vocabulary (signed, fingerspelled, spoken, and written). Teachers would all be fluent signers and understand their critical role in providing linguistic and interactional environments for fostering long-term language and literacy development. They would challenge the children to think, would understand the developmental nature of literacy and the role of extended conversation in supporting it, and would expect children who are deaf to become bilingual children achieving at or above grade level. Signing hard of hearing and hearing children would be welcome in these preschools in which all languages and ways of being in the world were valued as precious linguistic and cultural resources. By including these children, natural environments promoting spoken language use among peers would be available during specific times of the day for those children able to take advantage of them.

Parents, siblings, and extended family members, deaf and hearing, would also be members of this educational community. As their deaf infants, toddlers, and preschoolers were thriving in a barrier free, educationally stimulating, bilingual, multicultural environment, they, too, would be growing. New horizons would be open to them as they learned a new way of communicating and were welcomed into a world of new experiences introduced to them by their deaf child. Special grants from the government would allow parents of newly identified deaf children to take paid leave from their employment in order to learn about this new world they would be entering and to begin intensive sign language classes designed to give them vocabulary and visual strategies to facilitate communication and interaction with their infant. An extensive program of sign language instruction for parents would follow the initial period with weekend and week-long family camps to support families in their bilingual lives.

Although this vision of the future may sound utopian to many, Scandinavian countries have already implemented many of these ideas with considerable success (Hansen, 1994; Wallin, 1994). With what is now known about language and cognitive development during the critical years from birth to 5 and the relationship of that development to later literacy, the importance of the earliest possible exposure to a natural sign language for children who are deaf can no longer be contested; the fact that deaf people are bilingual and should be recognized and supported as bilingual from the earliest months, is also clear. What is not known is how this vision will unfold in practice, how nonnative signing, predominantly hearing teachers and child care professionals can best be taught to nurture and teach young children in these bilingual environments, and how fluency in a natural sign language can be used most effectively to promote literacy in a written language. Research has begun to provide answers to some of these questions and that effort must continue. Deaf children cannot wait, however, and what is happening to them now, for the most part, is unacceptable. Change is possible; the only thing lacking is the will to make it happen.

REFERENCES

Akamatsu, C., & Andrews, J. (1993). It takes two to be literate: Literacy interactions between parent and child. *Sign Language Studies, 81,* 333–360.

Anderson, D., & Reilly, J. (2002). The MacArthur Communicative Development Inventory: Normative data for American Sign Language. *Journal of Deaf Studies and Deaf Education, 7*(2), 83–106.

Bahan, B. (1989). Notes from a "seeing" person. In S. Wilcox (Ed.), *American deaf culture* (pp. 29–32). Silver Spring, MD: Linstok Press.

Blackburn, L. (2000). The development of sociolinguistic meanings: The worldview of a deaf child within his home environment. In M. Metzger (Ed.), *Bilingualism and identity in Deaf communities* (pp. 19–254). Washington, DC: Gallaudet University Press.

Blumenthal-Kelly, A. (1995). Fingerspelling interaction: A set of deaf parents and their deaf daughter. In C. Lucas (Ed.), *Sociolinguistics in deaf communities* (pp. 62–73). Washington, DC: Gallaudet University Press.

Bouvet, D. (1990). *The path to language: Bilingual education for deaf children* (J.E. Johnson, Trans.). Philadelphia: Multilingual Matters. (Original work published 1982 as *La parole de l'enfant sourd,* Paris: Presses Universitaires de France)

Boyes Braem, P. (1973). *A study of the acquisition of the DEZ in American Sign Language.* Unpublished manuscript.

Boyes Braem, P. (1994). Acquisition of the handshape in American Sign Language: A preliminary analysis. In V. Volterra & C. Erting (Eds.), *From gesture to language in hearing and deaf children* (pp. 107–127). Washington, DC: Gallaudet University Press. (Original work published 1990 by Springer-Verlag)

Bruner, J. (1983). *Child's talk: Learning to use language.* New York: W.W. Norton.

Calderon, R. (2000). Parental involvement in deaf children's education programs as a predictor of child's language, early reading, and social-emotional development. *Journal of Deaf Studies and Deaf Education, 5*(2), 140–155.

Capirci, O., Cattani, P., Rossini, P., & Volterra, V. (1998). Teaching sign language to hearing children as a possible factor in cognitive enhancement. *Journal of Deaf Studies and Deaf Education, 3*(2), 135–142.

Chamberlain, C., Morford, J., & Mayberry, R. (Eds.). (2000). *Language acquisition by eye.* Mahwah, NJ: Lawrence Erlbaum Associates.

Commission on Education of the Deaf (1988). *Toward equality: A report to the President and the Congress of the United States.* Washington, DC: Government Printing Office.

Cummins, J. (2000). *Language, power, and pedagogy: Bilingual children in the crossfire.* Buffalo, NY: Multilingual Matters.

Daniels, M. (1996a). Bilingual, bimodal education for hearing kindergarten students. *Sign Language Studies, 90,* 25–37.

Daniels, M. (1996b). Seeing language: The effect over time of sign language on vocabulary development in early childhood education. *Child Study Journal, 26*(3), 193–208.

Dickinson, D.K. (2001). Putting the pieces together: Impact of preschool on children's language and literacy development in kindergarten. In D.K. Dickinson & P.O. Tabors (Eds.), *Beginning literacy with language: Young children learning at home and school* (pp. 257–287). Baltimore: Paul H. Brookes Publishing Co.

Dickinson, D.K., & Smith, M.W. (2001). Supporting language and literacy development in the preschool classroom. In D.K. Dickinson & P.O. Tabors (Eds.), *Beginning literacy with language: Young children learning at home and school* (pp. 139–147). Baltimore: Paul H. Brookes Publishing Co.

Dickinson, D.K., & Tabors, P.O. (Eds.). (2001). *Beginning literacy with language: Young children learning at home and school.* Baltimore: Paul H. Brookes Publishing Co.

Erting, C. (1978). Language policy and deaf ethnicity. *Sign Language Studies, 19,* 139–152.

Erting, C. (1980). Sign language and communication between adults and children. In C. Baker & R. Battison (Eds.), *Sign language and the deaf community: Essays in honor of William C. Stokoe.* Silver Spring, MD: National Association of the Deaf.

Erting, C. (1982). *Deafness, communication, and social identity: An anthropological analysis of interaction among parents, teachers, and deaf children in a preschool.* Doctoral dissertation, The American University, Washington, DC. (Published in 1994 as *Deafness, communication, social identity: Ethnography in a preschool for deaf children.* Silver Spring, MD: Linstok Press.)

Erting, C. (1992). Partnerships for change: New possible worlds for deaf children and their families. In *Bilingual considerations in the education of deaf students: ASL and English.* Washington, DC: Gallaudet University Press.

Erting, C., Johnson, R., Smith, D., & Snider, B. (Eds.). (1994). *The Deaf way: Perspectives from the international conference on Deaf culture.* Washington, DC: Gallaudet University Press.

Erting, C., Prezioso, C., & Hynes, M. (1990). The interactional context of deaf mother-infant communication. In V. Volterra & C. Erting (Eds.), *From gesture to language in hearing and deaf children* (pp. 97–106). New York: Springer-Verlag.

Erting, C., Thumann-Prezioso, C., & Benedict, B. (2000). Bilingualism in a deaf family: Fingerspelling in early childhood. In P. Spencer, C. Erting, & M. Marschark (Eds.), *The deaf child in the family and at school: Essays in honor of Kathryn P. Meadow-Orlans* (pp. 41–54). Mahwah, NJ: Lawrence Erlbaum Associates.

Forrester, M. (1993). Affording social-cognitive skills in young children: The overhearing context. In D. Messer & G. Turner (Eds.), *Critical influences on child language acquisition and development.* New York: St. Martin's Press.

Gallaudet Research Institute. (2001, January). *Regional and national summary report of data from the 2000–2001 annual survey of deaf and hard of hearing children and youth.* Washington, DC: Author.

Goodwin, M. (1991). *He-said-she-said: Talk as social organization among black children.* Bloomington: Indiana University Press.

Grosjean, F. (1992). The bilingual and the bicultural person in the hearing and in the deaf world. *Sign Language Studies, 77,* 307–320.

Grosjean, F. (2001). The right of the deaf child to grow up bilingual. *Sign Language Studies, 1*(2), 110–114.

Hansen, B. (1994). Trends in the progress toward bilingual education for deaf children in Denmark. In C. Erting, R. Johnson, D. Smith, & B. Snider (Eds.),

The Deaf way: Perspectives from the international conference on Deaf culture (pp. 605–614). Washington, DC: Gallaudet University Press.

Hart, B., & Risley, T.R. (1995). *Meaningful differences in the everyday experience of young American children.* Baltimore: Paul H. Brookes Publishing Co.

Hart, B., & Risley, T.R. (1999). *The social world of children learning to talk.* Baltimore: Paul H. Brookes Publishing Co.

Heath, S. (1983). *Ways with words: Ethnography of communication, communities, and classrooms.* Cambridge: Cambridge University Press.

Hoffmeister, R. (1978). *The development of demonstrative pronouns, locatives and personal pronouns in the acquisition of American Sign Language by deaf children of deaf parents.* Unpublished doctoral dissertation, University of Minnesota, Minneapolis.

Israelite, N., Ewoldt, C., & Hoffmeister, R. (1989). *Bilingual/bicultural education for deaf and hard-of-hearing students: A review of the literature on the effective use of native sign language on the acquisition of a majority language by hearing-impaired students.* Toronto: Ministry of Education.

Jamieson, J., & Pedersen, E. (1993). Deafness and mother-child interaction: Scaffolded instruction and the learning of problem-solving skills. *Early Development and Parenting, 2,* 229–242.

Johnson, R., & Erting, C. (1989). Ethnicity and socialization in a classroom for deaf children. In C. Lucas (Ed.), *The sociolinguistics of the deaf community* (pp. 41–83). New York: Academic Press.

Johnson, R., Liddell, S., & Erting, C. (1989). *Unlocking the curriculum: Principles for achieving access in deaf education* (Gallaudet Research Institute Working Paper 89-3). Washington, DC: Gallaudet Research Institute.

Kannapell, B. (1974). Bilingual education: A new direction in the education of the deaf. *The Deaf American, 26*(10), 9–15.

Koester, L., Papousek, H., & Smith-Gray, S. (2000). Intuitive parenting, communication, and interaction with deaf infants. In P. Spencer, C. Erting, & M. Marschark (Eds.), *The deaf child in the family and at school: Essays in honor of Kathryn P. Meadow-Orlans* (pp. 55–72). Mahwah, NJ: Lawrence Erlbaum Associates.

Lane, H., Hoffmeister, R., & Bahan, B. (1996). *A journey into the DEAF-WORLD.* San Diego: Dawn Sign Press.

LaSasso, C. (1999, October). *A national survey of bilingual-bicultural programs serving deaf children in the United States.* Poster session presented at the William C. Stokoe and the Study of Signed Languages conference, Gallaudet University, Washington, DC.

Lederberg, A., & Everhart, V. (2000). Conversations between deaf children and their hearing mothers: Pragmatic and dialogic characteristics. *Journal of Deaf Studies and Deaf Education, 5*(4), 303–322.

Locke, J. (1993). *The child's path to spoken language.* Cambridge, MA: Harvard University Press.

Maxwell, M. (1980). *Language acquisition in a deaf child: The interaction of sign variations, speech, and print variations.* Unpublished doctoral dissertation, University of Arizona, Tucson.

Maxwell, M. (1984). A deaf child's natural development of literacy. *Sign Language Studies, 44,* 191–224.

Mayne, A., Yoshinaga-Itano, C., Sedey, A., & Carey, A. (2000). Expressive vocabulary development of infants and toddlers who are deaf or hard of hearing [Monograph]. *The Volta Review, 100*(5), 1–28.

Meadow, K., Greenberg, M., Erting, C., & Carmichael, H. (1981). Interactions of deaf mothers and deaf preschool children: Comparisons with three other groups of deaf and hearing dyads. *American Annals of the Deaf, 126*(4), 454–468.

Meadow-Orlans, K., MacTurk, R., Prezioso, C., Erting, C., & Day, P. (1987, April). *Interactions of deaf and hearing mothers with three- and six-month-old infants.* Paper presented at the biennial meeting of the Society for Research in Child Development, Baltimore, MD.

Meadow-Orlans, K., MacTurk, R., Spencer, P., & Koester, L. (1991). *Interaction and support: Mothers and deaf infants* (Final Report). Washington, DC: Gallaudet Research Institute.

Mehler, J., Jusczyk, P., Lambertz, G., Halsted, N., Bertoncini, J., & Amiel-Tison, C. (1988). A precursor of language acquisition in young infants. *Cognition, 29*, 143–178.

Meier, R., & Newport, E. (1990). Out of the hands of babes: On a possible sign advantage in language acquisition. *Language, 66*, 1–23.

Moeller, M. (2000). Early intervention and language development in children who are deaf and hard of hearing. *Pediatrics, 106*(3), 1–9.

Newport, E., & Ashbrook, E. (1977). The emergence of semantic relations in American Sign Language. *Papers and Reports on Child Language Development, 13*, 16–21.

Newport, E., & Meier, R. (1985). The acquisition of American Sign Language. In D. Slobin (Ed.), *The crosslinguistic study of language acquisition: Vol. 1. The data* (pp. 881–938). Mahwah, NJ: Lawrence Erlbaum Associates.

Nover, S. (1993, June). *Our voices, our vision: Politics of deaf education.* Paper presented at the biennial conference of the Convention of American Instructors of the Deaf, Baltimore, MD.

Padden, C. (1996). Early bilingual lives of deaf children. In I. Parasnis (Ed.), *Cultural and language diversity and the deaf experience* (pp. 99–116). New York: Cambridge University Press.

Papousek, H., & Papousek, M. (1987). Intuitive parenting: A dialectic counterpart to the infant's precocity in integrative capacities. In J.D. Osofsky (Ed.), *Handbook of infant development* (2nd ed., pp. 669–720). New York: Wiley.

Prinz, P. (Ed.). (1998). ASL proficiency and English literacy acquisition: New perspectives. *Topics in Language Disorders, 18*(4).

Raimondo, B. (2000). Perspective. *Infants & Young Children, 12*(4), ix–xii.

Rogoff, B. (1990). *Apprenticeship in thinking: Cognitive development in social context.* New York: Oxford University Press.

Schieffelin, B., & Gilmore, P. (Eds.). (1986). *The acquisition of literacy: Ethnographic perspectives. Vol. XXI: Advances in discourse processes* (R.O. Freedle, Series Ed.). Norwood, NJ: Ablex.

Schlesinger, H., & Meadow, K. (1972). *Sound and sign: Childhood deafness and mental health.* Berkeley: University of California Press.

Scribner, S., & Cole, M. (1978). Literacy without schooling: Testing for intellectual effects. *Harvard Educational Review, 48*, 448–461.

Slobin, D. (Ed.). (1985). *The crosslinguistic study of language acquisition: Vol. 1. The data.* Mahwah, NJ: Lawrence Erlbaum Associates.

Snow, C. (1983). Literacy and language: Relationships during the preschool years. *Harvard Educational Review, 53*, 165–189.

Snow, C., Barnes, W., Chandler, J., Goodman, I., & Hemphill, L. (1991). *Unfulfilled expectations: Home and school influences on literacy.* Cambridge, MA: Harvard University Press.

Snow, C.E., Tabors, P.O., & Dickinson, D.K. (2001). Language development in the preschool years. In D.K. Dickinson & P.O. Tabors (Eds.), *Beginning literacy with language: Young children learning at home and school* (pp. 1–25). Baltimore: Paul H. Brookes Publishing Co.

Spencer, P. (2000). Every opportunity: A case study of hearing parents and their deaf child. In P. Spencer, C. Erting, & M. Marschark (Eds.), *The deaf child in the family and at school: Essays in honor of Kathryn P. Meadow-Orlans* (pp. 111–132). Mahwah, NJ: Lawrence Erlbaum Associates.

Strong, M. (1995). A review of bilingual/bicultural programs for deaf children in North America. *American Annals of the Deaf, 140,* 84–94.

Strong, M., & Prinz, P. (1996). A study of the relationship between American Sign Language and English literacy. *Journal of Deaf Studies and Deaf Education, 2*(1), 37–46.

Supalla, S. (1994). Equality in educational opportunities: The Deaf version. In C. Erting, R. Johnson, D. Smith, & B. Snider (Eds.), *The Deaf way: Perspectives from the international conference on Deaf culture* (pp. 584–592). Washington, DC: Gallaudet University Press.

Swisher, M. (2000). Learning to converse: How deaf mothers support the development of attention and conversational skills in their young deaf children. In P. Spencer, C. Erting, & M. Marschark (Eds.), *The deaf child in the family and at school: Essays in honor of Kathryn P. Meadow-Orlans* (pp. 21–39). Mahwah, NJ: Lawrence Erlbaum Associates.

Tabors, P.O., Roach, K.A., & Snow, C.E. (2001). Home language and literacy environment: Final results. In D.K. Dickinson & P.O. Tabors (Eds.), *Beginning literacy with language: Young children learning at home and school* (pp. 111–138). Baltimore: Paul H. Brookes Publishing Co.

Tabors, P.O., Snow, C.E., & Dickinson, D.K. (2001). Home and schools together: Supporting language and literacy development. In D.K. Dickinson & P.O. Tabors (Eds.), *Beginning literacy with language: Young children learning at home and school* (pp. 313–334). Baltimore: Paul H. Brookes Publishing Co.

Taylor, D. (1993). *From the child's point of view.* Portsmouth, NH: Heinemann.

Thomas, R., Tillander, M., & Bergmann, R. (1994). Bringing up our children to be bilingual and bicultural. In C. Erting, R. Johnson, D. Smith, & B. Snider (Eds.), *The Deaf way: Perspectives from the international conference on Deaf culture* (pp. 552–561). Washington, DC: Gallaudet University Press.

Traxler, C. (2000). The Stanford Achievement Test, 9th Edition: National norming and performance standards for deaf and hard of hearing students. *Journal of Deaf Studies and Deaf Education, 5*(4), 337–348.

Wallin, L. (1994). The study of sign language in society: Part two. In C. Erting, R. Johnson, D. Smith, & B. Snider (Eds.), *The Deaf way: Perspectives from the international conference on deaf culture* (pp. 318–330). Washington, DC: Gallaudet University Press.

Wertsch, J. (1985). *Vygotsky and the social formation of mind.* Cambridge, MA: Harvard University Press.

Woodward, J. (1972). Implications for sociolinguistic research among the Deaf. *Sign Language Studies, 1,* 1–7.

Early Acquisition of American Sign Language

*Michael Bello, The
Learning Center for Deaf Children*

As an administrator and educator, I can attest to the success of the model program as described in this chapter.

Our school, The Learning Center for Deaf Children (TLC), has fostered early access to American Sign Language (ASL) for families and their deaf children since the late 1980s. At that time, the school implemented a schoolwide systemic change in communication policy and language usage. The school adopted a bilingual educational approach for all students. Early childhood acquisition of ASL was a primary goal and particular attention to creating a fully accessible language environment at school and in the home were and continue to be the cornerstones of the new pedagogy of TLC. The Parent–Infant Program (PIP; birth to 36 months) now provides early, accessible ASL for infants and toddlers, and facilitates the instruction of ASL for parents and provides frequent social and structured interactions between Deaf parents and hearing parents. We have witnessed a dramatic change in our children's readiness for age appropriate preschool and kindergarten activities as a result of this parent–infant programming model. Because of the success of the PIP in helping toddlers acquire a useable language, we have also changed our preschool curricula to include cognitive, linguistic, and literacy goals, which are developmentally similar to that which is taught to 3- and 4-year-old hearing children. The early language acquisition work, which traditionally did not begin until deaf children entered pre-school at age 3, is already accomplished for participating PIP students. Children with a rich language foundation who are already beginning to think are ready for school and are not in need of continued, clinical, early intervention.

Our task does not end in the PIP. When 3-year-old children enter preschool, which is a full day program at our school, they must continue to be taught by professionals who are fluent users of ASL. Our preschool teachers and the children become conversational partners in a discovery learning process. Erting, through a review of the Home–School Study of Language and Literacy Development research, points out the importance of extended conversation at this developmental period for children. Preschool should not be characterized by didactic, teacher-centered instruction. Children at this age need to discover their world through engagement in exciting hands-on cognitive activities, which result in mediated conversations with their teachers and peers. A common, accessible language is necessary to implement this kind of approach during the preschool years; therefore, early ASL acquisition is critical. Through daily participation in a rich language-based classroom, preschoolers develop critical thinking abilities and continued language and literacy development. This program requires the energies of highly skilled teachers who are deliberate and intentional in their preparation of activities. The teachers must be prepared for the engaged, extended conversations that are generated spontaneously by these classroom activities. In addition, a classroom that is alive with a visually accessible language allows deaf children an opportunity for natural incidental learning by "overseeing" conversations of others. A language-accessible environment, an intentional cognitive curriculum, and a program that emphasizes social competency skill development during preschool prepare a child for reading and literacy skill acquisition at the kindergarten level.

In recent years, our school and, in particular the PIP, has served children with cochlear implants. These children, as visual learners, have also benefited greatly from early access to ASL and the resulting extended linguistic interactions that they are then capable of having. With an understanding of the pragmatics of language usage coupled with age-appropriate cognitive development, these children begin to take advantage of their cochlear implants quickly. Their language experience in ASL prepares them to better interpret the auditory information they receive through their implants as meaningful linguistic exchanges. Though we do not have research data, our observations lead us to believe that parents who are planning implant surgery for their children should strongly consider establishing ASL as the first language for their infants and toddlers. As Erting points out, a deaf child is a "seeing child" and the only guaranteed way for a seeing child to learn is through a visual language.

Why gamble during the first few years of a child's life while waiting for an implant? If, as research suggests, the first 3 years of life are the "critical period" for language development, surely one would not want to sacrifice one to two thirds of this period with little understandable linguistic stimulation and potential delay of cognitive development while waiting for the implant surgery and activation. A strong foundation of visual language development coupled with a supportive environment for cognitive development prepares children for second language learning whether it is through audition or writing.

I was pleased to read Erting's suggestion that the proposed bilingual early education centers would include deaf, hard of hearing, and hearing children and adults. The suggested model would provide opportunities to acquire ASL and English in a supportive environment. Our school is piloting a new preschool program this year. The program serves deaf and hard of hearing children as well as children with cochlear implants and children who have normal hearing. The hearing children are sons and daughters of deaf adults or signing siblings of deaf children. Though only several months old, this program is providing a natural environment for both ASL and spoken English interaction for our students.

It is important not to confuse this model with what is typical when a young deaf child is placed in a mainstreamed classroom with hearing peers. The proposed model does not depend on interpreters or any other classroom modification for the deaf children to attain full access to the curriculum and to social, linguistic exchanges with hearing peers. The deaf children in our program and in Erting's suggested model have equal access to both ASL and spoken English and an ability to be full, active participants in all classroom activities. An active participating child is critical at these preschool ages. Passive learning with "pull out" re-teaching is a methodology that all too often characterizes mainstream approaches.

Erting's chapter is significant in its emphasis on language, literacy, and cognition as the building blocks for an early educational program. She and the research she summarizes differentiate between the acquisition of intelligible speech from the more critical acquisition of language. Though I am sure Erting values speech intelligibility for deaf children, she recognizes that it is not the only tool crucial to successful early learning. Improvements in hearing aid and implant technology have generated considerable new research. This research has been primarily focused on evaluating access to sound and speech intelligibility but is relatively silent regarding language acquisition. As an educator, I am concerned that the distinction between meaningful language development and intelligible speech will be a concept increasingly more difficult for parents and medical professionals involved in early identification and referral to understand. As a result, early education programming may be chosen with little or no consideration for the deaf child as a "seeing child" who needs a visual language.

Now more than ever before, the early educational model envisioned by Erting is crucial for the successfully educated deaf child. This model is deserving of more financial support and research. I applaud her efforts to bring it to our attention.

CHAPTER THIRTEEN

Technology

Its Impact on
Education and the Future

JANICE C. GATTY

A parent of a child who had a severe hearing loss was a graphic artist by profession. She was asked to design a brochure that described an evaluation program for infants and toddlers who were deaf and hard of hearing and their families. For the cover of the brochure she selected a photograph of a hearing aid held in a child's open hand. The child's hand lay in the open hand of an adult. When asked why she chose this picture, she said that she thought the hearing aid symbolized the attachment that she initially felt was threatened when she found out her son had a hearing loss. It was the sign of how she and her baby were different from each other. It was also a way to give him access to her world and to join him in his. Comfort, ease, and acceptance of the sensory aid became a touchstone for her acceptance of her son's hearing loss and celebration of his humanness.

For many years I have served as an educator on a team of professionals who work to minimize the negative effects that hearing loss can have on a child's development and maximize the level of the child's involvement in his or her family. The team includes audiologists, speech pathologists, psychologists, and, in some cases, surgeons. Often, my team's role has been to interpret the meaning of a child's behavior in order to make decisions with regard to a particular sensory aid or mode of communication. In some cases, our role has been to help parents understand a particular technology about which they will make a decision for their child. In many cases I mediate among team members with regard to family values and lifestyles, professional knowledge and ethics, and the emotional response that is generated by adults presented with a young child whose future growth and development is affected by the decisions they make. The job is interesting, the situation is usually complicated, and the critical factor is seldom exclusively *technology*.

Practitioners who work with children who are deaf need to be knowledgeable about the availability and efficacy of current technologies in their field. Parents count on professional knowledge. There are several excellent, well-written resources that describe hearing aids and cochlear implants, and the reader is encouraged to consult them. They are written by speech and hearing scientists who have been involved in the study, development, and evaluation of sensory aids (Boothroyd, 1997; Seewald, 1999). The perspective of this chapter, however, is broader. First, this chapter reviews the nature of hearing loss and some generally accepted principles that guide technological research. A brief historical overview of technology is followed by a description of sensory aids: how they work, their benefits and limitations, and a discussion of factors that influence efficacy. The final sections will address the following questions: Who makes decisions about sensory aids and how are they made? What other assistive devices can aid very young children? Where is technological research going? What ethical issues does current technology raise? What does the future hold?

THE NATURE OF HEARING LOSS AND
PRINCIPLES THAT GUIDE TECHNOLOGICAL RESEARCH

There are some basic truths about hearing loss, human nature, and the development of sensory perception and language acquisition that have guided the development of technological devices to aid children who are deaf and hard of hearing. The organ of hearing is small, but the consequences of differences in development in it are large. Without intervention, perceptual, language, cognitive, social, and emotional development can be compromised to an extent that depends, in part, on the severity of the hearing loss.

Our native language, which begins with the birth cry, is acquired in a social-emotional context by interacting with people in our culture who are already fluent. Most children who are deaf and hard of hearing have hearing parents with little or no experience interacting with people who have hearing loss. The language of the family and home is spoken. Without access to sound, and particularly the sounds of the human voice, children who are deaf and hard of hearing do not engage with their parents in the initial stages of the development of spoken language. Trust between the infant and caregiver is based on reciprocity and predictable behavior. Trust can be damaged, putting attachment at risk, if the infants are not responsive to their parents.

Sensorineural hearing loss is not primarily a medical concern, yet hearing parents will generally first turn to doctors for advice, guidance, and treatment. It takes time for parents to understand that deafness is primarily a developmental and educational concern. Increasing accessibility to the environment requires not only sensory assistance but also changes in the child's acoustic, experiential, and language environment. These adaptations should increase accessibility to sound and language in order to reduce the impact of hearing loss on development. Principles of neurological development suggest that consistent accessible sensory input is required to construct a perceptual system, while mastery of a language system requires that the symbols of the language be accessible to the user, as well as daily, consistent, regular use of that language for meaningful purposes.

Educators who specialize in working with children who are deaf and hard of hearing have long believed in the benefits and importance of getting an early start in working with families who have deaf children. In addition to early sensory stimulation and linguistic interaction, parents need time to adjust to the diagnosis of deafness, to become familiar with deafness, and to acquire information about technology, approaches to education, and language acquisition. They must also find out what works best for their family. All of this takes time. There is now empirical evidence that supports the efficacy of early identification and intervention, as well as a body of knowledge in the areas of infant and early neurological stimulation (Moeller, 2000; Yoshinaga-Itano, Sedey, Coulter, & Mehl, 1998). Because of this evidence, efforts have been directed to developing equipment and techniques to measure and optimize hearing status as early as possible in life.

HISTORY

Since the early 19th century, scientists and educators have made systematic efforts to reduce the effects that deafness can have on a child's development in a world in which most people hear. The greatest risk for children who were deaf in the early 19th century was not acquiring their native language. To minimize that risk, some form of sensory assistance was necessary. Most of the tools that resulted from early efforts in this direction worked to substitute the senses of vision and touch for that of hearing. Once the nature and value of residual hearing was recognized, however, acoustic listening devices were also used. These needs and early tools set the stage for technological advances both in auditory enhancement and in the tools that measure hearing (Bentler & Duve, 2000).

Advancements in electronics, computer technology, and telecommunications have offered a wide range of tools to transmit linguistic information to children with imperfect hearing or with no hearing at all (e.g., sensory aids, TTYs). These advancements, together with knowledge about infant development; the benefits of early intervention; and the social, political, and economic climate of education for children who are deaf and hard of hearing in the United States, make the choices for parents and educators much more complicated than they were in the early 1990s.

SENSORY AIDS AND PERCEPTUAL DEVELOPMENT

Sensory aids are devices that attempt to make the sounds of speech accessible through the ears or sometimes the skin. Recent technological efforts to improve the quality of life for infants who are deaf and their families include programmable and digital hearing aids, ear level FM systems, vibrotactile and frequency transposition aids, and cochlear implants.

Hearing Aids and FM Systems

Hearing aids function as small public address systems. They make sound louder to compensate for the loss of sensitivity imposed by sensorineural deafness. One of the effects of sensorineural deafness is that there is also a loss of clarity associated with auditory perception. Hearing aids do not compensate for the loss of clarity. This loss of clarity increases with increasing degree of hearing loss.

Hearing aids contain a microphone that detects sound in the environment. The sound is transmitted to the hearing aid. The circuitry turns sound into electrical information, amplifies it, turns it back into sound, and delivers it to the ear in almost real time. The research and development of hearing aids has been directed as much to making them smaller and less conspicuous as it has to improving the quality with which they deliver sound to the ear. These efforts have led to the availability of behind-the-ear hearing aids for most types of hearing losses and in-the-ear hearing aids for some. Programmable and digital hearing aids have been developed that can provide children with an acoustic signal that remains relatively stable in spite of changes in talker, talker effort, talker distance, and room acoustics. When worn consistently, and in environments that emphasize the use of hearing, modern hearing aids provide many children with moderate and severe degrees of hearing loss with enough auditory information to acquire spoken language through the sense of hearing. Unfortunately, however, hearing aids tend to amplify all sounds, which can make it difficult for the wearer to differentiate a speaker's voice in the presence of background noise.

Another amplification device is the FM system. An FM system consists of a hearing aid receiver, worn by the listener, and an FM microphone transmitter, worn by the speaker. FM systems, like hearing aids, make sound louder, but they have an additional feature to enhance the speech signal at the expense of interfering noise. An auxilliary microphone that works by frequency modulation (FM) transmission can be engaged so that the wearer or listener perceives the voice of the speaker to be in close proximity of the ear, reducing the effects of background noise and increasing the loudness level of the voice. FM systems are good for improving listening conditions in speaker-directed group situations, as the input level of the speaker's voice is increased or made louder while reducing the interference from surrounding noise and reverberation (Boothroyd & Iglehart, 1998).

Group FM systems are used most appropriately in traditional teacher-directed classroom situations when the distance between the teacher or speaker and the children varies or is far, and the children are all learning the same thing at the same time. Use of the FM component in preschool classrooms or open classrooms, however, where there are a number of learning centers and instructors with children engaged in individualized independent instruction, is less appropriate. In such cases the FM feature should only be used when the child is receiving instruction from the person wearing the FM microphone.

With the availability of ear level FM systems, infants and toddlers are being increasingly fit with small personal FM systems. Some parents report that they find this feature is helpful when the children are separated from the talker, as they might be in a car seat. Parents of toddlers, who are more mobile, have found that the FM feature is helpful on outings such as a trip to the zoo, the grocery store, or the park, where the nature of the activity means that the distance of the child and speaker may vary considerably. In general, however, the interaction between caregivers and infants puts them in close physical proximity. Examples include feeding, changing diapers, or rocking. In such situations, an FM system in unnecessary and may even be counterproductive.

It is important to note that conventional amplification devices address only the loss of sensitivity to sound—in other words, even when a hearing aid or FM system produces sounds loud enough for people with profound hearing losses to perceive, they may not always perceive these sounds clearly.

Vibrotactile and Frequency-Transposition Aids

A vibrotactile aid transmits speech sound through vibrators that are worn on the skin. The aid consists of a microphone to detect the sounds of speech and a vibrator or an array of vibrators that vibrates in response to those sounds. The listener can learn to use the vibrotactile patterns on the skin as an aid to interpreting lip movements in speechreading. A frequency-transposition aid functions like a hearing aid except it transposes acoustic information from the area of the speech spectrum in which the child does not have residual hearing to areas where the child seems to have some residual hearing. Both types of sensory aids are recommended for children who have limited low-frequency or no measurable residual hearing (about 10% of the severely or profoundly deaf population). These are the same children who usually receive little benefit from conventional hearing aids. Vibrotactile and frequency-transposition aids have been shown to provide limited benefit to children with minimal residual hearing in research and clinical settings (Kirk et al., 1995; Oller, 1995). They do not, however, offer dramatic benefits in practical application and are not widely used. In fact, a child who does not benefit from conventional amplification would probably receive greater benefit from a cochlear implant than a vibrotactile or frequency-transposition aid.

Cochlear Implants

Cochlear implants can provide most children who have profound and total hearing losses with greater auditory access to spoken language than they would obtain from hearing aids (Christiansen & Leigh, 2002). A cochlear implant is a device consisting of an electrode array that is surgically implanted in the cochlea. The internal device serves as a receiver for acoustic information about speech that is provided by a device worn on the outside of the body. The external device contains a microphone worn at ear level and is connected by a wire to a processor. Both the external and the internal devices have coils that allow sound to be transmitted from the outside to the inside of the head. The two coils are held in close proximity by tiny magnets. The microphone detects sound and sends it to the processor that contains a small computer program. The processor analyzes the sounds and decides how to direct them to the electrode array in the cochlea. These decisions are based on a *map*, which is a set of instructions based on information about the characteristics of the individual child's electrical hearing. The results of this process are sent up to the coil worn on the outside of the head. The information is transferred through the skin to the coil in the internal device and the appropriate electrodes are stimulated. The process takes place almost in real time.

Surgeons report that the procedure for implanting the internal device is relatively straightforward and takes anywhere from 2 to 5 hours. Some children go home the day of surgery. They can return to most daily activities about 1 week after surgery. The external device is fit when the incision is healed completely and swelling is reduced. In young children, this period of time is about 4 weeks. The computer program, or map, on the external processor is set by the audiologist on the cochlear implant team according to the perceptual needs of a particular child. The map is changed periodically as the child becomes adjusted to the sound and as the body adjusts to the presence of the implant. Readjustment of the map occurs frequently early in the process and less often as auditory perception develops. The need for adjustment of the map is often indicated by changes in the child's auditory behavior. As a result, auditory performance needs to be monitored carefully by adults who are good observers. They must also be knowledgeable about the child and about the potential for auditory development as implant users since objective ways to measure an infant's reaction to stimulation are not reliable.

Research has resulted in dramatic improvements in both the internal and external components of cochlear implants. Behind-the-ear processors eliminate the need for a long wire. Arrays with multiple electrodes, positioned close to the nerves of hearing, increase both sensitivity and clarity. Reverse telemetry, a process by which the internal device is able to send information back about the integrity of the electrodes and also about the responses of the auditory nerve to electrical stimulation, allows clinicians to assess how well the internal device is working. There have also been improvements in the speed of the processor and stimulator processing strategies to simulate speech patterns that are more easily detected and recognized by the user. It should be noted that the cochlear implant was designed primarily for speech perception. It can provide the wearer with access to environmental sounds, but research efforts and performance measures are usually defined by the user's ability to perceive speech.

The multichannel cochlear implant first received FDA approval for children in July 1990. Greater experience with and widespread use of the implant have altered the candidacy criteria. Currently, candidates for cochlear implants are children older than 12 months of age, who have worn traditional amplification full-time for 4–6 months in environments in which hearing is a priority, and who show little or no change in auditory behavior. Children without secondary disabilities with an average capacity for social, emotional, cognitive, and language development, and families who will support use of the device are the best candidates.

Perceptual Development

Hearing aids, FM systems, vibrotactile and frequency-transposition aids, and cochlear implants are designed to make the sounds of speech more accessible to children who cannot hear normally. None of these devices restore a normal sense of hearing, but under the right conditions the devices may provide children with enough auditory information to acquire spoken language through hearing. Initially, the sound provided by a sensory aid may not be meaningful, particularly if the child has previously had little or no access to sound. Auditory development requires auditory experience and takes place over time.

Piaget (1952) described the first 2 years of life as the period of sensorimotor development. According to Piaget, the major task of all infants during this stage is to organize sensory impressions, some of which they create into a perceptual scheme that becomes the basis for further cognitive development. Using this perceptual scheme the children come to know and understand the world around them. They learn to associate sensory impressions with each other and with experiences and events that produce them (e.g., the sight and smell associated with looking at a flower; the sight, smell, sound, and touch of playing with a dog; the sight, smell, sound, touch, and taste of "mother" from the experience of nursing). The process of developing a perceptual scheme, such as that of acquiring a native language, is natural, informal, and automatic. It takes place internally and results from interacting with people, objects, and events. During the process, the brain requires that reliable information be delivered consistently by the sense organs. The infant learns to detect, identify, and recognize particular patterns of sensory impressions. When associated with the events that produce them, they become meaningful. The infant then learns to anticipate events based on the sensory impressions associated with them. For example, the infant hears the sounds of footsteps, first quietly, then increasing in intensity with proximity. With experience, the infant begins to differentiate the sounds of footsteps produced by a man, woman, or child. As the sounds of the footsteps get louder and closer, the infant begins to anticipate the sight of a familiar parent, caregiver, or sibling. The preceding sensory events allow infants to prepare for this social experience. They begin to anticipate and prepare for the next set of events: the familiar facial pattern is associated with the sound of a particular voice and maybe a particular greeting.

Perceptual development requires sensory stimulation to be accessible and consistent. Inaccessible or intermittent sensory stimulation inhibits development. Full-time use (i.e., all waking hours) of amplification is required for the brain to develop a perceptual scheme that includes sound. A sensory aid that does not make sound sufficiently salient for a child to hear is obviously ineffective. Intermittent or inconsistent auditory stimulation will not be included in perceptual development. Children who wear hearing aids for only part of the day, children with chronic otitis media that prevents amplified sound from being delivered to the cochlea, or children who are in environments in which sound is not consistently accessible and meaningful, are not likely to receive full benefit from amplification (Pisoni, 2000a).

WHAT FACTORS AFFECT EFFICACY OF DIFFERENT SENSORY AIDS?

Understanding the process of perceptual development offers some insight into how technological assistance can provide children who are deaf and hard of hearing with enough sensory information to allow them to adapt effectively to their environment. The complexity of child development; the variety of environmental factors that are known to affect that course; the influence of the social, political, and economic climate of a particular time and place; and children's families all contribute to the effective use of sensory aids. There is, therefore, no simple formula to determine which sensory aid would provide the greatest benefit to an individual child. Although research efforts may not provide simple answers to questions about efficacy, they have provided a body of knowledge that allows isolation and identification of factors that are known to contribute to the effectiveness of sensory aids used by children who are deaf and hard of hearing. Understanding these factors can provide the information educators and clinicians need to use the tools provided by modern technology.

Hearing Status

Degree of deafness can affect how much benefit a child receives from a hearing aid or cochlear implant. Children with a unilateral or a mild hearing loss (15–30 dB HL) generally have enough access to conversational speech through the sense of hearing that speech and language develop without sensory aids. Hearing status and language development, however, should be monitored to ensure stability and age-appropriate acquisition of auditory and language skills.

Children with moderate hearing loss (31–60 dB HL) who wear hearing aids can usually develop auditory skills and acquire spoken language through the sense of hearing alone. Children with severe hearing loss (61–90 dB HL), who wear appropriate programmable or digital hearing aids and receive special instruction in how to use the information provided by the hearing aids, may learn to understand speech by hearing alone. They may be able to speak on the telephone and their speech should have good rhythm, tone, and articulation. As they mature, these children are described as "hard of hearing" and function as if they are partially hearing. (See Chapter 8 for an in-depth presentation and discussion of the child who is hard of hearing.)

The greatest variability in auditory potential and performance is found in children who have profound hearing loss (91–120 dB HL). Some children with hearing losses of 95 dB are able to function much like a child who is hard of hearing, but many do not. Children with hearing losses of 105 dB, with hearing aids, may be able to perceive the rhythm and tone of speech and may learn to recognize vowels and be able to differentiate some consonants through their sense of hearing. The information provided by a hearing aid is significant, but secondary to other factors such as vision or use of didactic speech instruction in their acquisition of spoken language skills. Research and clinical results (Boothroyd, 1997) increasingly support cochlear implants as the preferred sensory aid in providing children who have profound hearing loss with enough sensory information to adapt to their hearing environment and particularly to acquire spoken language skills.

About 10% of the children who have hearing losses are totally deaf (greater than 120 dB HL) and show no measurable benefit from wearing hearing aids. Children with this degree of hearing loss may be able to perceive the rhythm of speech through the sense of touch and may learn to recognize some environmental sounds such as footsteps or a door closing using a hearing aid. The benefit of a hearing aid is very limited in terms of helping children who are totally deaf to adapt to their environment. Children with total hearing loss have been shown to receive limited benefit from vibrotactile and frequency transposition aids and significant benefit from cochlear implants (Kirk et al., 1995).

Etiology can have an effect on a child's ability to use a sensory aid. Children who are not born deaf but have acquired hearing loss as a result of illness (e.g., meningitis) or ototoxic medications (e.g., chemotherapy) often develop an auditory perceptual system and language before losing their hearing. Their previous experience with sound gives them an advantage with regard to learning to use new sensory information provided by an aid. Etiologies that may involve insult to higher areas in the neurological system such as meningitis, rubella, cytomegalovirus, or Rh-incompatibility can cause a central processing disorder in addition to deafness that may make it more difficult for the child to integrate sensory information from any source into an inclusive perceptual system (Pisoni, 2000a).

The structure or physiological integrity of the cochlea can have an effect on the efficacy of a cochlear implant. The cochlear implant was designed and engineered to fit into the structure of a well-formed cochlea. There are many causes of deafness that affect the hair cell function in the cochlea but leave the structure of the cochlea intact (e.g., a recessive gene such as Connexin 26). In such cases, the prognosis for cochlear implantation is good. There are other causes of hearing loss, however, that can affect the structure of the cochlea, such as absence of a cochlea or meningitis. In such cases, the use of a cochlear implant or hearing aid may be ineffective.

Communication Modality

Sensory devices are designed to make the sounds of speech accessible to people who do not hear. None restores the sense of hearing completely, so the children wearing them must learn to recognize and interpret the auditory information provided by the device and integrate it with other sensory information presented simultaneously during the act of speaking. There is, therefore, a relationship between the efficacy of the sensory aid and the mode of communication used with the child. Children who use cochlear implants in oral programs perceive and produce speech better than do children in total communication programs (Boothroyd, Hannin, & Eran, 1996; Pisoni, 2000b). Children in programs that use sign language emphasizing speech development, however, are likely to evidence increased speech perception and production (see http://clerc center2.gallaudet.edu/KidsWorldDeafNet/e-docs/CI).

The cost and invasiveness of the cochlear implant has led to research to identify factors that affect efficacy. Research on efficacy of cochlear implants demonstrates greater use and effectiveness when worn by children in settings that give high priority to the accessibility of hearing and the development of spoken language. In such environments, attention is given to consistent use and maintenance of the device and to controlling the signal-to-noise ratio in acoustic environments to improve listening conditions. These are usually speech-immersion environments in which teachers and children are expected to rely on spoken language as the primary mode of communication. Knowledgeable adults monitor the child's auditory behavior and performance carefully.

There are, however, dramatic differences of auditory performance among children with implants even within oral programs (Boothroyd, 1997, 1998). Some of these differences may reflect age at implantation. There is growing evidence to support the conclusion that implants and hearing aids are more effective in children who receive them at a young age (Tait, Lutman, & Robinson, 2000; Yoshinaga-Itano & Sedey, 2000). This conclusion follows logically from results of early animal research (Knudsen, Esterly, & Knudsen, 1984; Knudsen, Knudsen, & Esterly, 1984), infant brain research (Raymond, 2000), and studies on early identification and intervention with regard to hearing loss (Calderon & Naidu, 2000; Moeller, 2000; Yoshinaga-Itano et al., 1998), all of which support the perceptual benefits of early sensory stimulation.

There is a need for research on children who have implants and are in bilingual/bicultural programs in which American Sign Language (ASL) is the primary mode of communication. Children in these environments are and will more commonly be using cochlear implants. Children with cochlear implants who are not able to acquire language auditorally may benefit from sign language or another visual modality, such as Cued Speech (Christiansen & Leigh, 2002). It will be important to learn more about the benefits of the device in these environments.

Developmental Factors

The effects of hearing loss on development are more predictable when the capacity for development in all other areas (i.e., motor, cognitive, social-emotional, and language development) are within the typical range. There are deaf children whose language delays can be attributed more to limited cognitive abilities rather than their hearing status. Some deaf children with atypical social-emotional development do not engage in face-to-face communication or use other nonverbal linguistic cues as a source of information. Delays in language acquisition may be as much a result of an inability to establish a social context for language learning as a result of inaccessibility to linguistic symbols. Deaf children who have severe gross or oral motor delays may have delays in language acquisition because of their limited capacities to explore the world or because of their inability to gain control of the speech mechanism. In all of these cases, the efficacy of a sensory aid may be predicted with less confidence. When the sole reason for delay in language acquisition can be explained by a lack of sensitivity to sound, the effectiveness of a particular device can be predicted within limited parameters. Sensory aids only make the child who is deaf more sensitive to sound. When factors other than hearing loss affect development, the potential benefit of the sensory aid is limited (Pisoni, 2000a).

MOLLY

Molly, a 6-year-old girl who has a profound hearing loss, had a developmental assessment. Results suggest that her cognitive and social skills are equivalent to that of a 2-year-old. Her communication skills are equivalent to that of an 18-month-old. Autism and limited cognitive capacity are suspected to contribute to delays in language acquisition as much as her hearing loss. Molly has participated in an ASL immersion program for 4 years. The diagnostic question for parents and professionals is whether Molly will benefit from a cochlear implant. The question is one that must be addressed at several levels. First, will she receive auditory benefit from the device? Probably. With experience and practice she will probably be able to produce consistent, observable responses to sound. She may produce a repertoire of sounds. Will she use the device to acquire spoken language? Probably not. Her ability to acquire language in a program designed for children who do not hear, using a language mode that is fully accessible through vision, has been limited. In addition, other developmental capacities have been identified as contributing factors in language acquisition. Would it be wise to place this child in an oral program designed for deaf children who use implants to acquire spoken language? Probably not. This child has made progress, albeit limited, in the educational program in which she has participated. Her social, emotional, cognitive, and general developmental needs take precedence over the sensory (i.e., auditory) needs associated with learning to use a particular sensory aid. In cases such as Molly's the implant may provide some sensory benefit and parents should pursue evaluations for candidacy with the understanding that sensory information from the device will probably not contribute to language acquisition.

TECHNOLOGICAL DECISIONS:
WHO MAKES THEM AND HOW ARE THEY MADE?

The single greatest risk for children who are deaf with hearing parents is that of not acquiring adequate language skills. Language gives access to the minds of others. Without it, language, social, emotional, and cognitive development are severely compromised. For very young children, the goal of choosing an appropriate sensory aid is to assist them in acquiring language. Quite simply there is no single technology that is equally effective for all children who are deaf and hard of hearing. The technological nature of hearing aids, the medical nature of the cochlear implant, and the educational nature of hearing loss require a team of people to make decisions about specific technological devices.

In theory, a *team approach* is the most respectful way to make choices about how to encourage the development of a child who is deaf or hard of hearing. The factors that contribute to choosing a mode of communication, an educational approach, and an educational setting are numerous. Knowledge of the child's developmental abilities and parents' values and wishes contribute to effective implementation of any decision. The same is true when selecting a particular technology or sensory aid.

In practice, however, a team approach to selecting a sensory aid can make parents and some practitioners feel ignorant, excluded, and judged by more technologically knowledgeable members of the team. Some parents have reported a perceived ineffectiveness of the team approach, and there is some evidence of this in professional literature (Hanson & Bruder, 2001).

Who Is on the Team?

Initially a team may consist of the parents, an audiologist, early intervention professionals, such as an educator of the deaf and/or speech pathologist, and any others who may have significant information about a child's medical or developmental conditions. When families are considering a cochlear implant, the team may be joined by a cooperating hospital's cochlear implant team, which usually includes an audiologist and otolaryngologist.

How Do Teams Get Started?

Best practice for establishing candidacy for a cochlear implant requires the child to establish full-time use of a conventional hearing aid for a diagnostic period of 4 to 6 months before being evaluated for a cochlear implant (NIH Consensus Statement, 1995). This period of time is important for everyone on the team. The child gets experience wearing a prosthetic device and experience in listening to sound. The parents get practice in maintaining and coming to terms with the benefits and limitations of a sensory aid and observing their child's behavioral changes in response to sound. The managing audiologist and early intervention specialists can observe the child's response to sound, abilities in acquiring communication skills, and learning style. In addition, the team learns to work together. If the team decides that the child is a candidate for a cochlear implant, then the managing team needs to coordinate services and exchange of information with a cochlear implant team. If the child receives an implant, the audiologist on the cochlear implant team usually assumes subsequent audiological management.

Who Leads the Team?

The process of choosing a particular technology or sensory aid is similar to the process of choosing an approach to communication or education: parents are making decisions that will affect the course of their child's development and future. The successful implementation of a particular technology or device will be affected by a family's lifestyle, values, and expectations; their approach to communication and education; and their available resources.

For example, cochlear implants provide the greatest sensory assistance when used in environments that emphasize hearing and spoken language; cochlear implants provide less benefit to the child who is in an environment where language is not spoken and hearing is not valued. In addition, the implant is a high maintenance device. After initial stimulation the child often participates in intensive one-to-one therapy to learn to use the new sensory information provided by the device. The child's auditory behavior must be closely monitored and recorded to provide data on how the device is working so that appropriate adjustments can be made in the map of the external processor. Implant teams are usually located in medical centers in urban areas. Often, support services are not available in rural areas. Frequent trips to the implant center are required early in the process to establish candidacy, prepare for surgery, and ensure an appropriate map and use of the device. Replaceable parts for implants are less accessible partly because of the individualized nature of the device but mostly because it is used less frequently than conventional hearing aids. Processors can break and implant centers usually have mechanisms for relatively quick repair and replacement. It is unlikely, however, that a local audiologist would have a loaner stock of external processors that simplify the repair process. Of great concern to parents is the stability of the internal device. Failure of the internal device requires surgery for replacement and repair. In short, successful use of the cochlear implants usually requires that families have resources in the form of time, energy, transportation, available services, and in some cases, money, to ensure effective, consistent use of the device.

Implementation of any technology or sensory aid requires great support from the home environment. The expectations that parents have of their child's behavior when wearing a sensory aid (e.g., full-time use,

use of sensory input for speech production) influence the child's performance with the aid. It makes sense, then, that the decision about what
technology to use should be family-centered and that the parents should
be the leaders of the decision-making team.

In American culture, parents are seen as the decision makers in
most aspects of their child's life. Special education laws, such as the
Education for All Handicapped Children Act of 1975 (PL 94-142) and
the Education of the Handicapped Act Amendments of 1986 (PL 99-
457), were written so that parents make the decision regarding the
services they may accept or reject. There are other cultures, however,
where parental autonomy is not highly valued, and adults have different
views on the boundaries of their control as parents. In such cultures,
parents may see themselves as nurturers and caregivers of young children
but view education as the responsibility of teachers, habilitation as the
responsibility of therapists, or deafness as a medical disability in which
advice from the doctor is valued above that of other professionals. In
such cultures, parents may have a hard time seeing themselves as leaders
of the team and may look to someone else to assume that role. Some
professionals may want to assume this role "for the sake of the child's
development." Others may see this behavior as fundamentally in conflict
with a commitment to family-centered intervention. Ultimately, this situation can cause great angst and frustration among team members and
affect communication with the family and the quality and effectiveness
of intervention for the child. If the issue of locus of control is identified as
a factor in providing effective intervention, it can be aired and discussed
directly and openly among professionals and the family. Such discussions
can lend insight into the perspective and values of the family as well as
team members. It is only after these viewpoints are recognized and
respected that the team has a chance of making good choices for the child.

When Is a Decision Appropriate?

The role of the professionals on the team is to educate parents about
the benefits and limitations of a particular technology and the factors
that contribute to efficacy and consequences so that they are informed
and confident in the decisions they make. Counseling and educating
parents and assisting them in developing realistic expectations without
undermining their hopes and aspirations for the future of their child's
development is difficult to do well. A team of professionals will know
that they have done this part of their job well, and that a particular
decision is appropriate, when the child and family are comfortable with
the choice of sensory aid: The child wears the sensory aid during all of
his or her waking hours and uses it to develop a perceptual system that

aids in the acquisition of language, the parents participate fully in their child's acquisition of language, and they enjoy the process of their child's growth and development as a complete and unique individual.

When Should a Decision Be Re-evaluated?

There are a variety of behaviors that suggest that the process of choosing a sensory aid is not working. Clear indicators would include the following: a family's interest in but inability to make a choice of a sensory aid, a child's refusal to wear a sensory aid, an adult's reluctance to put the aid on the child, or attention focused more on the sensory aid itself rather than on language development. Practitioners can support parents through this process by re-evaluating the choices of the aid, the educational program, communication options, and the role of other factors in efficacy.

What if Auditory and Language Skills Fail to Develop?

The timetable for perceptual development and language acquisition is different for all children. The rate at which individual children acquire perceptual and linguistic skills is affected by many variables: the accessibility of sensory input, the richness of the sensory and linguistic environment, the integrity of the neurological system, the temperament of the child, and the child's native ability or potential for development in these areas. Observation, monitoring, and re-evaluation of decisions made with regard to the sensory aid and mode of communication should be ongoing among members of the educational team, minimally every 6 months to make sure the child is acquiring language skills at an appropriate pace.

OTHER ASSISTIVE TECHNOLOGIES

Assistive technologies refer to all of the devices, aids, or procedures that can improve the quality of life for people who are deaf and hard of hearing. In addition to sensory aids, assistive technologies include other kinds of devices and diagnostic procedures for identification of hearing loss in newborns and identification of genes associated with deafness.

Assistive devices, other than sensory aids, refer to those devices that make environmental sounds accessible through the sense of vision or touch. Some devices include flashing lights connected to doorbells, telephones and alarm systems, vibrating alarm clocks, telephones for the deaf with a printed display of the conversation among parties (e.g., TTY), closed captioning devices, CART (captioning in real time) reporting, augmentative communication boards, voice activated computers, pagers, and so forth. Most assistive devices are used by school-age children and adults as adaptive devices to permit greater access and autonomy in the home and school environment. Installation of assistive devices, such as flashing lights to indicate the telephone is ringing or that someone is as the door, are helpful in providing young children with information about environmental activities usually associated with acoustic events and allowing them to anticipate the events that follow. A strong case can be made for using television captioning with preschool children who are deaf and hard of hearing as a way of highlighting and promoting early literacy.

GENETIC AND HAIR CELL REGENERATION RESEARCH

Genetic and hair cell regeneration research are made possible by advances in computer and biomedical technology. Both are likely to lead to a greater understanding of deafness and the way genes and the cochlea function.

Genetic research has made it possible to isolate and identify several nonsyndromic recessive genes that are associated with deafness. About two thirds of hereditary deafness is nonsyndromic, suggesting that children will exhibit no other clinical concerns in addition to hearing loss (Palacio, 2000; Rehm, 2000). Parents who have no family history of deafness can find out if there is a genetic predisposition for having children who are deaf by results from a blood test.

Hair cell regeneration research on rats, mice, and birds suggests that hair cells in the cochlea can be regenerated using tissue transplants. The function of these cells, however, is as yet undetermined (Cotanche, 2000). Although this research is currently being conducted on animal and adult human populations, the preliminary results lay groundwork for the restoration of the nerve fibers in the cochlea, thus restoring the capacity to hear (Seppa, 2000).

Both of these research areas, as well as neonatal identification of deafness, raise ethical considerations for parents and professionals regarding the use of knowledge from this kind of research.

ETHICAL CONSIDERATIONS

The threads of ethnocentrism, a belief or attitude that one's own group is superior to another, are deeply rooted in human nature. Tribal wars in South America and Africa, the Civil War in our own country, and World War II, were largely the result of fear, bigotry, and discrimination associated with ethnocentric beliefs. At the beginning of the 21st century, travel and media have made cultures around the world more familiar to everyone. The politics of education in America attempt to address the richness that diversity among cultures adds to the mainstream. Legislation (e.g., the Individuals with Disabilities Education Act Amendments of 1997, PL 105-17) has addressed the issues of accessibility in populations whose linguistic, cultural, or physical status would limit their access to resources in the mainstream culture. It is possible for many families to have real choices in the decisions they make for their children, and when their children who are deaf and hard of hearing grow up, they can take pride in the uniqueness of their hearing status, their language, and their culture.

Ethnocentrism is rooted so deeply in human nature that it has affected the course of research in education of the deaf for the past 200 years. A systematic, scientific search for truth is acceptable unless the results begin to threaten those beliefs that we consider to be essentially human about our species. The emergence of the Deaf culture and the identification of a deaf person as culturally Deaf (the roots of which can be traced to the case of *Brown v. Board of Education*) has contributed greatly to the mainstream culture's understanding of deafness in a way that research efforts have not.

Nothing threatens the structure of Deaf culture and undermines the identity of the Deaf as much as technology (National Association for the Deaf, n.d.). The use of cochlear implants in very young children, hair cell generation research, and even genetic research and counseling can be seen by some as attempts to restore the sense of hearing and eliminate the Deaf culture. One couple, for example, approached a physician about the possibility of using genetic engineering to ensure that their second child would not be born deaf. The physician was shocked and commented on the ethics of such a request, but this likely is not an isolated case.

Parents imagine their children in their own image. They look for likeness to themselves in their offspring from the time they are born. Most deaf children have hearing parents with little or no direct experience with deafness. It should not be surprising that they want their child to hear as they do; that they want their child to speak as they do. Without any direct experience with deafness, it is difficult for them to imagine how their child will grow and develop.

The benefits of early identification depend on the timely establishment of an appropriate program of early intervention for the child and family. Part of that process means choosing a sensory aid and a mode of communication at a time in development when the infant has limited ways of giving feedback as to what is likely to be successful. Parents are making decisions about sensory aids that will be used by their newborn infants before they know the infant or much about the nature of deafness.

In addition, the infant's response to sensory stimulation may not be easily observed depending on the degree of hearing loss, the neurological integrity of the child, and the device in question.

The challenge of early intervention will be to keep the focus broad. The rate at which parents acquire knowledge and understanding about deafness and the decisions they make about priorities and allocation of resources varies greatly among families. Families need professionals to support them in their efforts to decide which sensory aids and communication systems will work best for them and their child. Early intervention programs, regardless of their methodological affiliation or technological preferences, have a moral and ethical responsibility to present options in an unbiased manner and to evaluate the effectiveness of their approach with the children and families in their programs. They should take pride in the success of their efforts only when every participant is reaching his or her potential for development. This means that professionals must be prepared to support and guide families to alternative programs whose approach to habilitation, education, or sensory management may be more congruent with a child's learning style or an adult's style of parenting.

SUMMARY

The wonders of modern technology can offer deaf children greater accessibility to the world around them. We must not lose sight of the fact that technology has never offered and is still not a simple solution to the challenges of being deaf in a world in which most people hear. Technology provides professionals and parents with some tools to identify and quantify deafness in very young children and to make the auditory and linguistic environment more accessible to them. But solutions that ensure the fullest development—and fullest life experience—for deaf children will have to come from the people who understand both the possibilities and the limitations of technological solutions: It is educators and clinicians who must learn how best to use the tools provided by modern technology so that they can share this information with families of children who are deaf and hard of hearing.

REFERENCES

Bentler, R., & Duve, M. (2000). Comparison of hearing aids over the 20th century. *Ear & Hearing, December,* 625–639.

Boothroyd, A. (1997). Auditory capacity of hearing-impaired children using hearing aids and cochlear implants: Issues of efficacy and assessment. *Scandinavian Audiology, 26*(Suppl. 46), 17–25.

Boothroyd, A. (1998). Evaluating the efficacy of hearing aids and cochlear implants in children who are hearing-impaired. In F.H. Bess (Ed.), *Children with hearing impairment: Contemporary trends* (pp. 249–260). Nashville: Vanderbilt Bill Wilkerson Center Press.

Boothroyd, A., Hannin, L., & Eran, O. (1996). Speech perception and production of children with hearing impairment. In F.H. Bess, J.S. Gravel, & A.M. Tharpe (Eds.), *Amplification for children with auditory deficits* (pp. 55–74). Nashville: Vanderbilt Bill Wilkerson Center Press.

Boothroyd, A., & Iglehart, F. (1998). Experiments with classroom FM amplification. *Ear and Hearing, 19,* 202–217.

Brown v. Board of Educ., 347 U.S. 483 (1954).

Calderon, R., & Naidu, S. (2000). Further support for the benefits of early identification and intervention for children with hearing loss [Monograph]. *The Volta Review, 100*(5), 53–84.

Christiansen, J., & Leigh, I. (2002). *Cochlear implants in children: Ethics and choices.* Washington, DC: Gallaudet University Press.

Cotanche, D. (2000, July 9). Hair cell regeneration and the development of a biological cochlear implant. In *Biotechnology and the cochlea.* Research Symposium for Non-Scientists conducted at the A.G. Bell 2000 International Convention, Philadelphia.

Hanson, M., & Bruder, M. (2001). Early intervention: Promises to keep. *Infants and Young Children, 13*(3), 47–58.

Individuals with Disabilities Education Act Amendments of 1997, PL 105-17, 20 U.S.C. §§ 1400 *et seq.*

Kirk, K., Osberger, M., Robbins, A., Riley, A., Todd, S., & Miyamoto, R. (1995). Performance of children with cochlear implants, tactile aids, and hearing aids. *Seminars in Hearing, 16*(4), 370–381.

Knudsen, E., Esterly, S., & Knudsen, P. (1984). Monaural occlusion alters sound localization during a sensitive period in the barn owl. *Journal of Neuroscience, 4,* 1001–1011.

Knudsen, E., Knudsen, P., & Esterly, S. (1984). A critical period for the recovery of sound localization accuracy following monaural occlusions in the barn owl. *Journal of Neuroscience, 4,* 1012–1020.

Moeller, M.P. (2000). Early intervention and language development in children who are deaf and hard of hearing. *Pediatrics, 106*(3), 1–9.

National Association of the Deaf. (n.d). *Cochlear implants in children: A position paper of the National Association of the Deaf.* Silver Spring, MD: Author.

NIH Consensus Statement. (1995, May 15). *Cochlear implants in adults and children.* 13(2), 1–30.

Oller, D.K. (1995). Tactile Aids for the hearing impaired: An overview. *Seminars in Hearing, 16*(4), 289–295.

Palacio, M. (2000, August 14). The new genetics of deafness. *Advance for Speech-Language Pathologists & Audiologists,* 7–10.

Piaget, J. (1952). *The language and thought of the child.* London: Routledge & Kegan.

Pisoni, M. (2000a). Cognitive factors and cochlear implants: Some thoughts on perception, learning, and memory in speech perception. *Ear and Hearing, 21*(1), 70–78.

Pisoni, M. (2000b, November 20). In search of pre-implant predictors for pediatric patients with cochlear implants. *Advance for Speech-Language Pathologists & Audiologists,* 7–8.

Raymond, J. (2000) The world of the senses. *Newsweek Special Issue: Your Child,* 16–18.

Rehm, H. (2000, November–December). The genetics of deafness. *Volta Voices*, 10–16.

Seewald, R. (1999). Assistive hearing technologies. In D. Luterman (Ed.), *The young deaf child* (pp. 149–184). Baltimore: York Press.

Seppa, N. (2000). New inner early hair cells grown in rat tissue. *Science News*, *157*, 342.

Tait, M., Lutman, M., & Robinson, K. (2000). Preimplant measure of preverbal communicative behavior as predictors of cochlear implant outcomes in children. *Ear and Hearing*, *21*(1), 18–24.

Yoshinaga-Itano, C., & Sedey, A. (2000). Early speech development in children who are deaf or hard of hearing: Interrelationships with language and hearing [Monograph]. *The Volta Review*, *100*(5), 181–211.

Yoshinaga-Itano, C., Sedey, A., Coulter, D., & Mehl, A. (1998). Language of early- and later-identified children with hearing loss. *Pediatrics*, *102*, 1161–1171.

Suggestions for Further Development

Jennifer Rosner, mother of a child who was diagnosed at birth with a severe hearing impairment

The technological aspect of hearing impairment can be daunting and mysterious, and Gatty's chapter presents information about technological options that can be very useful.

There are four topics that I would have liked to see discussed in more depth and detail (of course, I recognize that length constraints are an issue):

- New parents of deaf and hard of hearing children unwittingly enter a highly charged political climate and it can be quite difficult to navigate through. Nearly every perspective turns out to be politically laden, and very few consider the individual child's unique situation to be the primary guide to choosing modes of communication, education, and technological aid. Sometimes the politicization is subtle, and it can be exhausting and difficult for parents to sort out the influences that affect the advice and information that they receive.

- Parents of newborns have to make decisions for their children at a time when their children's identities are undeclared, underdetermined, and hence unknowable. This can be a burden of great proportion to thoughtful parents because every choice creates but also forecloses on a variety of options and opportunities.

(When I told someone that we decided to pursue an oral approach for my daughter who was then just 4 months old, the person said, "Why don't you let her be who she is?" to which I replied, "Who is she?")

- There are nonobjective aspects of audiology (leading to choices of technology) that go unrecognized in the field. Different audiologists interpret the auditory brainstem response (ABR) test information differently. We have been given three different opinions as to the degree and exact specification of my daughter's hearing loss (each obtained in close time proximity at leading institutions: the University of California at San Francisco, Stanford University, and Children's Hospital in Boston). Hearing aids are digitally programmed according to one interpretation and we continue to wonder whether it is the "right" one. It would be refreshing to have "aired" some of the subjectivity and basic unclarity parents encounter.

- Most educators, audiologists, and social workers (and parents!) are not hearing impaired, and the advice and information parents receive from them is not based in personal experience of hearing impairment. Deaf adults who have used the technology and communication modes are one of the most important sources of information.

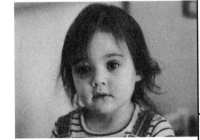

Research
Models

CHAPTER FOURTEEN

Redefining Family-Centered Services

Early Interventionist as Ethnographer

LAURA A. BLACKBURN

"I need more!" and "How do I know I'm making the right choice for my child?" are common statements made by the mother of the deaf child described in this chapter. This mother, however, is not alone in her bewilderment—parents of children who are deaf frequently ask these questions, which are rarely viewed as unusual by service providers. The most significant question for early interventionists who work with these children and their families is, When will these questions be answered and by whom?

Early interventionists working with children who are deaf have made good progress toward answering these questions, providing recent groundbreaking answers from the fields of linguistics and education. For example, linguists have provided conclusive evidence that American Sign Language (ASL) is a true language in its own right. At the same time, some educators have expanded those findings to describe the ease of ASL acquisition among hearing family members (Singleton, Supalla, Litchfield, & Schley, 1998), as well as the significant role ASL has in supporting deaf students' full acquisition of print English in the classroom (Supalla, Wix, & McKee, 2001). Another possible solution is to redefine the professional roles and responsibilities of early interventionists who work with children who are deaf and their families. This chapter proposes a model that expands on the traditional roles of early interventionists and family members by incorporating anthropological research methods into the picture of family-centered service delivery. Selected early intervention practices are explored with recommendations for how to enhance these processes, using case study excerpts to demonstrate these redefined practices (Blackburn, 1999). Examples show how early interventionists, evolving into "ethnographic interventionists," can become more effective parent advisors and educators by using an anthropological backdrop for service delivery. The benefits to the children and family members engaged in the process also are highlighted.

THE PERSPECTIVE OF THE DEAF CHILD

Regardless of the language or modality that hearing and deaf family members use to communicate with one another, family members with different hearing status generally view the world in different ways (Blackburn, 1999, 2000). This arrangement can create an intrinsic tension that can lead to cultural conflict among deaf and hearing family members (Erting, 1982/1994). Deaf and hearing people generally organize their thoughts and actions in everyday life quite differently. Erting describes being biologically deaf or hearing as one of the central organizing conditions of the human experience. People who are deaf shape their understanding of the world primarily through visual experiences alone, while individuals who can hear shape their understanding of the world through visual and auditory channels simultaneously (Erting, 1982/1994).

Take, for example, the task of cooking dinner. A person who hears might cook dinner for his or her family while simultaneously listening to the evening news, attending to the activities of the home (i.e., the children playing in the next room and the oven timer), and chopping vegetables for the salad. Hearing children would be accustomed to their caregiver listening to them and would expect to hear their caregiver's voice coming from the kitchen with comments such as, "Play nicely with your sister!"

A person who is deaf might choose to do all of the same tasks but would most likely complete them consecutively rather than simultaneously. The caregiver's work environment would be arranged differently so that he or she is positioned to see (rather than hear) his or her children playing. The children would expect frequent eye contact with their caregiver and would anticipate visual directives about their play behavior while he or she is preparing the meal. The deaf caregiver's in-kitchen activities would differ in that his or her eyes would quickly glance from the oven timer to the captioned television screen and back to the chopping block. Although seemingly stark in contrast, these two scenarios present the foundational element of the deaf child's unique learning and growing circumstances.

The deaf child's situation is further shaped by the fact that most children who are deaf (90%) are born into hearing families, creating multiple home environments in which cultural tension can occur among the deaf child and his or her family members (Blackburn, 1999, 2000; Erting, 1982/1994). The idea of cultural conflict existing between parent and child may seem odd or even incomprehensible to those who are new to the idea. How could parent and child, who in many cases possess the same biological history, live in the same environment, eat the same foods, and breathe the same air, experience cultural conflict?

Ethnographers study these intersections of culture by observing the artifacts that individuals bring to their physical environment as well as human language use and behavior (Spradley, 1979, 1980). An artifact is an object (often material and containing some sort of writing that serves as a channel for language and/or communication) that is unique to a group or society of people. Artifacts exemplify or symbolize what the people from that society value and find important for their survival or success. For example, typical artifacts in the home of a person who is deaf would be a printed conversation from a teletext telephone communication device (TTY), flashing lights attached to the doorbell, or a hearing aid. Cultural differences and ensuing conflicts are systematically observable when people use different languages, when the ways they orient themselves socially or linguistically cause them to behave differently, or when they use different artifacts or use the same artifacts differently for success (i.e., survival) in the same environment.

Families with both deaf and hearing members are more likely to misunderstand communicative interactions with one another because of differences in language use (i.e., signed language versus spoken language), sometimes misinterpreting intent or missing the meaning entirely (Blackburn, 1999). For example, maintaining eye contact is a critical part of using signed language effectively and politely with individuals who are deaf. People who are learning signed language as a second language frequently insult individuals who are deaf when communicating because they become distracted by a noise in the environment or a spoken language conversation and break eye contact with the person who is deaf in mid-conversation. Breaking eye contact or gazing away from a conversation with a friend who is deaf is as destructive as turning one's back on a friend in the midst of a spoken language conversation to speak with someone else without warning or proper closure.

These language and modality differences also produce differences in behaviors as family members move about the home (i.e., people using signed languages must communicate with one another face-to-face although people using spoken languages can communicate face-to-face or from another room). The physical arrangement of the house or devices such as doorbells, telephones, TTYs, and open captions on the television may serve either to contribute to or reduce cultural conflict in the home until the perimeters of their use are properly defined.

FROM EARLY INTERVENTIONIST
TO ETHNOGRAPHIC INTERVENTIONIST

The deaf child's unique situation presents the need for several changes in early intervention supports that expand the traditional model. For example, because we know that children who are deaf grow up in families with other deaf and hearing members, in which both visual and combined visual/auditory channels of communication are prevalent, it seems that an ethnographic intervention model would better serve young deaf children who require intervention, as there are cultural tensions present that need to be resolved. Changing and expanding the traditional intervention model requires changing the roles and titles of the professionals working with deaf children and their families. What if the early interventionist became the ethnographic interventionist, including ethnographic methods as a critical piece in the early intervention process? Although the traditional intervention model may provide introductory information for parents about the medical conditions or the language and communication needs of their deaf child, this proposed ethnographic intervention model supports family interactions and educating the individuals involved about cultural behaviors. Table 14.1 highlights the distinctions between the traditional intervention model and the proposed ethnographic intervention model.

The vignettes in the following sections are true stories about a young child who is deaf and his hearing family members who voluntarily participated for 2 years in an ethnographic intervention model. The names and some demographic information have been changed so that the family's privacy is protected. Henry Camillo is a 4-year-old deaf child whose first language is ASL. He is the second born of six children, all under the age of 7. Henry's five siblings and parents are hearing. His family uses spoken English at home but is committed to learning and using ASL as well. They often invite members of the Deaf community into their home for special dinners, school projects, and family celebrations. The

Table 14.1. A traditional intervention model versus an ethnographic intervention model

Traditional intervention model	Ethnographic intervention model
Individual needs of the child and family members are addressed separately within the context of the family.	Individual needs of the child and family members are addressed within the context of family interactions.
The curriculum is designed to restore the loss of sound and the ability to hear in the child's life and environment (e.g., therapeutic and medical emphasis).	The curriculum is designed to enhance the child and family's understanding of language and cultural interactions (e.g., linguistic and cultural emphasis).
The majority of "service provision" time is spent in school/clinical settings.	The majority of "service provision" time is spent in the home setting.
Data gathered are used for diagnosis and progress-reporting purposes.	Data gathered are used regularly for educational purposes (i.e., parents view videotaped observations and interviews with the ethnographic interventionist so they can learn and reflect on their own actions and comments).
Maximizes use of intervention strategies that focus on intervening in the child and family system in order to identify and pull in outside resources that can provide support.	Maximizes use of self-assessment and observation strategies to focus on teaching the family to understand and strengthen its own existing infrastructure.
The curriculum can be sound based and/ or language based.	The curriculum is primarily language based.

following scenarios are examples of what cultural conflict looks like in the home of a 4-year-old deaf child whose immediate and extended family members hear.

A DIFFERENT LANGUAGE
MODALITY LEADS TO CULTURAL CONFLICT

Henry's mother Sara expressed concern to the early interventionist because she felt Henry was too needy of her time and attention. She shared that Henry demanded more of her time than the hearing children in the family did because communicating with him required face-to-face contact. Sara asked the early interventionist, "Why does he bother me at the most inopportune times? He always interrupts me when I'm on the telephone to ask me who I'm talking to. And yesterday I had my hands full with frozen meat when I was cleaning out the freezer. He insisted that I stop to explain what I was doing! Wasn't it obvious what I was doing if the freezer door was open and my arms were full of frozen meat?"

Sara received several recommendations regarding this family challenge. The most popular solution recommended was for Sara to spend more face-to-face communication time with all of her children in order not to show favoritism and to reinforce the idea that one-to-one conversations between parent and child are a positive step that can reduce their need for individual attention. When the early interventionist was asked why she had chosen this particular strategy to solve Sara's problem, she justified her choice because of the limited amount of time Sara spent with the family and because the plan met the needs of all the children, thus making it a family-centered recommendation. Sara, however, found the recommendations to be impractical—with six children under the age of 7 years, Sara simply did not have time to converse one-to-one with each child everyday. Sara felt that the interventionist based her recommendation on Sara's statements alone and did not take the time to "walk in her shoes" and view the situation through Sara's eyes in an attempt to solve the problem. Sara had hoped for practical recommendations that she could apply specifically to her family of eight, rather than general advice that was more applicable for families with two or three children. It is possible that Henry and Sara's mutual frustrations persisted until, in her opinion, he "outgrew his needy stage and learned to figure things out for himself."

Imagine if there were a way for early interventionists to provide parents with tools that would allow them to solve problems on their own without consulting professionals for opinions or ideas. What if families could learn to be more systematic and efficient when assessing their family's situation, identifying and solving their own cultural tensions before they became conflicts? By preparing early interventionists as ethnographers, there is a solution to this scenario that is more family centered and empowering than the services and approaches that are currently available.

In this case, the real-life scenario had a positive outcome, as the ethnographic interventionist was able to extend the early interventionist's services and continue to work with Sara to solve her problem. They began with the foundational understanding that Henry did require one-to-one attention from his mother, as did his other five siblings. However, they expanded this developmentally appropriate information to a cultural level of understanding. Sara learned about the differences in how deaf and hearing individuals access information in their environment (i.e., deaf people via a visual channel and hearing people via both a visual and an auditory channel). Regarding her interactions with her children, Sara felt that Henry was demanding more of her attention because his signed language requires her direct eye contact to engage in every conversation. Sara learned that she isn't consciously aware of having numerous spoken language conversations with her hearing children while being involved in a variety of other activities because she is not required to stop what she is doing and redirect her eye gaze.

The ethnographic interventionist taught Sara this information by leading her through an activity that involved making lists about her daily activities with her children and learning to systematically observe her interactions with them. First, Sara was asked to make a concrete list of all the interactive situations when she became frustrated with Henry's needy behavior (i.e., he interrupts telephone conversations, he dominates conversations at the dinner table, his topics of conversation are very "me" oriented). Next, Sara had to compare Henry's view of the situation (visual only), his sibling's view (visual and auditory), and her own (also visual and auditory) in these specific situations.

In this circumstance, the task of the ethnographic interventionist effectively expanded the traditional role of early interventionist. Teaching her more insight about Henry's behavior solved Sara's problem. Next she was taught how to contrast Henry's way of viewing things with the views of her other (hearing) children. This process is an ethnographic procedure that encourages the examination of cultural barriers and how they are broken down. Providing parents with these new types of strategies for interaction and communication serves to reduce cultural tensions within the home and build increasingly family-centered environments. The acquisition of these skills helped Sara apply her new knowledge about cultural conflict to interactions with all family members, not just her interactions with Henry.

DISCREPANT BEHAVIORS LEAD TO CULTURAL CONFLICT

The Camillo family is packing their car for a weekend day-trip to visit cousins. Henry is fully dressed at 7:30 A.M., positioning himself on the staircase landing that overlooks the living room, kitchen, upstairs hallway, and front porch steps. Henry's older brother and younger sister are packing and carrying items to the car for the trip. His mother is in the kitchen making bottles and snacks for the trip—verbally directing the packing activities of her husband and Henry's hearing siblings. Henry's father, Mark, asks him several times to go to the basement to get toys for the infants to play with in the car. Each time Henry nods that he understands and even asks his father what toys he should get (i.e., a teething book for Luke and a wind-up toy for Mary). However, as departure time draws nears, Henry does not move from the steps. He glances at the basement door, asks his brother how much time is left before they leave ("10 minutes," then "5 minutes"). As the family heads out the door to get in the car, Henry gets into trouble because he has not left his perch on the stairs to retrieve toys for the infants from the basement. Mark asks the inevitable question with irritation, "What toys did you pick out for the infants?" Mark puzzles to Sara as they drive, "Does Henry understand our directions or is he choosing not to follow them?"

At his cousin's house there is a swimming pool. Henry hasn't learned to swim yet, but he loves to be in the water. He brings matchbox trucks that he lines up along the water's edge in the shallow end of the pool. While his cousins and siblings chatter and splash around him, Henry plays with his trucks. Mark spends the entire day in the pool with the children. He pretends to be a whale, a shark, a dolphin, and alternates giving all of his children rides on his back. When it's Henry's turn he tells his father, "Be a shark now Dad! Dive underneath and attack cousin Cody!" Observers could hear Henry's grandmother saying to Sara, "Oh bless his heart—Henry's having such a good time with his father! What are they saying to each other?"

Later that week when Sara meets with the ethnographic interventionist, they discuss how to improve communication between Henry and his immediate and extended family members. Sara shares her feelings and observations honestly, "Well, we are a signing family. My husband and I sign—the infants sign—we sign all the time! This weekend we went and visited my sister and her kids. My parents were there—they don't sign as well as my sister and her husband, but everyone is always asking good questions such as what's the sign for this or that? I really think we've come a long way in the 4 years since Henry was born."

The ethnographic interventionist is now in a position in which she has identified a discrepancy in what she is being told about the Camillo family's signed language use and what they are demonstrating in their actions. Although they indeed have good intentions about using signed language all the time and have increased the amount of time they are signing at home, they are not signing all the time and with everyone in the immediate and extended family. The professional has an obligation to take Henry's family further in their learning experience. The Camillo's view of their signed language use is typical of homes in which more hearing than deaf family members reside. Ensuring that family members learn to become fluent users of signed language is a critical component of their early education experience. Once again, the foundational concepts introduced by the traditional early interventionist can be extended to include ethnographic intervention methods.

APPLYING THE TOOLS OF ETHNOGRAPHY AND REDEFINING ROLES: IMPLICATIONS AND POSSIBILITIES

An ethnographer's work is similar to that of an early interventionist in that he or she is sent to learn from ordinary people about their everyday lives by interacting with and talking to them over a period of time (Spradley, 1979). Note the emphasis on the phrase *learn from*. It is this slight distinction of "learning from others" that distinguishes the ethnographer from the early interventionist. The ethnographer approaches people from a perspective of discovery and naiveté although the early interventionist enters as the expert. Ethnographers don't just observe and study people. Instead, they learn and are taught about people via their participation and observations while being in the midst of people and their interactions. Spradley suggested that questions such as "What concepts do my informants use to classify their experience?" and "How do my informants define these concepts?" (1979, p. 30) should always be at the forefront of the ethnographer's mind when learning about people in the community being studied.

To expand on their specific work objective, ethnographers also have three strategies that help them gather information systematically while they are taught about different aspects of the human condition: 1) participant observation, 2) video- and audiotaped observation, and 3) ethnographic interviews. The act of participant observation can be likened to home visits conducted by early interventionists. Another name for participant observation is fieldwork, and ethnographers consider fieldwork to be the hallmark of their profession. Fieldwork involves going to where the people to be studied live and observing them while participating in their customary activities (e.g., eating, washing clothes, play).

One benefit of good fieldwork is that the ethnographer learns rather quickly how the community establishes priorities and, consequently, what the members of the community value. An early interventionist who enters a home with ethnographic objectives would schedule long periods for home visits and plan the visits at different times so that he or she could learn about and experience a wide range of family activities. The early interventionist acting as ethnographer would learn more about the family's needs through hands-on experiences with the family rather than by observing only or using more traditional interview techniques. To the greatest extent possible, the ethnographic interventionist would strive to become an active participant in the family's environment while gathering information about daily routines before extending that data into educational plans and services.

Early interventionists often use video- and/or audiotape equipment for assessment purposes, while ethnographers use audiotapes and videotapes to document interactions and conversations among people in the community being studied. The way that both types of professionals use media equipment can be tied together in order to benefit young children and their families in this expanded model. For example, there are several ways that ethnographers rely on previously taped information to continue learning about their informant's lives. First, they may review the tapes from time to time to remind themselves of the specific parts of conversations and events that were captured in the past. One powerful assessment strategy an early interventionist could use is the gathering of audio- and/or videotaped information over time, not only to document for their own purposes but also to share with the children and their families. Sara Camillo, the mother from the previous vignettes, had the opportunity to observe her informal interactions with Henry on a weekly basis. She used the tapes for a variety of constructive purposes including to self-evaluate her signed language skills, to review conversations and lessons with the early interventionist, and to target concepts that needed to be discussed or re-taught to Henry's siblings and/or extended family members.

Lastly, the use of ethnographic interview strategies applied by a knowledgeable early interventionist could be very effective in either scheduled (in a formal social context in front of a video camera) or unscheduled (questions asked informally during fieldwork) contexts. The questions developed for ethnographic interviews are "people centered" and should be developed in advance of the interview in order to build on previously learned information. Ethnographic interview questions do not focus on the child's hearing loss, demographic information, linguistic background, and so forth. In contrast, ethnographic interview questions are often designed to be open-ended and exploratory such as "Tell me the story of the day that Henry was born" and "Tell me about some of the life-changing events (both positive and negative) that have happened to your family in the past 10 years."

We are left with the hope that by redefining the traditional early intervention model to include ethnographic perspectives, Sara Camillo's distressing questions regarding her ability to meet Henry's needs will permanently be alleviated. Although there are significant distinctions between the roles of early interventionist and ethnographer, ideal family-centered support systems can be created for the deaf child and her family if the work objectives and tools of both professions are merged. Ethnographic intervention programming will teach parents to draw from their own insights and experiences, finding personal family-centered meanings in the recommendations made by outside people. This newer model of intervention is preferred to individual families trying to make sense of general intervention information and how it applies to their personal lived experiences.

Ethnographic intervention programs would also become more culturally sensitive because they possess a unique focus on how people with different worldviews behave when they interact using different forms of languages and communication. Consequently, this model is not only sensitive to deaf children but also will impact children of deaf adults, individuals who are in some ways the "reverse" of the typical child who is deaf but who experience similar cultural conflicts in their day-to-day lived experiences.

REFERENCES

Blackburn, L.A. (1999). *Linguistic and cultural interactions among deaf/ hearing family members: Implications for family partnerships in early education.* Unpublished doctoral dissertation, Gallaudet University, Washington, DC.

Blackburn, L.A. (2000). The development of sociolinguistic meanings: The worldview of a deaf child within his home environment. In M. Metzger (Ed.), *Bilingualism and identity in deaf communities* (pp. 219–254). Washington, DC: Gallaudet University Press.

Erting, C. (1982). *Deafness, communication, and social identity: An anthropological analysis of interaction among parents, teachers, and deaf children in preschool.* Unpublished doctoral dissertation, American University, Washington, DC. (Published in 1994 as *Deafness, communication, social identity: Ethnography in a preschool for deaf children.* Silver Spring, MD: Linstok Press.)

Singleton, J., Supalla, S., Lichfield, S., & Schley, S. (1998). From sign to word: Considering modality constraints in ASL/English bilingual education. *Topics in Language Disorders, 4,* 16–29.

Spradley, J.P. (1979). *The ethnographic interview.* New York: Holt, Rinehart & Winston.

Spradley, J.P. (1980). *Participant observation.* New York: Holt, Rinehart & Winston.

Supalla, S.J., Wix, T.R., & McKee, C. (2001). Print as a primary source of English for deaf learners. In J. Nicol (Ed.), *One mind, two languages: Bilingual language processing*. Oxford, England: Blackwell Publishers.

CHAPTER FIFTEEN

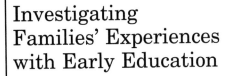

Investigating Families' Experiences with Early Education

A Team Approach

MARILYN SASS-LEHRER,
KATHRYN P. MEADOW-ORLANS,
AND DONNA M. MERTENS

Many changes have occurred in the education of young children with hearing loss since the early 1990s. For example, children and families are more diverse, requiring more diverse educators; children enter intervention programs at younger ages; and cochlear implants and improved hearing aids have expanded available technological options. Because educational research has not kept pace with these new technological and demographic developments, early education programs are struggling to provide appropriate services to young children with hearing loss and their families. Through an investigation of parents' reactions to services provided, this chapter describes one effort to address some of these issues and summarizes key results.

THE NATIONAL PARENT PROJECT

Gallaudet University's National Parent Project (NPP) was conceptualized in the spring of 1996 to review how individual differences among children with hearing loss and their families influence services provided, how well these services are received, and how effective they are (Meadow-Orlans, Mertens, & Sass-Lehrer, 2003; Meadow-Orlans, Mertens, Sass-Lehrer, & Scott-Olson, 1997; Mertens, Sass-Lehrer, & Scott-Olson, 2000). A research team that included a social scientist (Meadow-Orlans), a program evaluation specialist (Mertens), and an early childhood teacher educator (Sass-Lehrer) collaborated on the overall study, design, and analyses. Graduate students were important members of the team, actively participating in all aspects of the project.[1] Parents were also vital to the process, providing critical advice on the content and format of the study. The project proceeded in three phases: a national survey, individual parent interviews, and focus group interviews. Quotations in this chapter are excerpts from interviews collected from parents during the course of the project.

Background and Rationale for the Study

One of the most important findings from research on early intervention is that family participation is extremely important to the early development of the young deaf child (Calderon, 2000; Moeller, 2000). The Individuals with Disabilities Education Act (IDEA), reauthorized in 1997, emphasizes the importance of family involvement in early intervention and the

[1]Special thanks to Kimberley Scott-Olson, Selena Steinmetz, Susan Medina, and Jennifer Pittaway, who served as graduate student assistants in various phases of the research.

role of professionals in establishing partnerships with families. Families who are responsive to the needs of their children and support their social-emotional, communicative, and cognitive development witness greater progress in these areas. A lingering question for practitioners is how best to connect with families to provide information, support, and resources to enhance parents' and caregivers' abilities to promote their child's development. Professionals can suggest strategies for improving relationships with families and the quality and usefulness of services only after they have an understanding of families' experiences and responses to services provided.

Historically, approaches to research in early intervention have focused on such questions as, Which communication modality is most effective? Is earlier initiation of services more effective than later intervention? How do the needs of children with deaf parents differ from those of children with hearing parents? How do parent–child interactions influence language development? Researchers have begun to investigate the complexity of family functioning and accommodation, along with the role of social support in the overall development of the child with a hearing loss (Calderon & Greenberg, 1997). Research studies examining the differential effects of intervention approaches with individual children and unique family situations can provide deeper understandings of what works best for individual children and their families (Calderon & Greenberg, 1997; Meadow-Orlans & Sass-Lehrer, 1995). The NPP was designed to examine the complex relationships between family and child characteristics and professionals and services. For example, experiences with early intervention were considered from the perspectives of families with different hearing status or ethnicity and children with and without disabilities.

The NPP began with a review of the literature that provided basic demographic information on the population of children with hearing loss younger than 5 years old (Schildroth & Hotto, 1993; Strong, Clark, Barringer, Walden, & Williams, 1992), age of identification of hearing loss (Elssmann, Matkin, & Sabo, 1987; Harrison & Roush, 1996), the gaps between age of suspicion and identification, and gaps between age of identification and initiation of early intervention services (Elssmann et al., 1987; Harrison & Roush, 1996; Mace, Wallace, Whan, & Steinmachowicz, 1991). These data raised many questions: How are the experiences of families with children who are hard of hearing, deaf, or those with co-occurring disabilities different? How do hearing status, race, ethnicity, and socioeconomic status of parents relate to confirmation of hearing loss and provision of services? How does age of identification of hearing loss affect families and the services they receive? How do professionals influence parental feelings and actions? What services are most helpful?

The team deliberated on research strategies that would provide answers to these questions.

The literature review also revealed an absence of the voices of families from many studies investigating early intervention approaches. Professionals, rather than families, typically define the focus of research and script the research questions without family participation, which controls and often limits the richness of their findings. A study examining the impact of early intervention is less meaningful without input from families. Therefore, the NPP was designed to obtain information directly from parents by eliciting descriptions of their experiences, evaluations of the effectiveness of services, and recommendations for improvement. Parents provided important insights throughout the project from the design of the survey and interview protocol, to the analyses and implications of the findings, to a review of the completed report (Meadow-Orlans et al., 2003; Meadow-Orlans et al., 2000; Sass-Lehrer, Meadow-Orlans, Mertens, & Scott-Olson, 1999; Sass-Lehrer, Meadow-Orlans, Mertens, Scott-Olson, & Steinmetz, 1999).

The National Survey

The first phase of the project involved the collection of data on families' experiences from the time they suspected their child had a hearing loss through their child's preschool years. A four-page questionnaire was designed for parents of children between 6 and 7 years old to ensure that most later-identified children were included. By this age, parents would also have had the opportunity to reflect on the early years with a degree of perspective, while still able to recall events accurately. The questionnaire was intended to explore the following questions:

- How and when are children who are deaf and hard of hearing identified in various regions of the United States? When does early intervention begin?

- What intervention approaches are available, recommended, and accepted by parents? Are options requested and available?

- Are special services offered for population sub-groups (e.g., deaf parents, parents who are non-Anglo, parents with children who have co-occurring disabilities, parents with children who are hard of hearing)?

- What is the participation level of mothers, fathers, and other family members or caregivers in various subgroups?

- What are the responses of family members to the child's hearing loss?

- What is the level of parental satisfaction with services received?

- Who provides support for families?
- How do families gauge their levels of stress?
- How do parents assess their child's social adjustment and language progress?

A listing of programs that enrolled children who were deaf and hard of hearing was obtained from Gallaudet University's Center for Assessment and Demographic Studies (CADS). Questionnaires were distributed through program supervisors based on a sampling plan designed to represent geographic regions, program types, and program sizes. Questionnaires were completed by 404 parents of children enrolled in 137 programs in 39 states. Although African American and Hispanic families were somewhat under-represented, other demographic characteristics reflected those reported by CADS. (See Meadow-Orlans et al., 2003, for a detailed description of the sampling method, questionnaire, and characteristics of respondents.) Codes were constructed for 147 different pieces of information from the survey questionnaire, data were entered on a computer, and analyses were conducted by means of the Statistical Program for the Social Sciences (SPSS). A summary of survey results was mailed to all parents who had requested it, and program summaries were mailed to administrators of programs with 10 or more respondents.

Responses from the survey confirmed that children with hearing loss and their families are very diverse, thus requiring services that are truly individualized in order to address their priorities, resources, and concerns. More than one third of the participating parents had children with a special need in addition to a hearing loss, and many of these families encountered difficulties obtaining services. Some families waited almost 1 year from the time of identification of the hearing loss until they were enrolled in an early intervention or preschool program. Once in these programs, families generally expressed satisfaction with the services and with their children's progress and were highly appreciative of support from teachers and therapists. However, some families, particularly those who are non-Anglo, of mixed race, or deaf, were less satisfied with their services.

Interviews

A semi-structured interview was designed to encourage parents to describe their personal experiences and to address specific issues that emerged from the data, such as the circumstances surrounding the diagnosis, parental concerns, services provided, advice for professionals, and advice for other parents (Meadow-Orlans et al., 2003). Interviews with hearing parents were conducted by telephone and interviews with deaf parents were conducted with a telecommunications device used for communication with individuals who are deaf (e.g., TTY) or with the support of interpreters. The interviews lasted between 30 and 60 minutes and were tape recorded with the permission of the respondent. Graduate students interviewed parents, transcribed and entered data on computer files, and worked with senior members of the research team to establish a coding system.

Forty families were selected at random from those parents who indicated a willingness in their questionnaires to be contacted for a telephone interview. Subsequently, 22 additional families were randomly selected from specifically identified groups, including families whose children have co-occurring disabilities, parents who are deaf or hard of hearing, parents of children with cochlear implants, and non-Anglo families. In order to understand more about the circumstances surrounding the discovery of hearing loss, one interview proceeded this way:

Interviewer: *It says here on the survey that the audiologist first suspected her hearing loss. . . . Can you tell me a little bit more about that?*

Parent: *Well, he tested her at 4 days old. . . . He said she had a 65 dB [hearing loss], so I treated her as a hard of hearing individual. I have a brother that has a 65 dB [hearing loss], and he speaks very clearly. And I just expected her to turn out like him. And when she was 12 months old, she had a fever of 103 for about 3 days, and I have noticed ever since then, she's never responded to anything. And before that . . . I had called her name and she turned to look at me. And she would wake up to the vacuum, you know, loud noises . . . then after . . . the fever, I've noticed that she's never responded to any sound. I don't know if she really did have that much dB or not, at the time.*

Interviewer: *Have you had her hearing tested again since then?*

Parent: *Yes, yes, and with hearing aids on she's like 115 dB.*

Interviewer: *So, was it standard procedure to have her hearing tested at 4 days or did you ask the audiologist to test her?*

Parent: *Oh, well, we have deafness in our family. . . . My husband is deaf, and his parents and grandparents are deaf and I have siblings that are deaf.*

Prior to each interview, the interviewer reviewed the survey form completed by the parent and referred to this information to guide the questioning. This is illustrated by the following discussion regarding a father's evaluation of services received by his hard of hearing daughter:

Interviewer: *I have here that you were very satisfied with the program she was in . . .*

    Parent: *Oh yeah, it was great.*

Interviewer: *What did you like so much about it?*

    Parent: *The one-to-one time spent with the kids. I mean there were kids there that had cerebral palsy, attention deficit disorder; there was one child that was blind and it was, you know—it was even. They didn't dote on any one kid . . . they spent quality time with every one of them. And there were hearing and speech therapists and audiologists that came in and helped and it was just a great program.*

Interviewer: *Was there anything at all that you felt you or your family needed that they didn't provide?*

    Parent: *No, there really wasn't. . . . We were very lucky there. . . . Everything went very well.*

In this particular interview, the interviewer then referred back to the form commenting that she understood that his daughter was in a program with hearing children and used both signs and speech for fluent communication, then followed up with questions regarding satisfaction with the child's communication progress and the family's decision about communication modalities.

Questions for the interviews were influenced by an assumption associated with the emancipatory research paradigm—that those with less power (generally parents) should have an opportunity to share their thoughts with those with more power (generally professionals) (Mertens, 1998). Banks (2000) suggested that it is the groups in our society with power who largely determine what bodies of knowledge become institutionalized as established concepts and practices. These "cultural facts" are accepted without challenge until the voices of affected individuals have the opportunity to articulate their experiences and express their perspectives.

An example of a "cultural fact" related to working with families is that information about hearing loss, development, communication, and educational options should not be presented in a manner that may be overwhelming to parents, create confusion, or increase parental anxiety (Luterman, 1999). Thus, it follows that professionals should gauge the parents' level of receptiveness and match the amount and extent of information they provide accordingly. In the interviews, however, some parents told us that they disagreed with this perspective. In the words of one parent,

I would much rather have been given, just inundated with all this informa-
tion of different methodologies, different . . . resources so that we could exper-
iment and try different things . . . I mean one might do better with one
method and one might do better with another and allowing the families to
have more information, I think would make the families feel more flexible.
(as cited in Mertens et al., 2000, p. 45)

Interview responses were coded after several reviews of the interview transcripts and an inductive analysis of the data. Categories of comments were identified and the team developed an initial codebook. The coding categories were discussed and modified numerous times as the coding proceeded (Mertens et al., 2000). Analysis was accomplished by searching for terms related to the themes that emerged during the coding process using Ethnograph, a computer-based program for qualitative data analysis that can find segments of text using one or more code words. Much more data were generated in this process than could be presented even in a book-length monograph, thus the published results are illustrative rather than comprehensive. The decision about what to include was based on the notion of providing information that could enhance understanding of the conditions surrounding diagnosis, social adjustment, or language development. See Table 15.1 for the four coding areas that summarized the results of the qualitative data.

Focus Groups

In addition to the telephone interviews, three focus groups were conducted with parents in large urban areas, designed to expand the number of Hispanic and African American families represented in survey and

Table 15.1. Four coding areas that summarized the results of the qualitative data

1. What characterized the nature of the relationship between parents and professionals at the time of suspicion and confirmation of hearing loss?

2. How do parents describe their concerns about their child's social-emotional development in terms of behavioral issues and their interactions with professionals related to this area?

3. How do parents describe their concerns about their child's linguistic and communicative development and their interactions with professionals related to this area?

4. What advice do parents have for increasing professionals' sensitivity (including those who provide medical, audiological, educational, and other related services) in their interactions with each other? What advice do parents have for other parents?

interview data. These group interviews were held with parents of children between the ages of 6 and 7 years enrolled in programs for deaf and hard of hearing children. Parents participating in the focus groups had not completed a questionnaire, so the focus group interview questions were similar to, but more general than, the individual interview questions. Discussion evolved from the information shared by the focus group participants eliciting comments about families' experiences, feelings, and concerns during the time of suspicion and confirmation of their child's hearing loss; the people or services that were most helpful; needs that were not addressed by early intervention services; the communication decision-making process; and advice families had for professionals and for other parents. The same coding process used for the interviews was used to code the focus group data.

Benefits of Multiple Research Methodologies

The combination of survey, individual interviews, and focus group interviews provides a broad perspective as well as an in-depth understanding of individual family situations. The personal family experiences obtained through interviews and focus groups offer a context for the quantitative data obtained from the survey. From the interviews and analyses of the survey data, patterns emerged regarding both general and individual responses to the early intervention process. For example, although most parents appeared to be very satisfied with their early intervention services, some groups were less satisfied than others. One group that rated early intervention services less satisfactory was deaf parents. The interview process elicited comments such as the following from one deaf parent:

I think a lot of the problem is that the hearing professionals that work with deaf infants are not proficient in sign. So, many of us . . . have interpreters because these people can't sign fluently.

This comment underscores the importance of accommodating to the communication needs of all parents. Families who were non-Anglo or of mixed race also were generally less satisfied with the services they received than nondeaf, Anglo families. Though in general the comments from these families reflected the same themes as those of other families, specific comments appeared to be influenced by their status as minority members in a majority White and English-speaking society. Interviews with these families suggest specific concerns about societal and educational barriers that may limit their children. Some families were limited by financial worries that prevented access to services. One mother described her frustration obtaining assistance for expenses for her child:

Right now, I'm still trying to get his social security thing going. . . . It has been difficult because they're not making it easy. I know a lot of people who've gotten social security for lesser things. It's not like he's faking his hearing loss and stuff like that. I'm still in the process of that. That has been very difficult.

Overall, parents believed that the professionals they met were knowledgeable and very helpful in obtaining services. However, families also encountered professionals who were uninformed, inaccessible, or biased in their opinions. Parents commented repeatedly on medical professionals who overlooked their child's hearing loss and/or did not listen to their concerns.

Challenges and Issues

One of the challenges faced by researchers doing survey research is that of obtaining a high response rate that is representative of the target population. Because the questionnaires were distributed by program directors, it was not possible to know how many actually reached parents. Fortunately, the researchers were able to establish the representativeness of their sample by comparisons with selected demographic characteristics reported in the Gallaudet University Annual Survey conducted by CADS (Schildroth & Hotto, 1993). Focus groups increased participation and inclusiveness. Child care, food, transportation, language interpreters, and a small stipend provided support that encouraged families to participate.

Collaboration among experienced researchers and students was both a strength and a challenge of the project. The team approach required frequent meetings to discuss and clarify the research process, resulting in more clearly focused procedures. Student contributions to team discussions regarding the meaning of interview data and motivations of families also were invaluable. Students' university responsibilities and schedules, however, often conflicted with project deadlines, and before each semester, the senior research team had concerns about students' continuing involvement. Fortunately, Gallaudet University Research Institute funding supported student participation. The data collection and processing could not have been accomplished without the energy and commitment of the student members of the team. Practicing professionals are encouraged to collaborate with university programs for both expertise and assistance in conducting research.

CONCLUSIONS AND APPLICATIONS

Professionals are best equipped to provide early intervention services to children and their families when they understand the individual backgrounds and characteristics of those children and families, as well as how families respond and integrate information about their child. NPP survey data provide a snapshot of the population of families and children with whom early intervention specialists work and the kinds of services they receive. The interviews and focus groups in this project provided a forum for families to share personal stories about their experiences with the early intervention process and the individuals with whom they worked (Mertens et al., 2000). These conversations revealed the struggles and frustrations as well as the successes and achievements that are part of the early identification and intervention experience for most parents.

A research team approach that includes professional researchers, practicing professionals, students, and family members adds richness to the research process that cannot otherwise be found. It is an added benefit when team membership is diverse and includes multiple perspectives and experiences. Senior research members in this project benefited from the talents and diversity of the students on the team. Students and senior researchers learned from each other, and everyone benefited from the opportunity to listen to families tell their stories. Although working with a team presents challenges, such as scheduling and prolonged discussions that extend the time and resources involved, the results are more useful, insightful, and representative of the views of research participants.

Despite professional guidelines and legislative recommendations for professionals to create partnerships with families and promote their involvement, many families do not have an opportunity to express their views. The benefits of early intervention are achieved only when families are meaningfully engaged, and the best way to improve practices is to ask families for their views. When asked if they had advice for professionals, many parents were ready and willing to participate. They agreed that the most effective professionals were those who listened to their concerns, were honest about their child's progress, respected their views and opinions, and were knowledgeable and willing to provide complete and accurate information to enable them to make their own decisions

(Meadow-Orlans et al., 2003; Mertens et al., 2000). This research reinforces the conviction that effective intervention must be responsive to parents, and research must be sensitive to the diversity of family perspectives and designed to include multiple views and experiences.

REFERENCES

Banks, J. (2000). The social construction of difference and the quest for educational equality. In R.S. Bradt (Ed.), *Education in a new era* (pp. 21–45). Alexandria, VA: Association for Supervision and Curriculum Development.

Calderon, R. (2000). Parental involvement in deaf children's education programs as a predictor of child's language, early reading, and social-emotional development. *Journal of Deaf Studies and Deaf Education, 5*(2), 140–155.

Calderon, R., & Greenberg, M. (1997). The effectiveness of early intervention for deaf children and children with hearing loss. In M. Guralnick (Ed.), *The effectiveness of early intervention* (pp. 455–482). Baltimore: Paul H. Brookes Publishing Co.

Elssmann, S., Matkin, N., & Sabo, M. (1987). Early identification of congenital sensorineural hearing impairment. *The Hearing Journal, 9,* 13–17.

Harrison, M., & Roush, J. (1996). Age of suspicion, identification, and intervention for infants and young children with hearing loss: A national survey. *Ear and Hearing, 17*(1), 55–62.

Individuals with Disabilities Education Act (IDEA) Amendments of 1997, PL 105-17, 20 U.S.C. §§ 1400 *et seq.*

Luterman, D. (1999). *The young deaf child.* Baltimore: York Press.

Mace, A.L., Wallace, K.L., Whan, M.Q., & Steinmachowicz, P.G. (1991). Relevant factors in the identification of hearing loss. *Ear and Hearing, 12,* 287–293.

Meadow-Orlans, K., & Sass-Lehrer, M. (1995). Support services for families of children who are deaf: Challenges for professionals. *Topics in Early Childhood Special Education, 15*(3), 314–334.

Meadow-Orlans, K., Sass-Lehrer, M., & Mertens, D. (2000, July). *Parent to parent: Advice for parents with young deaf or hard of hearing children.* Paper presented at the American Society for Deaf Children. Washington, DC.

Meadow-Orlans, K.P., Mertens, D.M., & Sass-Lehrer, M.A. (2003). *Parents and their deaf children: The early years.* Washington, DC: Gallaudet University Press.

Meadow-Orlans, K.P., Mertens, D.M., Sass-Lehrer, M.A., & Scott-Olson, K. (1997). Support services for parents and children who are deaf or hard of hearing: A national survey. *American Annals of the Deaf, 142*(4), 278–288.

Mertens, D. (1998). *Research methods in education and psychology: Integrating diversity and quantitative and qualitative approaches.* Thousand Oaks, CA: Sage Publications.

Mertens, D., Sass-Lehrer, M., & Scott-Olson, K. (2000). Sensitivity in the family-professional relationship: Developmental implications for young deaf and hard of hearing children. In P. Spencer, C. Erting, & M. Marschark (Eds.), *The deaf child in the family and at school: Essays in honor of Kathryn P. Meadow-Orlans* (pp. 133–150). Mahwah, NJ: Lawrence Erlbaum Associates.

Moeller, M.P. (2000). Early intervention and language development in children who are deaf and hard of hearing. *Pediatrics, 106*(3), e43.

Sass-Lehrer, M., Meadow-Orlans, K., Mertens, D., & Scott-Olson, K., (1999, July). *Families with young hard of hearing children.* Paper presented at the Convention of American Instructors of the Deaf, 59th Biennial Conference, Los Angeles.

Sass-Lehrer, M., Meadow-Orlans, K., Mertens, D., Scott-Olson, K., & Steinmetz, S. (1999, May). *Hearing and deaf parents of young deaf children: Challenges and advice.* Paper presented at the National Symposium on Childhood Deafness, Sioux Falls, SD.

Schildroth, A., & Hotto, S. (1993). Annual survey of hearing-impaired children and youth: 1991–92 school year. *American Annals of the Deaf, 138*(2), 163–171.

Strong, C.J., Clark, T.C., Barringer, D.G., Walden, B., & Williams, S.A. (1992). *SKI-HI home-based programming for children with hearing impairments: Demographics, child identification, and program effectiveness, 1979–1991: Final report to the U.S. Department of Education, Office of Special Education and Rehabilitative Services* (Project No. H023C9000117). Logan: Utah State University, Department of Communicative Disorders, SKI-HI Institute.

CHAPTER SIXTEEN

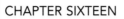

Signs of Literacy

An Ethnographic Study
of American Sign Language
and English Literacy Acquisition

CAROL J. ERTING

I thank Dr. Jane K. Fernandes and the Laurent Clerc National Deaf Education Center, the Gallaudet Research Institute, and the U.S. Department of Education for their support of this research. I would also like to thank the members of the Signs of Literacy research team, the parents, the children, the teachers, the administrators, and the Gallaudet undergraduate and graduate students who have collaborated with us over the years. Special appreciation goes to Carlene Thumann-Prezioso, Charles Reilly, Margaret Hallau, Michael Karchmer, Lynne Erting, Dennis Berrigan, Cynthia Neese Bailes, Dan Mathis, Marlon Kuntze, Beth Sonnenstrahl Benedict, Debbie Trapani, Debbie Cushner, Janet Weinstock, Steve Benson, and Tom Witte for their contributions to discussions regarding the challenges and benefits of collaborative research.

Collaborative interdisciplinary research involving deaf and hearing teachers and researchers is rare. Although many challenges arise from this approach, from the perspective of a qualitative and especially an ethnographic orientation, collaborative inquiry holds the promise of producing knowledge that teachers, families, administrators, professionals, and other researchers need in order to work together effectively on behalf of children who are deaf and hard of hearing. In 1992, researchers and teachers at Gallaudet University embarked on a collaborative effort to describe and document teaching and learning in six bilingual preschool classrooms. Several teachers at the demonstration school on campus had begun using American Sign Language (ASL) and written English as the primary languages of interaction and instruction with their students. These teachers, like most teachers of deaf children, had not received preservice education or in-service instruction to prepare them to teach in bilingual programs. Instead, their previous experience had prepared them to teach monolingually using simultaneous communication (sim-com), also known as Sign Supported Speech (SSS) (Johnson, Liddell, & Erting, 1989) wherein spoken English and signs are produced simultaneously.[1] With the transition to a new pedagogy came numerous questions from the teachers themselves, researchers, parents, and administrators. For example, what do teachers who use ASL and written English actually do in the classroom? What do they believe they should be doing and why? How do children from diverse backgrounds respond to this pedagogy? Are they acquiring the two target languages and making progress academically? What role does the family play in this process, and how do hearing families develop as Deaf bilingual entities?

This chapter briefly describes longitudinal research conducted by the Signs of Literacy team at Gallaudet University on teaching and learning in Deaf bilingual classrooms. The first phase of data collection occurred between 1994 and 1996, and the second phase of data collection began in 2001. This discussion focuses on what the team learned about the challenges and benefits of collaboration among deaf and hearing teachers and researchers in ethnographic classroom research.

CONTEXT OF THE STUDY

There is widespread recognition that the academic achievement of students who are deaf and hard of hearing is well below that of their hearing

---

[1]When using sim-com or SSS, the only language being produced is spoken English. The signed component of SSS consists of individual signs that have been disassociated from their linguistic context (i.e., American Sign Language). When produced as part of an SSS utterance, the resulting sign string is often meaningless, contradictory, or indecipherable (Johnson, Liddell, & Erting, 1989).

peers (Commission on Education of the Deaf, 1988; Traxler, 1999). Some claim that school programs are not making it possible for students who are deaf and hard of hearing to reach their academic potential. An increasing number of educators, researchers, and deaf community members argue that if students who are deaf and hard of hearing are provided with a visually accessible learning environment and given access to the curriculum through a natural sign language, their literacy levels and academic achievement will improve (Israelite, Ewoldt, & Hoffmeister, 1989; Johnson et al., 1989; Prinz, 1998). Since 1989, an increasing number of school programs serving deaf and hard of hearing children in North America have adopted a bilingual/bicultural perspective, introducing ASL into classrooms, schools, and homes as a primary language of instruction (LaSasso, 1999; Strong, 1995). Several studies conducted in the 1990s documented for the first time a significant relationship between students' proficiency in ASL and their English literacy skills (Padden & Ramsey, 2000; Prinz & Strong, 1998; Strong & Prinz, 1997). However, Strong's (1995) review of nine developing bilingual/bicultural programs for deaf children revealed that curricula and teaching methods were not well-defined for these programs and most of them did not have systematic research efforts underway to document their philosophy, curriculum, pedagogy, and the achievement of their students. After a survey of 80% of the residential and day schools listed in the 1998 American Annals of the Deaf, LaSasso (1999) reported there were 16 self-described bilingual programs serving approximately 4,000 students in the United States. Preliminary analysis of these data indicated that there was considerable variability among the programs in the following areas: reported ASL abilities of teachers and staff, how English was represented and conveyed, formal curricula, the age at which reading instruction was initiated, frameworks for reading instruction, and formal program evaluation.

As educators and researchers have become more interested in the potential of a bilingual approach to educate students who are deaf, questions have been raised about the ways in which a natural sign language such as ASL might support the acquisition of English literacy. Some writers have challenged the notion that ASL can directly support the learning of English (Mayer & Akamatsu, 1999; Mayer & Wells, 1996), while others have suggested that research is beginning to point to a number of strategies teachers may use to help students understand the relationship between the two languages, including the use of some form of English-like signing, fingerspelling and initialized signs, glossing, sign writing, and phonological and phonemic cuing systems (Neuroth-Gimbrone & Logodice, 1992; Padden & Ramsey, 1998; Prinz & Strong, 1998; Singleton, Supalla, Litchfield, & Schley, 1998; Supalla, Wix, & McKee, 2001).

In a review of research in the area of ASL proficiency and English literacy acquisition, Nelson pointed out that most deaf children are both language delayed and language deprived since a "very small minority of deaf children receive year-after-year excellent, processable language learning opportunities and use their excellent first language skills in ASL as the base for full acquisition of English literacy" (1998, p. 75). He argued, correctly, that future research must investigate how children who are deaf, especially those who do not come from families who use ASL, can achieve high first-language skills efficiently in ASL. Nelson argues future research must also investigate how to teach individual deaf students, taking into account not only what the child begins with at entry to formal schooling, but also what happens during instruction and learning, considering social-cultural-motivational factors along with the cognitive-linguistic factors that have been traditionally emphasized.

EARLY STAGES OF COLLABORATION

Through a series of planning meetings involving school personnel and researchers, the research team reached a consensus that the research should be voluntary, collaborative, and ethnographic, not quasi-experimental. Teachers expressed dissatisfaction with research they had participated in previously because they did not have a collaborative relationship with the researchers and their participation failed to benefit their own teaching practice. They were enthusiastic when a qualitative and ethnographic approach was suggested as the best way to address their concerns and begin to answer the initial research questions and, perhaps more important, to reveal what additional questions the team should be asking. The research team's goal was to capture and document the complexity of teaching and learning as it occurred in everyday classroom contexts and to chart individual children's progress over time (3 years initially).

WHY ETHNOGRAPHY?

Ethnography is the approach first developed by western anthropologists to describe and understand foreign cultures and their ways of life. Today, in a shrinking world with high-speed access to distant cultures and unfamiliar worldviews, anthropologists and other social scientists use ethnography to help make sense of the societies, cultures, and communities they participate in locally and at a distance (Bohannan & van der Elst, 1998). The underlying objective remains the same: to understand unfamiliar cultures on their own terms and, through systematic examination of alternative ways of living, to arrive at a more comprehensive definition of what it means to be human. Ethnographers participate in the cultural scenes they are studying at the same time they are observing those scenes, an approach that requires a considerable amount of time interacting with members of the culture in a variety of settings and fluency in the language or languages of that culture (Agar, 1980; Spradley, 1980; Wolcott, 1995). In order to accomplish their goals, ethnographers must overcome their own ethnocentrism and tolerate and learn from the emotional stress of culture shock.

Ethnocentrism is a product of enculturation so that as members of a particular culture grow from infancy to adulthood the worldview that is absorbed and adopted is unquestioned and taken for granted. That very particular worldview is treated as part of the natural order of things, when, in fact, it is learned, not given, and is only one of the many ways of seeing the world. Culture shock results when people encounter ways of seeing the world that differ from their own, forcing the questioning of the long-held assumption that their own cultural perspective is the only one or at least the best one with which to make sense of the world. While uncomfortable and sometimes even agonizing, ethnographers understand the critical role culture shock plays in the recognition of ethnocentrism and the development of more objectivity about one's own culture.

An important goal for the ethnographer is to understand why people believe and behave as they do. What assumptions and premises underlie the common understandings shared by a people? Once these kinds of questions are asked about others, one's own cultural assumptions can be seen more clearly, making them available for analysis and reconsideration. Ethnographers must beware of the temptation to view a culture as an objective reality rather than as a set of ongoing processes (Bohannan & van der Elst, 1998). Cultures are constantly changing, and no single member of a culture sees the world in exactly the same way another member does. Cultural practices are always situated—that is, they occur in particular local contexts under specific conditions. Boundaries between cultures are not fixed and members of contiguous cultures often share numerous cultural elements with their neighbors who often belong to other ethnic groups. Ethnographic description has a difficult time capturing this dynamic nature of culture because, like a frame of a video recording, it converts dynamic cultural process into still life. Ethnographers themselves complicate the situation further because their descriptions are situated in time and place as well as in their own unique perspectives.

In spite of these challenges, ethnography offers the best available antidote to ethnocentrism and oversimplification. By taking account of the complexity of cultural worlds including one's own, it is possible to open one's mind to the validity and utility of new perspectives. In this way, new possibilities emerge for the ethnographer's own repertoire of behaviors, beliefs, and attitudes.

ETHNOGRAPHY IN DEAF EDUCATION

When families, schools, deaf communities, and research teams are viewed as cultural systems, an important goal for participants is to gain insight into beliefs, values, and assumptions that are different from their own. Ethnographic research appealed to the planning team because ethnography provides the theoretical and methodological tools for uncovering, describing, and analyzing cultural systems. For example, in order for professionals to meet the needs of children and families, they must learn to see the world through deaf eyes, understanding what it means to be primarily visual in one's orientation to a world that is full of auditory information. In the case of classroom teachers, adopting a deaf perspective has implications for the structuring of classroom environments and school curricula. For example, hearing teachers who can communicate with spoken language in spite of visual barriers may not have considered the importance of arranging furniture in their classrooms to preserve unobstructed sight lines and therefore visual access for the children. Likewise, professionals seeking to help hearing families see the world through the eyes of their deaf child must first discover and understand the cultural systems of the diverse families they serve. When hearing parents discover their child is deaf, they have usually had no prior contact with deaf people. Their expectations for themselves as parents and for their child's future have been disrupted, and they usually need help in visualizing a future for their family that they can understand, accept, and work toward achieving. If professionals do not discover what parents believe and value, if they do not learn how particular families interpret their lives and specifically their new status as a family with a deaf member, it will be difficult, if not impossible, to serve that family effectively.

Deaf children, too, have to learn to understand perspectives other than their own. If they are to succeed in a world organized primarily for those who can hear, they must learn to participate effectively in cultural scenes—in the family, school, workplace, and community—that they cannot fully experience because they don't hear. Schools and families will need to teach children who are deaf about aspects of the larger culture that are usually not taught explicitly to hearing children. Enculturation usually takes place outside of awareness simply by having access to the sights and sounds in the environment, most important, the language of the cultural group. Because children who are deaf lack complete access to the auditory components of the culture, especially the language as it is spoken in everyday cultural settings, schools and families must consciously notice what the children are missing and provide them with this critical cultural capital (Hinchey, 1998). Looking and asking and using ethnography, participant-observers in homes and classrooms try to make sense out of cultural scenes they don't understand. They attempt to suspend their own cultural assumptions and beliefs to look at the scene through ethnographic eyes to ask, What's going on here? (Frank, 1999). What does this event mean from the perspective of each participant?

Further, because families, communities, and schools are dynamic, ever-changing systems, a longitudinal approach is important in order to understand the cultural processes involved. Prolonged engagement allows ethnographers to capture and document changes that occur, for example, in the children's language and literacy development, in the organization of the classrooms, in the teachers' thinking, and in teaching strategies as the classroom culture evolves (Lancy, 2001). Placing single snapshots of children or classroom practices within the context of change and development over time helps ensure interpretive validity. By carefully observing, videotaping, asking questions, and systematically analyzing the data over time, the research team can revise and refine the questions being asked and discover new ones, taking as a starting point the perspectives of participants in an attempt to avoid the ethnocentrism that plagues much of the existing research on deaf people, their families, and deaf education.

CONDUCTING THE RESEARCH

Commitment to collaboration and understanding participants' cultural perspectives meant that the Signs of Literacy research team first had to address the differences between the everyday worlds of teachers and university researchers. Teachers live in an environment in which immediate concerns and problem solving about the everyday lives of children in their care take precedence. Their daily schedules are constrained to a far greater extent than are the schedules of university researchers, with little time for activities that don't involve their students. In the culture of an elementary school, children's physical health and safety, social and emotional development, and their progress through the curriculum are primary. While participation in research is applauded and encouraged, there is usually no mechanism in place that allows teachers the necessary time to participate in a truly collaborative way. University researchers, however, do not expect research results to be immediately applicable to the classroom, and rather than thinking in terms of real children for whom they are responsible on a daily basis, they deal with children in the abstract. Their everyday schedules are flexible and to a large extent under their own control. Researchers often engage in solitary activity, reading academic literature, analyzing data, and writing up results in a university culture that tends to reward theorizing and publishing more readily than it does teaching.

Teacher–Researcher Collaboration

What did the teacher versus researcher cultural perspective mean for research design and implementation? First, the Signs of Literacy team agreed that the primary data for the project would be videotapes of naturally occurring, everyday interactions in the classrooms (not in research labs) collected biweekly for 3 academic years. During participant-observation and in interviews and video journals, researchers encouraged teachers to tell them what was important about the cultural scenes they were seeing and why. As Bohannan and van der Elst pointed out, "People's actions usually make sense *if you can manage to see what they see* in the world around them. It helps more than anything else if you just ask them" (1998, p. 56). When the research began, it was difficult to convince teachers that their perspectives were valued. These teachers reported that they had previously experienced educational researchers as aloof, arrogant, and intrusive, and they regarded the resulting research as irrelevant to classroom realities. In spite of such skepticism about the value of educational research, these educators were highly motivated to know more about how children learn and what changes they could make to their classroom practice that would help them reach their goals. It was only over time, with repeated demonstrations of interest in their expertise, that the teachers became convinced that the researchers respected their knowledge and regarded the collaboration with them as central to the success of the project.

Even though the teachers had volunteered to participate in the research, they were nervous about the videotaping and concerned about three cameras and four researchers in the classroom distracting the children and disrupting teaching and learning. Cables and wires hung from the ceilings and were strung across the classroom floors so that the three cameras could be connected to a central control station and time could be encoded on all three video recordings simultaneously. Not only was this arrangement obtrusive, it caused concerns about child safety that researchers had to address (with a lot of duct tape) and it created crowding in some of the classrooms. Experienced teachers and researchers who understood and valued the visual language and culture of Deaf classrooms worked together to solve these problems because all agreed that the sacrifices were worth the quality of the resulting video data. As the data collection proceeded, the teachers learned that the researchers, too, put the needs of children and teachers first. They were surprised at how little the children seemed to be affected by the researchers and their equipment and how quickly they, too, reached a level of comfort with the taping. From teacher reports it seems clear that this result was due to at least two factors: 1) the team's commitment to the research goals and 2) the sensitivity and ethnographic skills of the primary participant-observer and coordinator of data collection in the classrooms (Erting, Hallau, et al., 1997).

Time was always a factor in teacher-researcher collaboration during data analysis. There was not enough time for teachers and researchers to work together, and the problem was never adequately addressed or solved. Arrangements for released time for teachers during the school day were difficult to achieve, and plans to work together in the late afternoon after the children had left for the day often had to be set aside because other, more urgent matters that had arisen during the school day needed attention. Funds were allocated for 5 days of work per teacher during the summer months when the teachers could concentrate fully on the research, free from the daily demands of classroom life, and these days were among the most productive for collaborative work.

In order to address the need for flexibility during the school year, work was devised that the teachers could do alone, when researchers were not available. In most cases, asking teachers to sit alone in front of a video monitor to analyze data was not a very successful strategy. Teachers preferred to review tapes of their classroom with another team member. The interaction between teacher and researcher with their differing perspectives on classroom interaction proved to be stimulating and productive for both participants. Questions posed by the researcher often stimulated the teacher to see and reflect on classroom events in new and valuable ways. These sessions gave teachers the opportunity to attend to their own behaviors and teaching strategies from a different vantage point, as an observer. It also allowed them to focus on individual children interacting with teachers and peers, tracing one child's interactional path through one entire morning as well as through more extended periods of time. While researcher questions and comments during these sessions often derived from theoretical perspectives relating to language, literacy, or pedagogy, teachers' comments and questions emerged from their immediate and ongoing knowledge of and interest in the whole child. The knowledge produced through this kind of dynamic engagement of teacher and researcher perspectives was valuable to both partners. Researchers gained insights that helped them interpret the video data in new and more valid ways and teachers left these sessions with new perspectives on their own teaching and on individual children's learning needs and styles that were immediately applicable in the classroom (Erting, Hallau, et al., 1997).

Deaf–Hearing Collaboration

Partnership between deaf and hearing participants was central to the Signs of Literacy research in these preschool classrooms. In classrooms, deaf and hearing adults worked together to teach deaf and hard of hearing children, and in the homes of most of these children, deaf and hearing family members shared their lives. Likewise, the research team was a partnership among deaf and hearing teachers and researchers, and the work was bilingual. ASL was the language of everyday face-to-face discourse during participant observation, interviews, teacher journals, and data analysis, and written English was the language of e-mail correspondence, written documentation such as individualized education programs and other school records, teacher journals, data analysis, and academic reading and writing. For the hearing participants, ASL was learned as a second or foreign language in adulthood and spoken English was their native language. For most of the deaf participants, ASL was the first or native language while English was learned as a second or foreign language and primary access to it was by means of the written form. Team meetings were always conducted exclusively in the visual modality in ASL, presenting challenges for everyone even though hearing researchers and teachers were fluent signers. Deaf participants sometimes had to struggle to understand the nonnative signing of their hearing peers and frequently were required to repeat, rephrase, or sign more slowly so that hearing team members could understand them. Hearing researchers and teachers often found it difficult to express complex pedagogical or theoretical ideas in their second language (ASL) when they had acquired these concepts through education, reading, and discussion in their first language (English). In spite of these challenges that monolingual research teams are not required to address, there was never any question that the team would function bilingually, experiencing in its own work the challenges and rewards of bilingualism in the classrooms and the homes of the children they were studying (Blackburn, 2000; Erting, Cushner, et al., 1997; Erting, Thumann-Prezioso, & Benedict, 2000). This day-to-day experience helped to keep the visual nature of the deaf experience at the center of the inquiry while at the same time reminding team members that deaf–hearing interaction is an equally important aspect of the cultural scenes being studied.

CONCLUSION

This chapter has touched on some of the issues involved in planning and conducting ethnographic, longitudinal classroom research in preschool classrooms for deaf children with deaf and hearing teachers and researchers collaborating. At the end of the first phase of data collection, teachers and researchers agreed that while the experience had been difficult and challenging, it had been one of the best, most rewarding projects they had ever participated in during their teaching careers (Erting, Hallau, et al., 1997). The second phase of data collection, which began in the fall of 2001, builds on two important discoveries from the first phase. The first discovery is that educators are interested in knowing more about how individual children with differing social and cultural backgrounds, physical attributes, and learning styles progress through preschool to elementary grades and beyond. Educators want in-depth knowledge about the acquisition of ASL and English literacy by diverse deaf children followed from preschool through high school because they believe this knowledge will assist them in curriculum design and in individualizing instruction to meet the needs of individual students. The second discovery is that the children's experiences outside of the classroom, especially in the home, are critical. While the original research plan had included participant observation and interviews in the children's homes, that component of the preschool study was eliminated due to lack of resources. In the second phase, several children were selected for follow-up case studies and data collection will take place at school and at home. Parents joined teachers and researchers in this collaboration as all team members look forward to learning more about the kinds of home and school environments that support the ASL and English literacy acquisition of diverse deaf learners.

REFERENCES

Agar, M. (1980). *The professional stranger: An informal introduction to ethnography.* New York: Academic Press.

Blackburn, L. (2000). The development of sociolinguistic meanings: The worldview of a deaf child within his home environment. In M. Metzger (Ed.), *Bilingualism and identity in deaf communities* (pp. 219–254). Washington, DC: Gallaudet University Press.

Bohannan, P., & van der Elst, D. (1998). *Asking and listening: Ethnography as personal adaptation.* Prospect Heights, IL: Waveland Press.

Commission on Education of the Deaf (1988). *Towards equality. Final report to Congress.* Washington, DC: U.S. Government Printing Office.

Erting, C., Cushner, D., Erting, L., Thumann-Prezioso, C., & Trapani, D. (1997, July). *The challenges and advantages of deaf/hearing teaming.* Paper presented at the biennial meeting of the Convention of American Instructors of the Deaf, Hartford, CT.

Erting, C., Hallau, M., Benson, S., Berrigan, D., Chastel, G., Cushner, D., et al. (1997, July). *The development of language and literacy in preschool: Teachers and researchers collaborating.* Paper presented at the biennial meeting of the Convention of American Instructors of the Deaf, Hartford, CT.

Erting, C., Thumann-Prezioso, D., & Benedict, B. (2000). Bilingualism in a deaf family: Fingerspelling in early childhood. In P. Spencer, C. Erting, & M. Marschark (Eds.), *The deaf child in the family and at school: Essays in honor of Kathryn P. Meadow-Orlans* (pp. 41–54). Mahwah, NJ: Lawrence Erlbaum Associates.

Frank, C. (1999). *Ethnographic eyes: A teacher's guide to classroom observation.* Portsmouth, NH: Heinemann.

Hinchey, P. (1998). *Finding freedom in the classroom: A practical introduction to critical theory.* Washington, DC: Peter Lang.

Israelite, N., Ewoldt, C., & Hoffmeister, R. (1989). *A review of the literature on the effective use of native sign language on the acquisition of a majority language by hearing impaired students* (Research project no. 1170: Final report presented to Minister of Education, Ontario). York, Ontario: York University, Faculty of Education and Boston: Boston University, Center for the Study of Communication and Deafness.

Johnson, R., Liddell, S., & Erting, C. (1989). *Unlocking the curriculum: Principles for achieving access in deaf education* (Working Paper 89-3). Washington, DC: Gallaudet Research Institute.

Lancy, D. (2001). *Studying children and schools: Qualitative research traditions.* Prospect Heights, IL: Waveland Press.

LaSasso, C. (1999, October). *A national survey of bilingual-bicultural programs serving deaf children in the United States.* Poster session presented at the William C. Stokoe and the Study of Signed Languages Conference, Washington, DC.

Mayer, C., & Akamatsu, C. (1999). Bilingual-bicultural models of literacy education for deaf students: Considering the claims. *Journal of Deaf Studies and Deaf Education, 4,* 1–8.

Mayer, C., & Wells, G. (1996). Can the linguistic interdependence hypothesis theory support a bilingual-bicultural model of literacy education for deaf students? *Journal of Deaf Studies and Deaf Education, 1,* 93–107.

Nelson, K. (1998). Toward a differentiated account of facilitators of literacy development and ASL in deaf children. In P. Prinz (Ed.), *ASL proficiency and English literacy acquisition: New perspectives. Topics in Language Disorders, 18*(4), 73–88.

Neuroth-Gimbrone, C., & Logodice, C. (1992). A cooperative bilingual program for deaf adolescents. *Sign Language Studies, 74,* 79–91.

Padden, C., & Ramsey, C. (1998). Reading ability in signing deaf children. In P. Prinz (Ed.), *ASL proficiency and English literacy acquisition: New perspectives. Topics in Language Disorders, 18*(4), 30–46.

Padden, C., & Ramsey, C. (2000). American Sign Language and reading ability in deaf children. In C. Chamberlain, J. Morford, & R. Mayberry (Eds.), *Language acquisition by eye* (pp. 165–190). Mahwah, NJ: Lawrence Erlbaum Associates.

Prinz, P. (Ed.). (1998). ASL proficiency and English literacy acquisition: New perspectives. *Topics in Language Disorders, 18*(4).

Prinz, P., & Strong, M. (1998). ASL proficiency and English literacy within a bilingual deaf education model of instruction. In P. Prinz (Ed.), ASL proficiency and English literacy acquisition: New perspectives. *Topics in Language Disorders, 18*(4), 47–60.

Singleton, J., Supalla, S., Litchfield, S., & Schley, S. (1998). From sign to word: Considering modality constraints in ASL/English bilingual education. In P. Prinz (Ed.), ASL proficiency and English literacy acquisition: New perspectives. *Topics in Language Disorders, 18*(4), 16–29.

Spradley, J. (1980). *Participant observation.* Philadelphia: Holt, Rinehart and Winston.

Strong, M. (1995). A review of bilingual/bicultural programs for deaf children in North America. *American Annals of the Deaf, 140,* 84–94.

Strong, M., & Prinz, P. (1997). A study of the relationship between American Sign Language and English literacy. *Journal of Deaf Studies and Deaf Education, 2*(1), 37–46.

Supalla, S.J., Wix, T.R., & McKee, C. (2001). Print as a primary source of English for deaf learners. In J. Nicol (Ed.), *One mind, two languages: Bilingual language processing.* Oxford, England: Blackwell Publishers.

Traxler, C. (1999, April). *Measuring up to performance standards in reading and mathematics: Achievement of selected deaf and hard of hearing students in the national norming of the 9th Edition Stanford Achievement Test.* Paper presented at the annual meeting of the American Educational Research Association, Montreal, Quebec.

Wolcott, H. (1995). *The art of fieldwork.* Walnut Creek, CA: AltaMira Press.

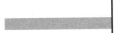

Recommended Resources

BOOKS, VIDEOTAPES, ARTICLES, AND PAMPHLETS

Batshaw, M.L. (Ed.). (2002). *Children with disabilities* (5th ed.). Baltimore: Paul H. Brookes Publishing Co.

Bronfenbrenner, U. (1975). Is early intervention effective? In B.Z. Friedlander, G.M. Sterritt, & G.E. Kirk (Eds.), *Exceptional infant: Assessment and intervention* (Vol. 3, pp. 449–475). New York: Brunner/Mazel.

Candlish, P.A.M. (1996). *Not deaf enough: Raising a child who is hard of hearing.* Washington, DC: Alexander Graham Bell Association for the Deaf and Hard of Hearing.

Christiansen, J., & Leigh, I. (2002). *Cochlear implants in children: Ethics and choices.* Washington, DC: Gallaudet University Press.

Christensen, K. (2000). *Deaf plus: A multicultural perspective.* San Diego: Dawn Sign Press.

Cole, E. (1992). *Listening and talking: A guide to promoting spoken language in young hearing impaired children.* Washington, DC: Alexander Graham Bell Association for the Deaf and Hard of Hearing.

Chute, P., & Nevins, M. (2003). *The parents' guide to cochlear implants.* Washington, DC: Gallaudet University Press.

Davis, J. (1990). *Our forgotten children: Hard of hearing pupils in the schools.* Bethesda, MD: Self-Help for Hard of Hearing People.

Duncan, G. (1997). *But what about my deaf child? A guide to special education in Pennsylvania for parents of children who are deaf or hard of hearing.* York, PA: Parent Education Network.

Estabrooks, W. (Ed.). (1994). *Auditory-verbal therapy for parents and professionals.* Washington, DC: Alexander Graham Bell Association for the Deaf and Hard of Hearing.

Estabrooks, W., & Marlowe, J. (2000). *The baby is listening* [Book and videotape]. Washington, DC: Alexander Graham Bell Association for the Deaf and Hard of Hearing.

Families with hard of hearing children: What if your child has a hearing loss? [Videotape]. (1997). Nebraska: Boys Town Press. (Available from the publisher, 14100 Crawford Street, Boys Town, Nebraska, 68010; 1-800-282-6657; fax: 402-498-1310; e-mail: btpress@girlsandboystown.org)

Ferrell, K.A. (1996). *Reach out and teach: Meeting the training needs of parents of visually and multiply handicapped young children.* New York: AFB Press.

Flathouse, V.E. (1979). Multiply handicapped deaf children and Public Law 94-142. *Exceptional Children, 45,* 560–565.

Garcia, J. (1999). *Sign with your baby: How to communicate with infants before they speak.* Seattle, WA: Northlight Communications.

Guidelines for evaluating auditory-oral programs for children who are hearing impaired. Washington, DC: Alexander Graham Bell Association for the Deaf and Hard of Hearing.

Harris, G. (1983). *Broken ears, wounded hearts: An intimate journey into the lives of a multihandicapped girl and her family.* Washington, DC: Gallaudet University Press.

Hart, B., & Risley, T.R. (1995). *Meaningful differences in the everyday experience of young American children.* Baltimore: Paul H. Brookes Publishing Co.

Hart, B., & Risley, T.R. (1999). *The social world of children learning to talk.* Baltimore: Paul H. Brookes Publishing Co.

Hart, V. (1973). *Beginning with the handicapped.* Springfield, IL: Charles C Thomas.

Hatry, H., van Houten, T., Plantz, M.C., & Greenway, M.T. (1996). *Measuring program outcomes: A practical approach.* Alexandria, VA: United Way of America. (Available from Effective Practices and Measuring Impact, 701 North Fairfax Street, Alexandria, VA, 22314-2045; 1-800-772-0008)

Helping your hard of hearing child succeed. Washington, DC: Alexander Graham Bell Association for the Deaf and Hard of Hearing.

The Home Team: Early Intervention Illustrated. [Videotape]. (2002). Seaver Creative Services.

Johnson, C.D., Benson, P.V., & Seaton, J.B. (1997). *Educational audiology handbook.* San Diego: Singular Publishing Group.

Joint Committee on Infant Hearing. (2000). Year 2000 Position Statement: Principles and guidelines for early hearing detection and intervention programs. *American Journal of Audiology, 9,* 9–29.

Jones, T.W. (1984). A framework for identification, classification and placement of multihandicapped hearing impaired students. *The Volta Review, 86,* 142–151.

Jones, T.W. (1998). Can a deaf student have a learning disability? The exclusion clause and state special education guidelines. In H. Markowicz & C. Berdichevsky (Eds.), *Bridging the gap between research and practice in the fields of learning disabilities and deafness* (pp. 113–118). Washington, DC: Gallaudet University Press.

Jones, T.W., & Ross, P.A. (1998). Inclusion strategies for deaf students with special needs. *The Endeavor, 37,* 2–22.

Lane, H., Hoffmeister, B., & Bahan, B. (1996). *A journey into the deaf world.* San Diego: Dawn Sign Press.

Lane, S., Bell, L., & Parson-Tylka, T. (1997). *My turn to learn: A communication guide for parents of deaf and hard of hearing children.* Surrey, British Columbia, Canada: The Elks Family Hearing Resource Center.

Linder, T.W. (1993). *Transdisciplinary play-based assessment: A functional approach to working with young children* (Rev. ed.). Baltimore: Paul H. Brookes Publishing Co.

Listen! Hear! For parents of children who are deaf or hard of hearing [Pamphlet]. Washington, DC: Alexander Graham Bell Association for the Deaf and Hard of Hearing.

Marschark, M. (1997). *Raising and educating a deaf child.* New York: Oxford University Press.

Marschark, M., & Spencer, P. (Eds.). (2003). *Deaf studies, language, and education.* New York: Oxford University Press.

Manolson, A. (1992). *It takes two to talk: A parent's guide to helping children communicate.* Toronto: The Hanen Centre.

Meadow-Orlans, K., Mertens, D., & Sass-Lehrer, M. (2003). *Parents and their deaf children: The early years.* Washington, DC: Gallaudet University Press.

Mindel, E., & Vernon, M. (1971). *They grow in silence: The deaf child and his family.* Silver Spring, MD: National Association of the Deaf.

National Association of the Deaf (NAD). *NAD position statement on cochlear implants.* Silver Spring, MD: Author.

National Association of State Directors of Special Education. (1994). *Deaf and hard of hearing students: Educational service guidelines.* Alexandria, VA: Author.

The non-hearing world: Understanding hearing loss [Videotape]. (1993). Princeton, NJ: Films for the Humanities & Sciences. (Available from Films for the Humanities & Sciences, P.O. Box 2053, Princeton, NJ, 08543-2053; 1-800-257-5126; fax: 609-275-3767; http://www.films.com)

Ogden, P. (1996). *The silent garden: Raising your deaf child* (2nd ed.). Washington, DC: Gallaudet University Press.

Paul, R. (1992). *Pragmatic activities for language intervention: Semantics, syntax, and emerging literacy.* Tucson, AZ: Communication Skill Builders.

Pearpoint, J., O'Brien, J., & Forest, M. (1994). *PATH: A workbook for planning positive possible futures.* Toronto: Inclusion Press.

Pollack, D., Goldberg, D., & Caleffe-Schenck, N. (1997). *Educational audiology for the limited hearing infant and preschooler: An auditory-verbal program* (3rd ed.). Springfield, IL: Charles C Thomas.

Price, S.C., & Price, T. (1994). *The working parents help book.* Princeton, NJ: Peterson's.

Rushmer, N. (1994). Supporting families of hearing impaired infants and toddlers. *Seminars in Hearing, 15*(2), 160–172.

Schleper, D. *Read it again and again* [Videotape and manual]. Washington, DC: Gallaudet University, Clerc Center.

Schleper, D.R. *Reading to deaf children: Learning from deaf adults* [Videotape and manual; available in English, Arabic, Chinese, Russian, Spanish, Tagalog, Vietnamese]. Washington, DC: Gallaudet University, Clerc Center.

Schlesinger, H. S., & Meadow, K. P. (1972). *Sound and sign: Childhood deafness and mental health.* Berkeley, CA: University of California Press.

Schuyler, V., & Sowers, J. (1998). *For families: A guidebook for helping your young deaf or hard of hearing child learn to listen and communicate.* Portland, OR: Hearing & Speech Institute.

Schuyler, V., & Sowers, J. (1998). *Parent-infant communication* (4th ed.). Portland, OR: Hearing & Speech Institute.

Schwartz, S. (Ed.). (1996). *Choices in deafness: A parent's guide to communication options* (2nd ed.). Bethseda, MD: Woodbine House.

Schwartz, S., & Miller, J.E.H. (1996). *The new language of toys: Teaching communication skills to children with special needs.* Bethesda, MD: Woodbine House.

Showers, P. (1993). *Ears are for hearing.* New York: HarperTrophy.

Sindrey, D. (1997). *Listening games for littles.* London, Ontario, Canada: Word Play Publications.

Solit, G., & Bednarczyk, A. (1999). *Issues in access: Creating effective pre-schools for deaf, hard of hering, and hearing children.* Washington, DC: Gallaudet University Press.

Solit, G., Taylor, M., & Bednarczyk A. (1992). *Access for all.* Washington, DC: Gallaudet University Press.

Sound hearing [Booklet and audiotape]. Portland, OR: Garlic Press.

Spencer, P., Erting, C., Marschark, M. (Eds.). (2000). *The deaf child in the family and at school: Essays in honor of Kathryn P. Meadow-Orlans.* Mahwah, NJ: Erlbaum Associates.

Staub, D. (1998). *Delicate threads.* Bethesda, MD: Woodbine House.

Stewart, D., & Luetke-Stahlman, B. (1999). *The signing family: What every parent should know about sign communication.* Washington, DC: Gallaudet University Press.

Taylor-Powell, E., Rossing, B., & Geran, J. (1998). *Evaluating collaboratives: Reaching the potential.* Madison: University of Wisconsin, Cooperative Extension. (Available from Cooperative Extension Publications, 630 W. Mifflin Street, Room 170, Madison, WI, 53703; 608-262-3346)

Vandercook, T., Tetlie, R.R., Montie, J., Downing, J., Levin, J., Glanville, M., et al. (1993). The McGill Action Planning System (MAPS): A strategy for building the vision. *Journal of The Association for Persons with Severe Handicaps, 14,* 205–215.

Watkins, S., Pittman, P., & Walden, B. (1998). The deaf mentor experimental project for young children who are deaf and their families. *American Annals of the Deaf, 143*(1), 29–34.

W.K. Kellogg Foundation. (1998). *Kellogg Foundation evaluation handbook.* Battle Creek, MI: Author. (Available from the author, One Michigan Avenue East, Battle Creek, MI, 49017-4058; 269-968-1611; http://www.wkkf.org)

Wolfensberger, W. (1975). *The origin and nature of our institutional models.* Syracuse, NY: Human Policy Press.

Yoshinaga-Itano, C., & Sedey, A. (Eds.). (2000). *Language, speech, and social-emotional development of children who are deaf or hard of hearing: The early years.* Washington, DC: Alexander Graham Bell Association.

ORGANIZATIONS AND COMPANIES

Alexander Graham Bell Association
for the Deaf and Hard of Hearing (AG Bell)

3417 Volta Place, NW
Washington, DC 20007
http://www.agbell.org
202-337-5220 (voice)
202-337-5221 (TTY)
202-337-8314 (fax)
bellmembers@aol.com (e-mail)

AG Bell provides hearing-impaired children with information and special education programs and acts as a support group for parents of deaf children. AG Bell publishes a newsletter and *The Volta Review* four times per year.

American Association of the Deaf-Blind (AADB)

814 Thayer Avenue
Silver Spring, MD 20910
http://www.tr.wou.edu/dblink/aadb.htm
301-495-4403 or 1-800-735-2258 (voice)
301-495-4402 (TTY)
301-495-4404 (fax)
info@aadb.org (e-mail)

AADB advocates children and adults who are deaf and blind and provides technical assistance to families, educators, and service providers.

American Evaluation Association (AEA)

16 Sconticut Neck Road, #290
Fairhaven, MA 02719
http://www.eval.org
1-888-232-2275 (voice/fax US/Canada)
508-748-3326 (voice/fax international)
AEA@kistcon.com (e-mail)

AEA is an international professional association of evaluators devoted to the application and exploration of program evaluation, personnel evaluation, technology, and many other forms of evaluation. Evaluation involves assessing the strengths and weaknesses of programs, policies, personnel, products, and organizations to improve their effectiveness.

American Society for Deaf Children (ASDC)

Post Office Box 3355
Gettysburg, PA 17325
http://www.deafchildren.org
717-334-7922 (voice/TTY)
717-334-8808 (fax)
1-800-942-ASDC (parent hotline)
ASDC1@aol.com (e-mail)

ASDC is an organization of parents and families that advocates for deaf or hard of hearing children's total quality participation in education, the family and the environment. *The Endeavor* is ASDC's news magazine published four times a year.

American Speech-Hearing-Language Association (ASHA)

10801 Rockville Pike
Rockville, MD 20852
http://www.asha.org
1-800-498-2017 (voice/TTY for professionals/students)
1-800-638-8255 (voice/TTY for general public)
actioncenter@ahsh.org (e-mail)

ASHA provides information about communication disorders for parents, family, media, and others. ASHA also provides resources and information for prospective students of audiology or speech-pathology, as well as practitioners, scientists, and researchers in the communication field.

Auditory-Verbal International

2121 Eisenhower Avenue
Suite 402
Alexandria, VA 22314
http://www.auditory-verbal.org/AVIcontact.asp
703-739-1049 (voice)
703-739-0874 (TDD)
703-739-0395 (fax)
audiverb@aol.com

The Auditory-Verbal approach is based upon a logical and critical set of guiding principles which enable children who are deaf or hard of hearing to learn to use even minimal amounts of amplified residual hearing or hearing through electrical stimulation (cochlear implants) to listen, to process verbal language, and to speak. The goal of the Auditory-Verbal approach is for children who are deaf or hard of hearing to grow up in typical learning and living environments and to become independent, participating citizens in mainstream society. The Auditory-Verbal philosophy supports the option for children with all degrees of hearing impairment to develop the ability to listen and to use verbal communication within their own family and community constellations.

Boys Town National Research Hospital

555 North 30th Street
Omaha, NE 68131
http://www.boystownhospital.org
http://www.babyhearing.org

The Boys Town National Research Hospital web site provides current research reports, a catalog of books and videotapes, and other helpful resources for interventionists as well as families with deaf and hard of hearing children.

Cochlear Implant Association International (CIAI)

5335 Wisconsin Avenue NW
Suite 440
Washington, DC 20015-2052
http://www.cici.org
202-895-2781 (voice)
202-895-2782 (fax)
info@cici.org (e-mail)

CIAI, formerly Cochlear Implant Club International, Inc., is a nonprofit organization for cochlear implant recipients, their families, professionals, and other individuals interested in cochlear implants. The Association provides support and information and access to local support groups for adults and children who have cochlear implants, or who are interested in learning about cochlear implants. CIAI also advocates for the rights of and services for people with hearing loss.

Council for Exceptional Children (CEC)

1110 North Glebe Road
Suite 300
Arlington, VA 22201-5704
http://www.cec.sped.org
703-620-3660 or 1-888-CES-SPED (voice)
703-264-9446 (TTY)
703-264-9494 (fax)

CEC focuses on all children with disabilities. The CEC web site leads you to divisions within the organization, including the Division for Early Childhood. CEC is also a funder of the Culturally and Linguistically Appropriate Services: Early Childhood Research Institute (http://clas.uiuc.edu/).

Deaf Advocacy Center (Orange County, CA)

2960 Main Street
Suite A100
Irvine, CA 92614
http://www.deafadvocacy.com
949-955-0054 (TDD and fax)
ocdac@deafadvocacy.com (e-mail)

Orange County Deaf Advocacy Center is a non-profit agency determined to educate the community of people with hearing disabilities that reside in Orange County, California. The Orange County Deaf Advocacy Center provides services such as information and referrals, interpreter referrals, advocacy, community counseling, community education, communication assistance, informational workshops, social activities for community seniors, and community social activities.

Deaf Education Web Site

http://www.deafed.net

Deaf Education is a comprehensive web site for families, students, teachers, teacher educators, and other professionals in the field of education of deaf and hard of hearing students. The site is designed to promote collaborative projects and sharing of information through discussion forums, topical expert forums, bulletin boards, and cyber mentor projects. The site contains job postings, a calendar of events, and announcements of new products that provide guidance in the field. The site also provides information and links to national organizations involved with the education of students who are deaf and hard of hearing.

Families for Hands & Voices

Post Office Box 371926
Denver, CO 80237
http://www.handsandvoices.org
303-300-9763 or 1-866-422-0422 (voice)
parentadvocate@handsandvoices.org (e-mail)

Families for Hands & Voices is a nonprofit, parent-driven national organization dedicated to supporting families of children who are deaf or hard of hearing. They are nonbiased about communication methodologies and believe that families will make the best choices for their child if they have access to good information and support. Hands & Voices membership includes families who communicate manually and/or orally.

Federation for Children with Special Needs

1135 Tremont Street
Suite 420
Boston, MA 02120
http://www.fcsn.org
617-236-7210 or 1-800-331-0688 (voice/TTY)
617-572-2094 (fax)
fcsninfo@fcsn.org (e-mail)

The national office of this parent education network can supply a list of contacts in your state.

Gallaudet University

Laurent Clerc National Deaf Education Center
800 Florida Avenue, NE
Washington, DC 20002
http://clerccenter.gallaudet.edu
202-651-5031 (voice/TTY)
clearinghouse.infotogo@gallaudet.edu (e-mail)

This site offers practices in educating deaf children and links to programs available for deaf children. The Laurent Clerc Center also hosts http://clerccenter2.gal laudet.edu/KidsWorldDeafNet, which provides a comprehensive list of organizations and other sources of assistance to families with deaf and hard of hearing children. Important resources within Kids World Deaf Net include *A Good Start: Suggestions for Visual Conversations with Deaf and Hard of Hearing Infants and Toddlers* (http://clerccenter2.gallaudet.edu/KidsWorldDeafNet/ e-docs/visual-conversations/index.html), *Cochlear Implants: Navigating a Forest of Information One Tree at a Time* (http://clerccenter2.gallaudet.edu/KidsW orldDeafNet/e-docs/CI/index.html), and *Early Beginnings for Families with Deaf and Hard of Hearing Children: Myths and Facts of Early Intervention and Guidelines for Effective Services* (http://clerccenter2.gallaudet.edu/KidsW orldDeafNet/e-docs/EI/index.html). The site also includes papers in easy-to-read format that provide information about parenting and educational issues.

Harris Communications

15155 Technology Drive
Eden Prairie, MN 55344-2277
http://www.harriscomm.com
952-906-1180 or 1-800-825-6758 (voice)
952-906-1198 or 1-800-825-9187 (TTY)

952-906-1099 (fax)
mail@harriscomm.com (e-mail)

Harris Communications provides children's books and signed videotapes.

Harvard Family Research Project (HFRP)

Harvard Graduate School of Education
3 Garden Street
Cambridge, MA 02138
http://gseweb.harvard.edu/-hfrp
617-495-9108 (voice)
617-495-8594 (fax)
hfrp@gse.harvard.edu (e-mail)

The HFRP is a useful source of information about the evaluation of community-based initiatives. The project's free quarterly newsletter, *The Evaluation Exchange,* deals with emerging strategies in evaluating child and family services. The HFRP web site has useful information and links for program evaluators.

Innovation Network, Inc.

Headquarters
1001 Connecticut Avenue, NW
Suite 900
Washington, DC 20036
http://www.innonet.org/
202-728-0727 (voice)
202-728-0136 (fax)
info@innonet.org (e-mail)

Supported by several major foundations, the Innovation Network, Inc., was launched to enable public and nonprofit organizations to improve the way they plan, implement, and evaluate their operations, programs, and services. Organizations can use the interactive "work station" on the web site to develop a strategic program map (similar to a program logic model), evaluation, and fundraising plans. InnoNet staff provide free feedback on plans.

John Tracy Clinic

806 West Adams Boulevard
Los Angeles, CA 90007
http://www.jtc.org/index/htm
213-748-5481 or 1-800-522-4582 (voice)
213-747-2924 (TTY)
213-749-1651 (fax)

The John Tracy Clinic provides free guidance and services to families with deaf and hard of hearing infants and young children. It has a venerable history of providing suggestions for activities and interactions with the children. This organization may be of most interest to families that want a focus on spoken language development, but it has information valuable to all.

Legal Information Online

http://www.nolo.com

Nolo provides articles on almost any legal topic and links to other helpful web sites. People who need more help can buy a book or software program, download a short "eGuide" or electronic Form Kit, or fill out a single legal form online.

LRP Publications

747 Dresher Road
Post Office Box 980
Horsham, PA 19044
http://www.lrp.com
1-800-341-7874 (voice)
215-658-0938 (TTY)
215-784-9639 (fax)

LRP has an extensive library of legal materials including special education publications and over 65 special education documents on-line, such as the text of the Individuals with Disabilities Education Act Amendments of 1997 (PL 105-17) and *The Special Educators* and *Special Education Law Monthly* newsletter.

Marion Downs National Center for Infant Hearing

University of Colorado at Boulder
Department of Speech, Language & Hearing Science
Campus Box 409
Boulder, CO 80309-0409
http://www.colorado.edu/slhs/mdnc

The primary mission of Marion Downs National Center for Infant Hearing is to assist states in developing statewide systems for screening, diagnosis and intervention.

National Association of the Deaf (NAD)

814 Thayer Avenue
Silver Spring, MD 20910-4500
http://www.nad.org
301-587-1788 (voice)
301-587-1789 (TTY)
301-587-1791 (fax)
NADinfo@nad.org (e-mail)

NAD advocates for the rights for deaf people and is a clearinghouse of information on deaf children and deaf people. It has a variety of information related to all different issues such as promoting equal access to communication, education, and employment. NAD has a law center branch on the site. Lists of organizations, services, and recreation are available to deaf citizens and NAD publishes a newsletter, *Broadcaster,* 10 times a year.

National Association for the Education of Young Children (NAEYC)

1509 16th Street, NW
Washington, DC 20036
http://www.naeyc.org
1-800-424-2460 (voice)
naeyc@naeyc.org (e-mail)

NAEYC offers information on early childhood research, reports, and legislative activities.

National Center for Hearing Assessment and Management (NCHAM)

Utah State University
2880 Old Main Hill
Logan, UT 84322
http://www.infanthearing.org
435-797-3584 (voice)
mail@infanthearing.org (e-mail)

NCHAM provides the latest information on infant hearing screening.

National Cued Speech Association (NCSA)

23970 Hermitage Road
Cleveland, OH 44122-4008
http://www.cuedspeech.org
1-800-459-3529 (voice/TTY)
cuedspdisc@aol.com (e-mail)

NCSA is a nonprofit membership organization that was founded in 1982 to promote and support the effective use of Cued Speech. NCSA raises awareness of Cued Speech and its applications, provides educational services, assists local affiliate chapters, establishes standards for Cued Speech, and certifies Cued Speech instructors and transliterators. The NCSA mission is to promote and support the effective use of Cued Speech for communication, language acquisition, and literacy.

National Early Childhood Technical Assistance Center (NEC*TAC)

Campus Box 8040
University of North Carolina–Chapel Hill
Chapel Hill, NC 27599-8040
http://www.nectac.org
919-962-2001 (voice)
919-843-3269 (TDD)
919-966-7463 (fax)
nectac@unc.edu (e-mail)

NEC*TAC supports the implementation of the early childhood provisions of the Individuals with Disabilities Education Act (IDEA) Amendments of 1997 (PL

105-17). The mission of NEC*TAC is to strengthen service systems to ensure that children with disabilities birth through 5 years and their families receive and benefit from high-quality, culturally appropriate, and family-centered supports and services.

National Information Center
for Children and Youth with Disabilities (NICHCY)

Post Office Box 1492
Washington, DC 20013
http://www.nichcy.org
1-800-695-0285 (voice/TTY)
202-884-8441 (fax)
nichcy@aed.org (e-mail)

NICHCY is a clearinghouse of information on children and young people with special needs. It has a variety of information for parents, including information about specific disabilities, "state sheets" listing points of contacts for organizations and agencies in each state, and briefing papers summarizing key topics regarding the laws of education for children with disabilities. NICHCY has the most comprehensive IDEA training packet that can be either downloaded or bought.

National Information Clearinghouse
on Children who are Deaf-Blind (DB-LINK)

http://www.tr.wou.edu/dblink/index.htm
1-800-438-9376 (voice)
1-800-854-7013 (TTY)
dblink@tr.wou.edu (e-mail)

The DB-LINK web site includes information about resources, family associations, and even recommendations for toys that benefit children with dual sensory loss. An electronic paper by D. Gleason, *Early Interactions with Children Who Are Deaf-Blind*, gives specific suggestions for effective communication and play strategies.

National Parent Information Network

University of Illinois at Urbana-Champaign
Children's Research Center
57 Getty Drive
Champaign, IL 61820
http://www.npin.org
1-800-583-4135 (voice/TTY)
217-333-3767 (fax)
npin@uiuc.edu (e-mail)

NPIN provides access to research-based information about the process of parenting and about family involvement in education. NPIN is funded by the U.S. Department of Education.

Parent Advocacy Coalition for Education Rights (PACER)

8161 Normandale Boulevard
Minneapolis, Minnesota 55437
http://www.pacer.org
952-838-9000 (voice)
800-537-2237 (in Minnesota only)
952-838-0190 (TTY)
952-838-0199 (fax)
pacer@pacer.org (e-mail)

PACER is an organization for families and advocates focusing on partnership for education, latest legislative actions, the Individuals with Disabilities Education Act Amendments of 1997 (PL 105-17) and rights, publications, articles, resources, and web site links. The PACER web site also hosts the Family and Advocates Partnership for Education (FAPE) (http://www.fape.org), which aims to inform and educate families and advocates about IDEA 1997 and promising practices.

Parent Soup

http://www.parentsoup.com

The Parent Soup web site includes topics on inclusion, individualized education programs, and types of disabilities and sponsors an expert message board and chat rooms for parents.

Raising Deaf Kids

3535 Market Street
9th floor
Philadelphia, PA 19104
http://raisingdeafkids.org
215-590-7440 (voice)
215-590-6817 (TTY)
215-590-1335 (fax)
info@raisingdeafkids.org (e-mail)

The Raising Deaf Kids web site was created by the Deafness and Family Communication Center (DFCC) at the Children's Hospital of Philadelphia. The DFCC gives clinical services for deaf and hard-of-hearing children and teenagers and does research on how hearing loss affects children, teenagers and their families. The Raising Deaf Kids web site provides information and resources on hearing loss.

Self-Help for Hard of Hearing People, Inc. (SHHH)

7910 Woodmont Avenue
Suite 1200
Bethesda, MD 20814
http://www.shhh.org
301-657-2248 (voice)
301-657-2249 (TTY)
301-913-9413 (fax)

National@shhh.org (e-mail)

SHHH is the United States' foremost association representing consumers (26 million people) who are hard of hearing. The goal of SHHH is to enhance the quality of life for people who are hard of hearing. SHHH has 250 affiliates, located in towns across the United States, that advocate on the behalf of, educate, and assist people with hearing loss.

The Special Education Advocate

Post Office Box 1008
Deltaville, VA 23043
http://www.wrightslaw.com
804-257-0857 (voice)
webmaster@nwrightslaw.com (e-mail)

The Special Education Advocate offers information on different types of disabilities, effective educational practices, progress measures, tests and evaluations, legal rights and responsibilities, and tactics and strategies in educating children with disabilities. Also available is *The Special Ed Advocate,* a free on-line newsletter. An advocacy package, information about books, conferences, and other projects can be obtained from this site.

Special Education Resources on the Internet (SERI)

http://www.seriweb.com

SERI is a collection of Internet-accessible information in the field of special education. This resourceful reference includes links related to early intervention, all types of disabilities, legal resources, parents and educator resources, special education discussion groups, and a reading list.

Index

Page references followed by t indicate tables;
those followed by f indicate figures.